MEDICINE AND CARE OF THE DYING

MEDICINE AND CARE OF THE DYING

A Modern History

Milton J. Lewis

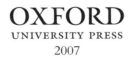

OXFORD

UNIVERSITY PRESS

2007

OXFORD
UNIVERSITY PRESS

Oxford University Press, Inc., publishes works that further
Oxford University's objective of excellence
in research, scholarship, and education.

Oxford   New York
Auckland   Cape Town   Dar es Salaam   Hong Kong   Karachi
Kuala Lumpur   Madrid   Melbourne   Mexico City   Nairobi
New Delhi   Shanghai   Taipei   Toronto

With offices in
Argentina   Austria   Brazil   Chile   Czech Republic   France   Greece
Guatemala   Hungary   Italy   Japan   Poland   Portugal   Singapore
South Korea   Switzerland   Thailand   Turkey   Ukraine   Vietnam

Published by Oxford University Press, Inc.
198 Madison Avenue, New York, New York 10016

www.oup.com

Oxford is a registered trademark of Oxford University Press

Library of Congress Cataloging-in-Publication Data
Lewis, Milton James.
Medicine and care of the dying : a modern history / Milton J. Lewis.
   p. ; cm.
Includes bibliographical references and index.
ISBN-13 978-0-19-517548-6

1. Terminal care—History. 2. Palliative treatment—History. 3. Euthanasia—History.
[DNLM: 1. Terminal Care—history. 2. Euthanasia—history. 3. History, 19th Century.
4. History, 20th Century. 5. Neoplasms—history. 6. Palliative Care—history.
WB 310L675m 2006] I. Title.
R726.8.L484   2006
616′.029—dc22   2006003085

9 8 7 6 5 4 3

Printed in the United States of America
on acid-free paper

ACKNOWLEDGMENTS

This study would not have been possible without the generous financial support of the Sisters of Charity Health Service, Sydney; the Uniting Church Aged Care Services, Sydney; the Corporation of the Little Company of Mary, Sydney; Anglican Retirement Villages, Sydney; Hope Healthcare, Sydney; and the Betty Garvan Cancer Research Bequest, University of Sydney.

Norelle Lickiss, former head of Palliative Care Services, Royal Prince Alfred Hospital, Sydney, and founder of the Sydney Institute of Palliative Medicine, has offered encouragement from the beginning of the project. The following people provided helpful comments on early drafts of some of the chapters: Stephen Leeder, Charles Kerr, Martin Tattersall, and Bruce Armstrong, Faculty of Medicine, University of Sydney; Peter Ravenscroft, Faculty of Medicine, University of Newcastle; and Jane Grattan-Smith, Sydney. Timothy Earnshaw and Rachael Fraher were tireless research assistants. As ever, the staff of the Fisher Library (especially the Interlibrary Loans Section), the Medical Library, and the Burkitt-Ford (Public Health) Library provided essential support. I would like to express my deep appreciation to all of these individuals, organizations, and institutions.

CONTENTS

MEDICINE AND CARE OF THE DYING

INTRODUCTION

In this book I examine the relationship between the approach of Western medicine to the care of the dying and its changing social, cultural, demographic, economic, and political context over the last two centuries in five Anglo-Saxon countries: the United Kingdom, the United States, Australia, Canada, and New Zealand.[1] According to Daniel Callahan, within contemporary medicine a struggle is taking place between the research imperative with its implicit goal of overcoming death itself and an old clinical obligation to make the process of dying as free from suffering as possible. The modern palliative care movement, par excellence, embodies that clinical imperative, but insofar as it focuses on the needs of the whole person, it is also a contemporary expression of a person-centered approach that has surfaced from time to time over the last century in reaction to mainstream, reductionist, scientific medicine (Lawrence and Weisz, 1998, 1–18; Callahan, 2000, 654–55).

A history of care of the dying should include not only an account of medical theory and practice—internalist history—but also contextual history (i.e., a description of the relevant aspects of the culture, society, economy, and polity in which modern medicine is located. Central to the cultural history is the rise of modern science and in particular the Baconian view that science would promote reliable knowledge of the natural world and thereby confer unprecedented control of it. Francis Bacon (1561–1626), the English philosopher who stands on the brink of the modern world, advocated a new learning that, while motivated by religion, was rational and secular. He in turn influenced the philosophers of the French Enlightenment, who themselves held certain core beliefs. They believed in the natural rather than the supernatural and in science rather than religion; in the use of reason to solve problems in human affairs; in the perfectibility of humankind; and in the rights of people. The decline of religious and associated moral discourses and the advance of scientific-professional ones is the larger cultural setting within which to understand medicine's care of the dying.

Although for very many people death has become overwhelmingly a medical matter, for many others it is still a significant religious matter also. In the incompletely secularized, late-modern societies of our Anglo-Saxon countries, a moral and religious pluralism means that controversy over voluntary euthanasia for the dying, like other bioethical disputes, is not likely to be resolved any time soon (Bierstedt, 1978, 5, 32; Wildes, 1996, 378–81; Sismondo, 2000, 65).

The development of modern urban–industrial society was marked by a demo-graphic transition and an epidemiological evolution—the first, from the high mor-tality and elevated fertility of traditional society to the lows of contemporary society, and the second, from a cause-of-death profile in which communicable dis-eases were primary to one dominated by chronic, degenerative maladies. Average life expectancy and the proportion of the aged in the population have climbed to hitherto unknown levels (Corr, 1999, 32–33).

People in modern societies tended to die from chronic ailments requiring pro-longed care. This, together with more effective life-maintenance systems, con-tributed to the fact that care of terminal patients became a salient issue in the sec-ond half of the twentieth century. Indeed, some sociologists have gone so far as to advance a typology of forms of death characteristic, respectively, of traditional, modern, and late-modern society. The archetypal death in the first is one due to infectious disease or trauma. There are extensive rituals that, in the face of death, celebrate the links between the worlds of the living and the dead; they also mark a shared metaphysical and moral framework that ties the individual closely to the collective, while religious intermediaries enjoy much authority as the interpreters of this framework.

In modern society, the archetypal death is that from cancer, and it is managed by doctors. Dying occurs in institutions, death tends to be almost a taboo subject, rituals are limited, and bodies are often cremated, not interred.

In late-modern society, the typical death results from any of a number of de-generative diseases. For many who have rejected organized religion as a source of existential meaning, the individual self's life journey has become a way in which to make sense of life and death. People commonly arrange for funeral rituals reflect-ing their particular identity and life experience. Rejecting the authority of medi-cine, they may attempt to control the dying process itself, even to the point of arranging euthanasia (Clark and Seymour, 1999, 13–14).

Eric Cassell has reminded doctors that the relief of suffering is as much an objec-tive of medicine as is the cure of disease. He has pointed out that medicine's success has caused doctors to forget that they are healers of the sick. The correctness of the scientific diagnosis and treatment is not a sufficient explanation of illness. The pa-tient has become isolated amid a plethora of tests, procedures, and teams of health professionals. Edmund Pellegrino maintains that healing requires of the physician both competence (i.e., scientific diagnosis and treatment) and compassion (i.e., the ability to maintain solidarity with the patient) (Browder and Vance, 1995, 1033). Anne Davis has noted in the care of the dying that the instrumental meaning of care must be replaced by that most deeply human aspect of caring, the expressive art of being fully present to another human being (Reich, 1995b). In the postwar era, U.S. medical schools made various attempts to introduce teaching about caring into the curriculum: first, through the behavioral sciences and history of medicine and later through the medical humanities and bioethics. The assumption that formal courses can influence attitudes and behavior is questionable, and there is little convincing evidence that such instruction has produced more caring doctors (Cassell, 1982,

639–45; Reich, 1989, 83, 106; Reich, 1995b, 331–36; Browder and Vance, 1995, 1032–38; Ludmerer, 1999, 304–5).

From about the mid-nineteenth century, deaths in our Anglo-Saxon countries became more institutionalized; increased numbers of poor and aged people died in hospitals, workhouses, benevolent asylums, lunatic asylums, and prisons. In the emerging urban-industrial society, it was becoming state policy that the sick poor should be concentrated in large institutions, often under degrading conditions: for example, in New South Wales, one of the two most populous of the Australian colonies, deaths in public institutions (excluding prisons) rose from 11 percent of the total in 1860 to more than 35 percent in 1920 (Jalland, 2002, 200–3).

In the nineteenth century, the state began to intervene in health care. It introduced the legal regulation of medical practitioners and of the funds that financed medical services for the lower-middle and working classes. The state became more concerned with the health status of the population (whether in order to produce a healthy workforce, healthy citizens to defend the nation or empire, or healthy mothers to reproduce the workers and soldiers or, more recently, to promote social justice).

Early in the twentieth century, the larger European countries were spending less than 1 percent of their gross domestic product on health, but by 1970 that had grown to 6–10 percent. Other indices reveal the growth of state financial support for health care in the United Kingdom and the United States. Medical expenditure per capita (in 1938 U.S. dollars) in the United Kingdom was $8.35 in 1890, $9.60 in 1930, and $56.90 in 1970; in the United States it was $8.40, $25.20, and $119.45 respectively. In these and the other Anglo-Saxon countries, a huge infrastructure of organizations in medical research, medical education, and health care delivery was built to support scientific medicine. In Britain, the great expansion in the central government's funding of the health care delivery system is reflected in the changes in the significance of different funding sources between 1901 and 1970: private individuals and insurance were down from 70.3 to 16.7 percent; public and private hospitals, 26.1 to 0 percent; local government, up from 3.6 to 5.6 percent; and central government, up from 0 to 77.8 percent.

Efforts to introduce a national health insurance plan in the United States failed in 1935 and again in 1948. The failure of President Clinton's national health initiative confirms there is almost insuperable opposition by corporate interests and ideological opponents. However, the 1960s saw a return to New Deal concern about access to health care, out of which came Medicare, which provides federal health benefits for the aged, and Medicaid, a federal-state plan to provide services for the poor (basically a form of public assistance). In the 1970s, in a fee-for-service medical system, spending on these plans fueled a steeply rising expenditure for health care that helped reinforce a sense of crisis in the affordability of medicine, which was also widely seen as technically impressive but too often incapable of providing compassionate care (Rogers Hollingworth, 1981, 271–72; Terris, 1999, 13–17; Anderson, Hurst, Hussey, and Jee-Hughes, 2000, 150–56; Webster, 2000, 125–38; Wildes, 2001, 71–72).

Significant state funding of medical research began earlier in the United Kingdom than in the United States, although Germany preceded both. In Britain the

Medical Research Council (established in 1913) channeled state funds into bio-medical research, while the private Wellcome Trust did not provide funds until the 1930s. In the United States, research laboratories were set up at the Rockefeller Institute for Medical Research as early as 1901. The contributions of science, including medical science, to the war effort from 1939 to 1945 convinced the governments of all of these countries to commit greater funds to research. Indeed, the U.S. government became the largest contributor to medical research funding; in the 1950s the budget of the National Institutes of Health more than doubled, from 28 to 60 million dollars in just five years.

The nineteenth-century German emphasis on basic sciences and laboratory research in university medical education was taken up in all of the Western countries. In the twentieth century, citizens encountered a growing array of increasingly effective technologies that were being used in hospital diagnosis and treatment. Diseases were clinically identified there before being investigated in the laboratory, and, if useful diagnostic and therapeutic knowledge resulted, it was applied to hospitalized sufferers. Hospitals were thus central to modern health care delivery in the biomedical model, so it is not surprising that U.S. hospitals greatly increased in number—from 178 in 1873 to 5,736 in 1960. Hospital beds per 1,000 people in England more than doubled between 1890 and 1970—from 628 to 1,335.

In the 1950s, after half a century of growth in its cultural authority and social status, powerful critiques of the efficacy and ethics of biomedicine began to appear. René Dubos claimed that social and political factors might have been more significant than biomedicine's antimicrobials in the reduction of mortality from communicable diseases. Thomas McKeown made an even more full-blooded attack on the contribution of biomedicine to the unprecedented reduction of all-cause mortality in the previous two centuries. He argued, plausibly, that nonmedical factors, especially better nutrition, had been more important than biomedical interventions. According to Ivan Illich, modern medicine created dependence in sickness and dying, undermining the individual's capacity to respond in a self-reliant way to sickness, pain, suffering, and death (Clark and Seymour, 1999, 116; Brandt and Gardner, 2000, 26–32).

Another powerful critique was one that developed in relation to the care of the dying by the pioneers of the palliative care movement.[2] The principles of hospice care that physician Cicely Saunders began applying at Saint Christopher's Hospice in London in 1967 were quickly adopted in other Anglo-Saxon countries. At the heart of Saunders's approach were pain control and compassionate care. As a result of her efforts, dying patients were freed enough from physical and emotional (and, for Saunders, spiritual) suffering to allow them to come to terms with their situation. If Saunders's ideas directly inspired the setting up of the first hospices in the United States, physician Elisabeth Kübler-Ross, the leader of the death and dying movement, turned hospices into a nationally known concept even though she herself was not active in planning those programs.

To establish wider access and financial viability, the hospice movement in the United States sought to make hospice an insurance benefit. In 1982 Medicare, Blue Cross/Blue Shield, and other insurers offered hospice as a benefit. However, the Medicare benefit was restricted to supportive, not medical, care and was available only to those with a diagnosis of six or fewer months to live. Moreover, hospice was disproportionately used by the educated middle class, while ethnic minorities and rural residents were underrepresented (Siebold, 1992, 61–74, 87–88, 109–13, 132–36).

The British model of the hospice also had an important influence on the early movement in Australia. Over time, however, a distinctively local mix of services evolved. In 1988 the federal government began funding projects aimed at improving the delivery of palliative care (Cavenagh and Gunz, 1988, 51–52; Kasap and Associates, 1996, ix). Canada and New Zealand responded in their own ways to the pioneering work in Britain. The first Canadian palliative care facilities opened in the mid-1970s. In 2000 a Canadian senate report called for a national strategy for palliative care (MacDonald, 1998b, 1710; Quality End-of-Life Coalition, 2003, 1–2).

The biases of scientific medicine that led it to focus on the cure of bodies rather than the care of people and to neglect important needs of the dying stem from deeper cultural sources. At the beginning of the modern scientific era, René Descartes (1596–1650) sought to anchor the new science in a secure ontology of the thinking self and a God who guaranteed the truth of sense experience. His metaphysical gifts to modern culture, especially modern science, were materialism, mind/body dualism, and reductionism (Little, 1998, 76–92). But the certainty he believed he had bequeathed to those in the late-modern era become problematic. Because the deep reflexivity of contemporary Western culture undermines systems of meaning and social order, the disappearance of belief in a divine order leaves the individual as the only source of meaning. This reflexivity is fed by an unprecedented number of analyses of society and nature. In sociologist Anthony Giddens's runaway world, as the security of the foundations of knowledge of the social and natural worlds becomes even more doubtful, the tensions of late-modern society are simply those of modern society in an exaggerated form (Bracken, 2001, 740). The search for meaning in a runaway world may rest particularly heavy on the individual when the self faces its own disintegration in the process of dying.

Chapters 1 and 2 are painted with a broad brush. Chapter 1 traces the interaction of medicine and religion in the development of hospitals and hospices for the dying; in particular, it highlights the significant role the nursing nuns, Catholic and Protestant (who cared for the body for the sake of the soul), played in the development of these institutions; it emphasizes the proliferation of medical specialties and technologies as hospitals became the bastions of scientific medicine. If secularization was the mark of modernity, then the decline of the role of spirituality in hospitals and hospices was by no means a simple matter. Even at the zenith of the authority of scientific medicine in the two to three decades after World War II, what might be termed a sacrilizing reaction occurred in the form of the British hospice movement.

Chapter 2 looks in detail at the rise of scientific medicine, discussing two significant, nineteenth-century models—the Paris hospital-based model and the German laboratory-based one. Recent critiques of the Cartesian heritage of modern medicine (in particular its dualism and reductionism), which is blamed for the depersonalization of the patient in its approach to sickness and dying, are discussed, as is the fact that medicine is unavoidably caught up in values. Other factors that have shaped modern medicine are discussed at some length: the rise of a medical research culture in each of our five countries; the demographic and epidemiological changes that have influenced modern and late-modern society; and the cultural, social, and political reactions to an aging population and in particular to the issue of death and dying in that group.

Chapter 3 has a narrower focus. It examines the history of medicine's approach to cancer. The approach is a paradigmatic example of medicine's great concern with advancing scientific knowledge, to which relief of the suffering of the dying has too often been subordinated.

The focus of Chapter 4 is the spread of the palliative care movement from the United Kingdom to the other Anglo-Saxon countries. As it has developed, palliative medicine has faced the dilemma of medicine in general—how to fruitfully marry technical expertise and humane care.

Chapter 5 is concerned with pain control. The phenomenon of pain sits at the juncture of human biology and culture, and, indeed, the prevailing theory (the gate control theory) of how pain operates allows for a modifying role for culture (for attitudes, beliefs, and values) in one's experience of pain. Modern palliative care could not function without effective pain control.

Chapter 6 examines the changing meaning of euthanasia. From the late nineteenth century, arguments in favor of euthanasia were no longer confined to the circles of philosophers. By the 1930s, a Euthanasia Society had sprung up in England and the United States and had begun lobbying for legalization. In Nazi Germany the implementation of an involuntary euthanasia program for people with disabilities discredited the euthanasia movement in the Anglo-Saxon world. Nevertheless, in the 1960s, the movement began to gain respectability. In the mid-1990s, Oregon legalized physician-assisted suicide, and Australia's Northern Territory legalized euthanasia. Many gay men with AIDS-related conditions have sought euthanasia. Indeed, there is evidence of an illegal euthanasia underground in cities with large gay communities.

The final chapter reviews subjects such as the effects of the heritage of medical reductionism on the care of the dying and the cultural sources of caring in "secular," late-modern societies such as these Anglo-Saxon countries.

Cartesian medical science has produced unprecedentedly reliable knowledge of, and powerful therapies for, disease, but it has also tended to detach medicine from its deep moral roots; the commitment to know (in order to cure) has tended to overshadow the pledge to reduce suffering even where cure is not possible. There is also a larger cultural problem—we lack a conception of the spiritual that might provide a sense of meaning for those secular-minded individuals who at times of extreme existential vulnerability are not satisfied by the answers provided by Christianity or other organized religions but are also not satisfied by those furnished by science. Secular humanism in the name of a reductionist, materialist science is dismissive of traditional religious conceptions of the spiritual, but so far it has not developed a widely appealing, nonreligious alternative that offers escape from our isolating, late-modern subjectivities. We seem to be in need of a convincing, humanistic spirituality that offer us a sense of solidarity in the face of life's extreme situations. In health care, especially in the care of the dying, a new ethics of care grounded in such a spirituality might help moderate the excessive emphasis on personal autonomy and existential control (through technology) inherited from the larger individualistic, scientistic culture, and it would advance the sense of human community needed in the face of death—that ultimate threat to the integrity of the person.

NOTES

1. I have used the term "Anglo-Saxon" for want of a better one to describe the cultural, political, economic, and social heritage shared by the five countries, four of which, of course, were once settlement colonies of Britain. This heritage includes important features such as the English language (clearly in Canada the French language and associated cultural traditions have also played a major historical role), the rule of law, representative democracy, freedom of worship, separation of church and state, a free-market economy that is subject (to a greater or lesser extent) to state intervention, social welfare and health systems that are publicly funded to varying degrees, high valuation of individualism (but also variable emphasis on communitarianism), secularism (but resurgent interest in organized religion, especially of a more fundamentalist or conservative type), appreciation of science and technology (or at least the benefits they confer), and, in more recent times, acceptance of multiculturalism.

Facing space constraints, I have tended to give greater coverage to Britain, the United States, and Australia. This is because British medical practices continued to influence medicine in Australia, Canada, and New Zealand well into the twentieth century and because Canada has been influenced more by U.S. medicine, and New Zealand more by Australian medicine than vice versa. It is not a judgment of the importance of developments in Canada and New Zealand.

2. While mentioning the palliative care of children from time to time, because of lack of space I have not given special treatment to pediatric palliative care and children's hospices. In a book on the history of palliative care as such, I would discuss at length particular issues concerning the care of children. There are discussions of developments in the United Kingdom, the United States, Australia, and Canada, respectively, by Dominica (1999, 1098–1100), Faulkner (1999, 1105–6), Stevens and Pollard (1999, 1102–5), and Davies (1999. 1100–2). Special issues relating to pediatric palliative care are discussed in Hilden, Himelstein, Freyer, Friebert, and Kane (2001, 161–98). The need for further development in pediatric palliative care in New Zealand is discussed in Jones, Trenholme, Horsburgh, and Riding (2002, 1–6).

1 THE RELIGIOUS AND THE MEDICAL

As the heir of Enlightenment theories of progress, nineteenth-century sociology assumed that social progress involved a process of secularization. However, the great pioneering figures of sociology, Max Weber and Émile Durkheim, conceptualized the change from traditional to modern society in different ways. For Durkheim, society was a moral force at the heart of which were values that were treated as sacred. Thus, society was the source of religion. For Weber, the focus of sociology was social action; one type was rational (economics and law), and the other nonrational (religion); the rationalization principle (everything is calculable) underlies modern society, and what was originally a religious phenomenon—the Protestant work ethic or hard work as the enactment of God's will—becomes a this-worldly end in itself as faith in God disappears; modernization entails the "disenchantment" of the world (Bell, 1977, 588; Carroll, 2001, 221).

Durkheimians insist that the Weberian idea of modernization, which involves a fundamental transformation from a "religious" to a "secular" society, is mistaken; rather, the transcendentalism of Christianity is manifested in new forms. Kenneth Thompson has suggested that a logical development of Durkheim's claim that the sacred persists is that a dialectical relationship exists between secularization and sacralization. Thus, modern features may generate sacralizing reactions such as religious fundamentalisms and the reinvigoration of ethnic and national identities (Thompson, 1990, 161–64; Alexander and Sztompka, 1990, 8–9).

The rise of scientific medicine was accompanied by the decline in our Anglo-Saxon countries of the role of institutional religion in the processes of death and dying. Yet, the late nineteenth century witnessed an upsurge of activity by Christians of different denominations to create special hospices for the care of the dying. Moreover, at the pinnacle of the triumph of scientific medicine in the 1960s, "a sacralizing reaction" in the form of the British hospice movement took place in relation to the care of the dying. The unclear role of spirituality (and, even more so, of Christianity) in modern palliative care points up the contested nature of the sacred and the sources of morality in late-modern society.

There are both religious and naturalistic explanations of religion, and they are not mutually exclusive. While religion may be shown to be culturally constructed, it may still be a means for expressing essential aspects of human identity. Yet, modern scientific medicine, as a highly reductionist form of naturalism, is not able to accommodate the transcendent realm of the spiritual; at the same time, the contemporary distinction between the spiritual and the religious presents its own problems. The recent rise of modern hospices and palliative care has reintroduced a public model of the good death. However, discussion of the role of spirituality is problematic because language moves uneasily between religious and psychological terminology, depending on whether the speaker has a religious or naturalistic worldview. Within clinical and scientific ways of knowing, spiritual need becomes identified with emotional need, and the spirituality of the patient is legitimate only when it serves clinical goals, not when it interferes with clinical processes (Rumbold, 2002, 6–19).

Pioneer of modern hospice care Cicely Saunders built on the tradition of care at Saint Joseph's, an inner-city Catholic hospice set up in London as part of the late nineteenth-century religious hospice movement. Her new facility, Saint Christopher's, which opened in the 1960s, included in its aims spiritual ones drawn from the Christian faith—expression of the love of God in skilled nursing and medical care, as well as in the use of every scientific means of relieving suffering, and in the formation of a community united by a sense of vocation (Small, 1998, 170–74).

THE DECLINE OF CHRISTIANITY?

Between about 1880 and 1980 in Britain, regular church attendance dropped off, and secular interpretations of the human and natural worlds advanced. The church's role as provider of social and educational services was taken over to a large extent by the welfare state. Yet, it has not been a case of steady decline but rather one of decline and recovery. The evangelical revival of the eighteenth century, the Anglican revival of the nineteenth, together with the Victorian expansion of Roman Catholicism and the dissenting churches, demonstrated the resilience of Christianity. Even in the twentieth century, a decline in institutional religion was punctuated by a modest revival in the 1950s and, more recently, by a resurgence in evangelical Christianity. New Age cosmologies and cults, not to mention the flourishing of fundamentalism in Christianity, Islam, and Judaism, indicate that belief in transcendent worlds has not disappeared.

The ambiguities of community attitudes toward spirituality have resonated within the modern hospice movement. In the mid-1980s Florence Wald, a pioneer of hospice in the United States, talked about a "basic flaw" in the perception of hospice in that country, the result of which was that the necessary blend of medical science and spiritual care that was Saunders's model was not widely appreciated. Indeed, the Christian basis of Saunders's Saint Christopher's was quite clear, but the spiritual aspect of hospice in the United States was vague. To address the issue, in 1986 Wald convened a colloquium. The divide the colloquium could not bridge was that between those who saw the Godhead as the necessary source of spirituality and those who did not. The participants struggled to find a common language (Small, 1998, 178; Foster and Corless, 1999, 11).

In Australia the great waves of religious millenarianism that washed over U.S. Protestants after the Great Awakening of the 1740s did not occur. Moreover, there were few groups who came to Australia for religious reasons. Strong antipathy to Christianity was thus rare; rather, apathy and other priorities kept people away from churches. The colonists were opposed to the established churches of Britain enjoying similar status in Australia because of memories of abuse of privilege or because they preferred churches to exercise spiritual, not legal, authority. While sometimes bitter sectarianism erupted, each church was kept busy building the institutional strength of its own people in a new environment. The greatest points of commonality with the United States and Britain were to be found in the rapidly growing cities of the late nineteenth century. The experience of Christianity in Sydney and Melbourne was like that in Chicago, Manchester, and Glasgow. Respect for freedom of conscience was strong, and the pluralism of Christianity in Australia itself generated a sometimes reluctant tolerance of other churches.

In the United States, the position of the clergy was weaker after the Revolution. Thomas Paine and other Deists had criticized orthodox Christianity, and anticlericalism was strong among Jeffersonian Democrats. In the early nineteenth century, in the southern states, public funds to support the established churches were no longer forthcoming, while in New England immoral acts such as uttering profanities were not being punished by law. In reaction to the anticlericalism, a Second Awakening spread across rural America. Between 1800 and 1835, church membership virtually doubled in size.

In the postbellum era, the effects of industrialization, urbanization, and immigration combined with intellectual critiques arising from Darwinian theory and higher biblical criticism to challenge orthodox Christianity profoundly. The failure to provide moral leadership over important, emerging issues like social justice further reduced the standing of the clergy. The churches strongly expressed their patriotism in World War I but, reflecting the general reaction against internationalism, were doubtful about whether the United States should participate when World War II broke out (Duffy, 1984, 4–15).

The mass unemployment of the Depression threatened liberal Christian optimism about unlimited progress in the United States. Church membership declined, recovering only in the mid-1930s, when the economy began to stabilize. Whereas in Britain church membership fell during World War II, in the United States, the growth of the later 1930s continued throughout the war and postwar years, from 49 percent of the population in 1940 to about 65 percent in 1970. The advent of the Cold War reinforced support since a Christian United States was seen to oppose an atheistic Soviet Union. About 1970 the growth of overall church membership faltered, but whereas membership in the mainstream denominations was particularly affected, that of conservative churches, such as the Southern Baptists, continued to expand. New spiritual groups drawing on Hindu and Buddhist religious or mystical principles and practices suddenly appeared. Against a background of rising consumerism, mainstream faiths—Protestant, Catholic, and Jewish—tended to offer a form of religion based on a psychologized and individualistic experientialism that relativized religious meaning and allowed nonreligious sources of meaning to flourish in significant areas of everyday life.

Beginning in the early 1960s, political alienation grew because of assassinations, racial tensions, widespread anger about the Vietnam War, and libertarianism among the college-educated young. Opposition to the established political and social order included rejection of the mainstream faiths.

Various responses to a loss of spiritual and moral certainty may be discerned. One was the search for individually affirming experience in the new mystical groups that drew on Asian traditions or in the transformative groups employing various psychotechnologies. Another was the retreat into countercultural lifestyles or the pursuit of personal meaning in family life. Yet another was the strong assertion of traditional, absolutist, religious values, of which a prime example was the claims of Moral Majority conservatism (Smith, 1986, 96–101).

From the beginning of the formal European occupation of Canada, French and then English governments had privileged one church. In the 1850s legal equality of the different denominations was established. Church membership was expanding faster than population growth as the British North American colonies became settled societies. However, the Protestant churches did not dominate as in the United States. So strong was Francophone Catholicism that, for the rest of the nineteenth century, the ratio of Protestants to Catholics continued to be about 6:4. Indeed, the Catholic church was widely recognized as the national church of those who had cofounded Canada.

Canadian Catholicism was, like Catholicism elsewhere, encouraged in its militancy by Ultramontanism and the belief of Pope Pius IX (1846–1878) that liberalism and Catholicism were not compatible. In the Ultramontane view, all aspects of a Catholic's life should come under church auspices; thus schools, hospitals, and other social agencies should be run by the church, although the state was obliged to provide funding. Many Protestants opposed state funding, and bitter disputes over Catholic schooling developed in the mid-nineteenth century. By the latter part of the century, newer Protestant churches such as the Salvation Army were appearing. Industrialization in the 1880s called forth the social gospel movement, with its concern for justice, in the United States and Britain. In Canada, the gospel influenced the main Protestant churches, producing a convergence that eventually led to the formation of the United Church in 1925.

The experience of the Great War, in which 60,000 Canadians died, destroyed overly naïve, social gospel beliefs, but it strengthened the commitment of many Protestants to the reconstruction of Christian society in a cooperative way. Initially concerned about communism, the Protestant churches in the later 1930s turned to the threat of Fascism, deploring Hitler's persecution of Jews but not formally supporting a campaign to allow refugees into Canada until early 1939. In line with Vatican policy, the Catholic Church defended Fascist Italy's 1935 Abyssinian adventure and did not publicly condemn Hitler's persecution of the German churches until 1938. With the outbreak of World War II, the Canadian churches sought to avoid the ultrapatriotism of the years between 1914 and 1918.

The strong desire to return to normalcy saw membership in the main Protestant churches grow impressively in the interwar years. Catholics sustained a high level of church attendance in the 1950s, but, by 1960, weekly attendance had fallen to 38 percent among Protestants, although in 1896 only 55 percent of Toronto's population attended church. The Evangelicalism and Ultramontanism that had dominated Protestantism and Catholicism respectively for more than a century ceased to shape cultural and social life. In the 1960s consumerism and immigration from non-European countries were affecting traditional values, and, as in other Anglo-Saxon countries, many young people were seeking answers to existential issues from exotic sources such as Asian religions.

French Canadians turned to a secular lifestyle: attendance at weekly mass fell from 88 percent in 1957 to 41 percent in 1975. The church ceased to enjoy hegemony over French-Canadian culture. In the 1960s the reforms of the Second Vatican Council brought greater lay involvement in church government and more openness to other Christian and non-Christian faiths. Not only did church attendance and membership in both Catholic and Protestant churches fall in the 1960s, but the number of people who claimed no religious affiliation also increased to 20 percent at the beginning of the 1990s. A 1993 national poll found that 80 percent of respondents believed in God and 66 percent in the death and resurrection of Christ, although much of this probably represents a residual adherence to traditional beliefs. However, some conservative Protestant groups such as the Pentecostals expanded their numbers more quickly than the general population increased. Religious tolerance is now a fundamental value, and diversity in religion, culture, and race a social reality (Clarke, 1996, 187–88, 223–96, 324–41, 354–57; Murphy, 1996, 361–69).

THE NURSING NUNS

The Counter-Reformation in France witnessed the formation of new charitable societies, of which the most successful was Vincent de Paul's Ladies of Charity, who worked among the sick poor. Louise de Marillac began to train women as nurses to work on behalf of the aristocratic ladies. In 1633 she was allowed to instruct them in spiritual as well as practical work, and so emerged the Daughters of Charity. Such communities of common women continued to grow in number until the Revolution, and they sparked an interest in Protestant countries. Napoleon Bonaparte fully restored the nursing sisterhoods. With their emphasis on practical responses to the needs of others, the Daughters of Charity became an influential example for subsequent Catholic communities, including those that established Saint Vincent Hospitals throughout the Anglo-Saxon world; for the founder of the Deaconess movement, Lutheran pastor Theodor Fliedner; for the founder of the Protestant Sisters of Mercy, English Quaker Elizabeth Fry; for the Anglican sisterhoods; and for Florence Nightingale, founder of modern nursing.

The nineteenth-century revival of Catholicism in Ireland was at least as impressive as that in France. At the start of the century, the Catholic church was oppressed down by the British penal codes. By its close, the Irish church had provided thousands of nuns and priests for the United Kingdom, North America, and Australasia.

In Protestantism, a woman's calling traditionally lay in the sphere of the home, but in the course of the nineteenth century the sphere was expanded to include some of the needs of the community. In 1838 Pastor Fliedner, inspired by the evangelizing work of the Daughters of Charity in Strasbourg, revived the female deaconate of early Christianity in the Rhenish town of Kaiserwerth. Within a short time, from Switzerland to Norway, the deaconesses were running Lutheran hospitals and doing extensive home nursing among the urban poor. In Britain, in contrast, no consensus was reached about what the Protestant version of the nursing nuns was to be; consequently, there was a range from deaconesses to Catholic-like religious communities.

In North America the women religious nursed the poor at home during the recurrent epidemics of the era and then established first-class charitable hospitals. Thus, in Detroit the Catholic Sisters of Charity devotedly nursed the victims of the Asiatic cholera epidemics of 1832 and 1834, and in 1845 the Sisters of Saint Vincent de Paul established the city's first hospital. These women intimately knew the economic and medical needs of the urban lower classes. They also cared for the dying both before and after the advent of modern, secular nursing (Drews, 1939, 767–76; Nelson, 2001, 17–31).

With the penal code repealed in 1829, the Irish Church faced the task of reconstructing Catholic institutions for the sick and the poor, as well as evangelizing the impoverished. The 1845–1850 famine saw millions of peasants leave the rural areas, and many emigrants, then and later, sought relief in Britain, the United States, Canada, and Australia. In British cities, the Irish, as among the poorest, were very hard hit by cholera and typhoid epidemics and were blamed for the heavy demands they made on public relief. The English Catholic church represented a refuge for the Irish immigrant masses, but, in contrast to the church in other Anglophone countries, its hierarchy was not taken over by Irish leaders. In 1839 in Bermondsey, London, the Dublin-based Sisters of Mercy established the first convent in England since the Reformation, and later, they worked in the first Catholic hospital in England since that time.

Both Catholics and Protestants believed not only that recruitment of the poor urban masses to a Christian way of life was a religious imperative but also that it would ameliorate the problems of crime, poverty, civil disorder, and ill health. Members of the English social elite were well acquainted with the work of Catholic charities on the Continent. In 1839 Quaker Joshua Hornby introduced home visiting in Liverpool. Inspired by the German deaconess model, Elizabeth Fry established the Protestant Sisters of Mercy in London in 1840. With their name changed to Institute for Nursing Sisters to avoid any identification with Catholicism, the Fry nurses did home nursing after first training at Guy's Hospital.

For the socially advantaged English woman, in the second half of the century the choice was deaconess or nun, with the former role appealing to low church Anglicans, Methodists, and Quakers. In 1861 Rev. William and Mrs. Catherine Pennefather established Mildmay Park according to the Kaiserwerth model, and two decades later it had produced 200 deaconesses and 1,500 associates. The North London Deaconess Institution was established along Kaiserwerth lines in 1862, and later the group took over nursing at the Great Northern Hospital. The Rochester Deaconess Institution, in contrast, trained women to work in the community by providing instruction in nursing, visiting, and the scriptures.

The Anglican sisterhoods were more successful at attracting upper-class women. In 1845 the Oxford Movement spawned the Anglican Order of the Holy Cross, or the Park Village Sisters, who cared for the sick poor at home. In 1848 Priscilla Sallon established the Sisters of Mercy in Devonport, and in 1855 the Devonport group absorbed the Park Village Sisters.

By the 1870s members of Saint John's House, the All Saints Sisterhood, the Sisters of the Holy Rood, and the Community of Saint Margaret were the best-trained nurses in Britain. The Order of Saint John the Evangelist took control of nursing at King's College Hospital, London, in 1856, Charing Cross Hospital in 1866, and the Nottingham Hospital for Sick Children in 1867. Saint John's House, as a hybrid model under which upper-class pious women trained nurses in teaching hospitals under the supervision of a council of religious and medical men, eventually foundered due to its failure to allow the women to exercise full authority. Within Anglicanism, the tensions between the high church and evangelicals, in Protestantism between Anglicans and Nonconformists, and in Christianity between Protestants and Catholics meant the liberal argument that state and civil institutions should be secular was rendered very persuasive. Florence Nightingale's solution better fitted an emerging view in a scientific and democratic country: while denominational religion could not be allowed to direct the institutions of education and government, a nondenominational Christian morality was essential to the production of good citizens (Nelson, 2001, 57–75).

Between 1829 and 1900, Catholic sisterhoods established 299 hospitals in the United States. Despite the power of anti-Catholicism, they established the foundations of the private system of hospital care that emerged in the twentieth century. Because they could offer financially attractive care for the sick poor, they won contracts with insurers, private companies, the federal government, and the army.

As early as 1807, Elizabeth Seton, a Catholic convert, founded the Sisters of Charity (later the Daughters of Charity). The Napoleonic wars prevented connection with the French Daughters. In 1823 the Sisters of Charity took over nursing at the Baltimore Infirmary, which was affiliated with the University of Maryland. In the face of episcopal interference in their affairs in New York, the sisters split in 1846. Those who chose to remain in the diocese of New York formed the Sisters of Charity of Saint Vincent de Paul of New York and created Saint Vincent's Hospital in 1849. In 1858, to buttress their independence, they also became the U.S. province of the French Daughters of Charity of Saint Vincent de Paul. However, not all were happy with this, and ultimately five separate communities were established. Despite their organizational problems, the Daughters of Charity established 44 hospitals throughout the United States between 1823 and 1898.

The fortitude of the sisters as they nursed the victims of epidemic cholera or yellow fever won them the admiration of many non-Catholics. Among the poorest who were dying in the city slums were Irish immigrants—the saving of whose souls was as important as the care of their ravaged bodies. Moreover, Protestant wariness of Catholics meant there was a dearth of charitable institutions in which poor Catholics might be cared for. The need for the Catholic nursing nuns to found and run hospitals was thus great.

The nursing nuns served on both sides during the Civil War. After the war, their involvement in the establishment of hospitals continued to increase, reaching a high point in the 1890s, when 89 new hospitals were founded by 59 communities. Diligent, disciplined, and technically skilled, the sisterhoods were knowledgeable about business enterprise and sources of private and government funding, and they were astute in their dealings with clergy and doctors alike (Nelson, 2001, 32–54).

In Germany, the success of the Catholic revival brought the church into conflict with both the Prussian state and liberalism. The Kulturkampf witnessed the state's persecution of Catholic clergy and religious communities and the migration of a million Germans to the United States between 1870 and 1880. Among the immigrants were Mother Odilia Bergen and a handful of nursing nuns, who, on arrival in Missouri, where many Germans resided, set up a community of the Sisters of Saint Mary. They opened a number of hospitals: Saint Mary's in Saint Louis (1877), Saint Joseph's in Saint Charles (1887), Saint Mary's in Chillicothe (1888), the Saint Louis Quarantine Hospital, and railroad hospitals in Saint Louis and Sedalia.

Between 1849 and 1900 no fewer than six Catholic sisterhoods established hospitals in New York and Brooklyn. The Sisters of Charity, Sisters of Saint Joseph, Dominican Sisters, Franciscans, Misericordia Sisters, and the Missionary Sisters of the Sacred Heart founded at least one hospital each; as a result, after New York and Brooklyn merged in 1898, altogether they were running about half of the city's charitable hospitals and associated institutions. Their hospitals were the site of their spiritual life, as well as their communal world, and patients were seen to be like them—sufferers in the mystical body of Christ. Moreover, the smallness of their hospitals compared with city-run health institutions helped preserve a strong sense of connection with patients.

Beginning in the Progressive Era, hospital reform, including the professionalization of nursing, challenged the role of the sisterhoods in New York hospitals. Although the Catholic hospitals did not close, in the face of the new salience of scientific and professional discourses, the reputation of the sisters as health care experts declined both inside and outside the church (McCauley, 1997, 289–308).

In Canada, the Catholic revival saw 57 new female communities formed between 1837 and 1914. They established missions on the frontiers of settlement, as well as in cities. Four Grey Nuns traveled from Montreal to Red River in 1844. Fifty years later, the Sisters of Providence (founded in Montreal in 1843) went north from Portland to Vancouver. They soon opened a 25-bed hospital, known as Saint Paul's Hospital. By 1907 they had opened a school of nursing at Saint Paul's (Perin, 1996, 212; Providence Health Care, 2006).

Women religious founded the first hospitals in New France, beginning with l'Hôtel-Dieu de Québec in 1639. As noted already, a new wave of hospital establishment occurred in the 1840s. By 1920, more than 100 had been established, and 10 years later there were 134 hospitals conducted by 29 different orders of nuns, of which the main ones were the Grey Nuns, the Sisters of Providence, the Sisters of Saint Joseph, and the Sisters of Misericordia. By the early twentieth century, the Methodist (later United) and Anglican churches, the Salvation Army, and other religious and charitable groups had also established hospitals (Agnew, 1974, 1–2, 40–41).

Seeing the huge need for hospitals in U.S. industrial cities, Pastor William Passavant persuaded Kaiserwerth to send four deaconesses to Pittsburgh in 1849. A hospital was provided, but the order had difficulties retaining members. In 1884 seven deaconesses led by Oberin Sister Marie Kruger migrated from Westphalia. Located in one of the strongest Lutheran centers in the United States, the Philadelphia group successfully adapted to the new conditions. In England, Australasia, and North America, Anglicans, Methodists, and various evangelical groups took up the deaconess model, although not all deaconesses everywhere focused on nursing as they did in the United States. In the late nineteenth century new waves of immigration from Scandinavia led to Norwegian, Swedish, and Danish Lutherans establishing deaconess houses and hospitals in the United States. Erik Fogelstrom founded the Immanuel Deaconess Institute in Omaha, and by 1890 enough trained women were available to open the Immanuel Hospital. Fogelstrom believed the spiritual alienation of pioneering life could be overcome through the caring work of the sisters (Nelson, 2001, 138–43).

When the first five Irish Sisters of Charity arrived in Australia five decades after the beginning of European settlement, Sydney was the seat of government for the whole vast continent, as well as for New Zealand. About half the population was of English origin, a quarter Irish (many convicts or ex-convicts), and the remainder mostly Scottish and Welsh. Reflecting the conditions of pioneer society, Australia's colonial population was heavily male. In 1840, per 100 population, there were almost 34 more males than females, and that difference was even greater in the earlier decades (Cumpston, 1989, 52–53, 92). Women convicts who were on assignment to settlers often became pregnant. The Female Factory at Parramatta housed pregnant and other female prisoners who were returned by settlers. The first Sisters of Charity came to care for the factory women and children. From 1788 to 1828, 40 percent of female convicts were Irish.

Mother Mary Aikenhead, who founded the Irish Sisters of Charity in 1815, believed the most efficient way to reach the largest number of impoverished sick people was by establishing a hospital. She thus opened Saint Vincent's in Dublin in 1834. In the same year, she agreed to send sisters to New South Wales (NSW) after John Bede Polding, the vicar apostolic of New Holland (New South Wales) and Van Diemen's Land (Tasmania), described the great needs of Irish women convicts. For almost two decades the Sisters of Charity did home nursing in Sydney, and then in 1857 they opened Saint Vincent's Hospital. Protestants and Jews, as well as Catholics, financially supported the hospital (Burns, 1968, 44–47; Nelson, 2001, 81–97).

The deaconess movement in Australasia remained small scale. A training house was set up in Melbourne in 1884. By 1890, the three deaconesses were involved in "rescue" and mission work in the slums. However, because they were unable to recruit, the house closed. In 1902 an interdenominational missionary college, Saint Hilda's House, was established, and two decades later it became an Anglican training center for deaconesses. The most influential deaconess institution was the Sydney Deaconess Institute, founded by Anglican Rev. Mervyn Archdall. The Sydney center focused on teaching, mission work, and welfare activities. While trained in nursing, the Sydney deaconesses did not run hospitals, although they helped pioneer specialist care of the dying in Australia and opened a home of peace for the dying in 1907 (Grierson, 1981, 101–2; Tress, 1993, 21–27).

In 1893 Edith Mellish from the London Deaconess Institution migrated to Christchurch, New Zealand, where she set up a deaconess community, later called the Community of the Sacred Name. The focus of its early work was on teaching and on nursing in the community. Sybilla Maude resigned as matron of Christchurch Hospital to develop a district nursing service with the Anglican deaconesses. The community continued to be a deaconess training center until the 1920s but then became an autonomous sisterhood with its own superior (Grierson, 1981, 105; Reed, 1987, 123).

In the same year as the Christchurch community was created, the Church of England Deaconess and Missionary Training House was established in Toronto, Canada, with the assistance of the English deaconess movement. As in the Kaiserwerth model, both nurses and teachers were trained. In the early years of the twentieth century, some deaconesses from the Rochester Deaconess Institutions migrated from England to Calgary, where they did both welfare and parish work. Some deaconesses worked on Indian reservations. Wilfred Stapleton, for example, spent fifteen years doing mission work with the Sioux in Manitoba (Grierson, 1981, 104–5).

Modern nursing emerged from a Christian pastoral mission to the nineteenth-century poor; the caring ethic of modern nursing was embedded in the evangelizing work of religious women. The nursing nuns were in charge of many hospitals in the Anglo-Saxon world when the modern acute-care hospital emerged. They were also in charge as professional training schools came into being. At the beginning of the nineteenth century, respectable nursing could be carried out only by nuns. Florence Nightingale was able to take the historical mission of the nursing nuns—nursing as moral and religious work—and confer it on a secular, professional group of women; by the close of the century the skills of this group were in more and more demand as hospitals ceased to be refuges for the sick poor and provided the most technologically advanced care for all in the community (Nelson, 2001, 151–63).

Sociologist Bryan Turner has argued that modern nursing is a perfect example of Weber's theory of the transition from religious to secular society. Modern nursing, as it emerged in the later nineteenth and early twentieth century, was a secular vocation, the religious origins of which ceased to matter. However, as Alison Bashford has pointed out in contrast to Turner, it is not simply a matter of secularization but a heritage of religious-moral legitimation in nursing that is noteworthy; this background has resulted in a continuing ambiguity in the location of nursing between religious/moral and secular/scientific fields of meaning.

Bashford argues that, as medicine became more reductionist, secular nursing perpetuated long-standing, nonreductionist ways of thinking about the body; moral meaning in health care was preserved, even if its status remained provisional. This latent religious-moral quality could be mobilized when needed or overlooked when the scientific face of nursing had to be paraded (Bashford, 1998, 43–61). The professional nurse as a carrier of religious-moral values was the Christian healer in modern form. Judith Godden and Carol Helmstadter argue further that the Nightingale construct of nursing privileged the woman's religious-moral character over her clinical knowledge, leaving "strength of understanding"—control of great clinical knowledge—to the male doctor (Godden and Helmstadter, 2004, 174).

HOSPICES FOR THE DYING

Hospitals and home nursing services were some of the fruits of resurgent Christianity. Another outgrowth of the Catholic and Protestant missionary surge was hospices for the dying. Again, France and Ireland did the pioneering work. In 1842 Jeanne Garnier established l'Association des Dames de Calvaire. In that hospice, which opened in Lyons in 1843, a calm and prayerful attitude in the face of death was to be observed. Although Garnier herself died in 1853, another six hospices were opened by the end of the century; the first of these was in Paris in 1874.

In 1845 the Sisters of Charity acquired a property in Harold's Cross, about a mile from Dublin Castle. Renamed "Our Lady's Mount," it was the motherhouse from 1845 to 1879, when the novitiate moved to Milltown. Sister Mary John Gaynor remained at Harold's Cross and founded Our Lady's Hospice there, which was officially opened in December 1879. Most of its dying patients came from tenement houses, and in the early years the majority suffered from tuberculosis. Later, cancer patients became common. Care of the soul was as much the aim as care of the failing body. An estimated 20,000 patients died in the hospice between 1845 and 1945 (*Our Lady's Hospice, Harold's Cross,* n.d., 19–25; *City Set on a Hill,* 1945, 20–25, 36; Clark, 2000a, 51).

The sisters used the term *hospice* because, like the medieval hospices, which provided food, lodging, and spiritual succor to pilgrims, the Dublin hospice was a stopping place for the soul on its journey to God. Palliation involved spiritual support, devoted physical care on the part of the staff, and stoicism on the part of the patient (Lamerton, 1980, 17; Kerr, 1993, 19). The environment was comfortable and, naturally, included Christian imagery and symbols.

Like European hospices, the earliest U.S. hospices provided what hospitals did not—comfortable accommodation. Unlike the European institutions, they focused on the care of cancer patients. In the 1890s Rose Hawthorne Lathrop became concerned for those of New York's poor who contracted cancer. At a time when cancer was commonly thought to be contagious, patients would often be left by family or friends to die, uncared for, in a poorhouse. Hawthorne Lathrop took a three-month nursing course at New York Cancer Hospital, and then in 1899 she and the women who had joined in her work as the Servants of Relief for Incurable Cancer opened Saint Rose's Hospice in lower Manhattan. She became Mother Alphonsa, and her organization, the Dominican Sisters of Hawthorne. The sisters established six more hospices in different cities (Siebold, 1992, 23; Joseph Sr., 2001).

In 1899, inspired by the work of the Dames de Calvaire, Annie Blount Storrs organized a small group of New York Catholic widows as the Women of Calvary to care for terminally ill, poor women in Manhattan. In 1915 Calvary Hospital was moved to the Bronx. There they were assisted by the Dominican Sisters of Blauvelt until 1958, and the work was subsequently carried out by the Dominican Sisters of the Sick Poor. In 1974 a lay administration took over (Cimino, n.d., 1–2; James E. Cimino, letter to Milton Lewis Calvary Hospital, Bronx, New York, from August 3, 2001, 1–2).

Few such homes for the dying were established in the late nineteenth and early twentieth centuries in the United States or indeed in any other Anglo-Saxon country, and their concerns were spiritual and moral, as much as the medical needs of the dying person.

In England, the need for specific institutions for the dying was recognized in part because, in the 1850s, institutions for the long-term incurable had already begun to be established. In the 1850s and early 1860s, both the *British Medical Journal* and the *Lancet* drew attention to the needs of the many terminally ill patients whose domestic circumstances prevented them from enjoying well-ventilated rooms, proper diet, and experienced nurses. One article pointed out that, in England, two-thirds of the more than 5,500 cancer deaths and 64,000 deaths from TB every year involved the incurable poor.

In the 1870s the Poor Law infirmaries cared for sick paupers, but the care was of poor quality and the stigma of pauperism ever present. In the 1880s, with the approach to TB becoming one of active treatment and prevention and with the public hospitals being unwilling to admit chronic cases, terminal TB sufferers had nowhere to go. Similarly, for those dying of cancer, institutional provision was woefully inadequate.

Two small London institutions did offer refuge to the respectable poor who were facing death: Saint Peter's Home, Kilburn, founded in 1861 by the Anglican Sisters of Saint Peter, kept a few beds for the dying; and the Hospital of Saint John and Saint Elizabeth, established in 1856, would accept dying patients (although only women and children before 1900). Outside London, institutional accommodation for the dying was equally sparse.

Frances Davidson founded the Friedenheim in Mildmay Park in 1885, primarily to accommodate people dying of TB. Although it initially provided only 8 beds, the number increased to 35 when it moved to a new location in 1892. While solicitous nursing and medical care were provided, the main object was spiritual support along Anglican lines. From 1890 to 1905, four new homes were opened in London: the Hostel of God (1892); Saint Luke's House (1893); the Home of the Compassion of Jesus (1903); and Saint Joseph's Hospice for the Dying (1905) (Goldin, 1981, 393–96; Humphreys, 1999, 24–50).

There is little information on the formative period of the Home of the Compassion of Jesus. However, it clearly shared the basic position of the other three homes. The Anglican Community of the Compassion of Jesus established it in Deptford in 1903, but by 1912 it had moved to Thames Ditton. It catered to the "superior" poor who were to receive care of both body and soul.

The other three hospice establishments were founded as part of the wider work of the religious organizations responsible for their foundation. Indeed, Saint Joseph's Hospice for the Dying was the third such institution established by the Irish Sisters of Charity.

The sisters were invited to work among the poor Catholics of Hackney because of the low level of religious observance among Irish immigrants. Saint Joseph's opened as a 12-bed hospice in 1905, expanding to 25 beds in 1907.

The Methodists had also become concerned about the problem of declining church attendance, and a "forward movement" was established to focus on social needs rather than the traditional concern with personal salvation. In 1887 the London Wesleyan Methodist Mission created the West London Mission, having already created central and east London missions. Its services included everything from youth clubs to a "poor man's lawyer" service. By 1888 it had a medical department headed by Dr. Howard Barrett. The West London Mission agreed to provide a home for the dying; named for Saint Luke, it opened with 15 beds in 1893. In 1911 the governing committee of Saint Luke's decided to become independent of the mission.

The Hostel of God opened in Clapham in May 1892. Named after the Hôtel-Dieu in Paris, it had 15 beds and was staffed by the Sisters of Saint James' Servants of the Poor, an Anglican sisterhood formed in the 1880s. In 1896 the Sisters of Saint Margaret of East Grinstead took over from the founding sisters. Formed in 1855, the Sisters of Saint Margaret had progressed from home nursing and pastoral care to establishing a variety of institutions and setting up branches throughout England and Scotland, as well as abroad.

These late Victorian homes for the dying all sought to provide a homelike ambience, the better to encourage spiritual reflection. They would not admit the chronic, the infectious, or the mentally disturbed. They functioned mostly in isolation from each other. They were reliant on charitable donations and subscriptions, but Saint Luke's came to depend on patient contributions more and more, just like the public hospitals.

All of the homes saw the dying person as having a body, mind, and soul and associated different types of pain and suffering with each of the three: physical pain, mental anguish, and agony of the soul. Pain and suffering served to bring the sufferer closer to Christ. However, beginning around 1915, care of the soul was no longer uppermost at Saint Luke's, even if spiritual concerns continued to preoccupy Saint Joseph's and the Hostel of God. Instead, there was equal emphasis given to the care of the body, mind, and soul. This shift had something to do with Barrett's retirement as medical superintendent in 1913 and perhaps with the general decline in interest in religion brought about by World War I. It also had to do with a change after 1917 in the function of Saint Luke's, which now became "Saint Luke's Hospital for Advanced Cases," a special public institution. Indeed, in 1925 it saw itself as a modern, fully equipped hospital.

From 1890 to World War II the Hostel of God retained a strong spiritual emphasis, and in accordance with Anglo-Catholic thinking, the sacraments were especially important in one's preparation for death. Saint Joseph's remained committed to ensuring a holy and happy death, but since many patients in the early 1920s were non-Catholic, they first had to be persuaded of the need to die as a Catholic (Humphreys, 1999, 50–72, 86–89, 109–12, 117–26).

In 1890 the success of the Dublin hospice of the Sisters of Charity encouraged them to establish another hospice on the other side of the world: the Sacred Heart

Hospice for the Dying, near their general hospital, Saint Vincent's, in inner-city Sydney. Demand for beds increased (in the first decade, almost 1,000 patients had been admitted), and the original 13-bed hospice (with its 3-bed isolation ward) was demolished. A two-story, sandstone and brick hospice was opened by Cardinal Moran in October 1901. It contained two general wards, six medium-sized wards, and six private wards. Moran warned of a utilitarian spirit abroad that coldly argued that an end should be put to the terminally ill. Rabbi Landau proposed a vote of thanks to the cardinal and to the sisters. Among the patients admitted in the first decade were, in addition to Catholics, Anglicans, Presbyterians, Methodists, Jews, Muslims, and Chinese. In the 1930s the sisters established Caritas Christi Hospice in Melbourne and Saint Joseph's Hospice in Lismore, New South Wales.

In Nottingham in 1877 Mary Potter founded the Little Company of Mary to care for the sick and save the souls of the dying. In 1885 a small group of nuns arrived in Sydney and immediately began nursing the sick and dying in their own homes. In 1889 they opened a small children's hospital. When women were admitted in 1892, its name became "Lewisham Hospital for Women and Children." The order opened Calvary Hospital in Adelaide in 1900. The original, special concern with the needs of the dying tended to be overshadowed by the huge task of developing surgical and medical nursing services in acute-care hospitals that, in the first half of the twentieth century in Australia, as in the other Anglo-Saxon countries, were increasingly caught up in the technological advance of medicine. In the 1960s the Little Company of Mary opened modern hospices for the dying in various cities across Australia (*Sydney Morning Herald,* 1901; MacMahon, 1973, 1–21; Wordley, 1976, 10–51; O'Carrigan, 1986, 66–67, 206; Harris, 1995, 11–13).

The population of Western Australia increased dramatically in the 1890s, and the need for institutions to care for the sick poor likewise increased. The Irish Sisters of Saint John of God served as nurses in the gold-mining district in 1896, establishing a hospital in Kalgoorlie. The Methodist Sisters of the People provided home nursing in Perth and in the gold-mining area for the chronically ill, for whom the few hospital beds were not available. In 1896 Lady Madeleine Onslow, wife of the chief justice, and other prominent Anglicans, supported by surgeon Athelstan Saw, opened the Anglican Home of the Good Shepherd for the chronic and terminally ill. Lacking funds, the home was forced to close in 1898. However, the Forrest government indicated it would provide public funds but only for a nondenominational facility. State aid to churches and religious schools had ceased in 1895.

The Home of Peace opened in 1902. Of the first 100 patients, a third had some form of paralysis, a third had cancer, and the remainder had chronic rheumatism, dementia, or spinal injury. The state government continued to subsidize the home. Since cancer was still considered contagious even by some doctors, general and private hospitals—even the Saint John of God hospital—would not willingly accommodate cancer patients for long periods. From 1903 to 1918, 500 cancer patients were admitted, most in an advanced state. The only treatment available was morphine for pain. By 1935 a total of 1,000 patients had been admitted, and of these, 616 were cancer sufferers. In 1939 Matron Ruth Bottle visited the Home for Incurables in Adelaide and the Austin Hospital in Melbourne and reported that the focus at the Austin had changed from the care of the incurable to rehabilitation of the chronically ill. In 1948 the name of the home became the Home of Peace for the Chronic Sick (Gare, 2001, 23–27, 55–76, 91–95, 128–31, 165–68).

Visiting a Catholic hospice for the dying, Archdeacon J. D. Langley was asked by a patient why the Anglican Church in Sydney did not have a similar institution. Working with Maude Ashe, superintendent of Deaconess House, and Dr. W. H. Crago, Langley amassed enough funds to purchase Eversleigh, a house in Petersham, a western suburb. In 1907 Eversleigh was opened as the first Anglican House of Peace for the Dying in Sydney. A matron and nurse could care for up to six patients at a time. By 1941 a total of 4,700 people had been admitted to the home. In 1947 the home qualified for state government funding. A second Home of Peace Hospital, Neringah, opened in 1955, and a third at Greenwich on the north shore a decade later (Dibley, 1991, 17; Tress, 1993, 16, 22–33; Breward, 1993, 85–87).

Susan Schardt, herself blind from birth, formed a committee to provide accommodations for people discharged from Sydney hospitals as incurable and with nowhere to reside, and in late 1901 a home was opened. In 1906, when new premises were urgently needed, the governor, Sir Henry Rawson, convened a public meeting to deal with the situation. In December 1906 Weemala in Ryde was opened, and in 1924 a 25-bed facility for cancer patients was established. In 1954 the Home for Incurables became Royal Ryde Homes, and in the 1960s the institution began to provide rehabilitation services (*Australasian Medical Gazette,* 1906, 291; Royal Rehabilitation Centre, 1995).

In Adelaide, the Home for Incurables, which opened in 1879, was the innovation of Julia Farr, wife of the headmaster of the Anglican Saint Peter's College. At the close of 1881, the home had 44 patients. In these early years, TB patients were admitted, as were cancer patients for a few years around the turn of the century. One hundred years after the first patients were admitted, the home accommodated 826 patients (*Australasian Medical Gazette,* 1912, 347; Kerr, 1979, 5–6, 11–16, 49).

In 1880 Elizabeth Austin, widow of a wealthy rancher, gave £6,000 to establish a hospital for incurables. About the same time, a letter appeared in the (Melbourne) *Argus* from a reader who called for an institution for incurables, pointing out that the ward for the terminally ill at the benevolent asylum was almost always full. In 1885 the governor's wife, Lady Loch, opened the new cancer wards (Second Annual Report of Austin Hospital, 1883–1884, 4, 6, 19; *Australian Medical Journal,* 1885, 139).

Just as cancer cases had been isolated in special wards, an area for tuberculosis patients was opened in 1891 because the TB sufferer with no means and barred from general hospitals had nowhere to go but jail. The hospital management committee noted that the rapid advance of medical science was offering hope to some incurables, but treatment was largely symptomatic, with morphine, blisters, or poultices for relief of pain.

Soon after Robert Koch introduced tuberculin injections, they were used at the Austin Hospital. In 1902 the committee undertook to increase the number of beds for TB patients from 41 to 100. Beginning in that same year, professional bedside nursing was offered by Isabel Marsh, the head nurse of the TB ward. In 1907 Matron Marsh applied this professionalism to nursing throughout the hospital (Gault and Lucas, 1982, 5–10, 21–22, 31–45, 52–57).

In the 1880s and 1890s, cancer patients could expect only radical surgery (at considerable risk) to remove the cancer and morphine to dull their pain. Many arrived in such an advanced state that they in effect came to die. The Melbourne and Alfred hospitals sent cancer patients on to the Austin, which also took patients from rural areas. In 1906 X-ray therapy was used on superficial cancers, and in 1924 the Syme Pavilion acquired a deep X-ray center. In 1926, 50 milligrams of radium were loaned to the hospital, and a committee member, Meyer Zeltner, paid for additional radium. In addition to TB and cancer, paralysis due to a variety of causes was another common reason for admission.

Spiritual support was provided by visiting chaplains. However, in the first few decades, religious services and entertainment alike had to be held in the wards. In 1917 Meyer Zeltner and his wife, both liberal Jews, offered to fund a hall for these activities.

In the late 1920s Hugh Trumble used surgery to treat pulmonary tuberculosis, inducing the collapse of the diseased lung to allow it to rest. In 1931 he carried out operations for thoracoplasty to achieve the same effect. From 1931 to 1939, 47 people were treated in this manner, with a death rate of 15 percent, and 18 people returned to work (Gault and Lucas, 1982, 57–74, 119–21).

From 1886 to 1890 the TB mortality rate in Victoria climbed to a peak of slightly more than 183 per 100,000 population but fell to just under 77 (Australia) between 1911 and 1915. In New South Wales, the Queen Victoria Homes operated two sanatoria (with 106 beds). Indigent, advanced cases were sent to the state asylums at Liverpool and Newington. In 1909 the state opened a sanatorium at Waterfall. By 1915 there were 474 total beds in New South Wales (i.e., less than half of the average annual deaths from TB). About 18.5 percent of patients died in sanatoria, and at best 7 percent of institutionalized patients recovered.

Victoria also had sanatoria run by the state and public organizations: Heatherton (with 90 beds) had been set up jointly by the state and local government authorities; Greenvale was run by the state; Amherst (with 62 beds) and the tuberculosis wing at the Austin Hospital (with 120 beds) were charitable institutions that received government subsidies. Victoria had a total of 372 beds in 1915. All of the early cases were encouraged to go into sanatoria, where they normally did not stay longer than three months, during which time they were shown how to care for themselves at home with minimal supervision from visiting nurses. The Austin Hospital took the terminal cases, although in the interwar period active treatment began to be pursued. The smaller states also had sanatoria. Queensland had three, all run by the government, with a total of 157 beds. Western Australia had 300 beds at Wooroloo. South Australia and Tasmania each had a charitable institution subsidized by the government. Consumptive homes attached to the principal general hospitals in Adelaide and Hobart took a few terminal cases (Thame, 1974, 85–89).

When Saint Vincent's Hospital opened in Sydney in 1857, the Sisters of Charity accepted TB cases. From 1882 to 1895 they admitted 416 TB patients, of whom 21 percent died, and, from 1895 to 1907, 532, of whom only 9 percent died. The latter were mainly early cases amenable to sanatorium-style care and, in some cases, tuberculin therapy.

In 1886, recognizing that the need for care was not being fully met, the sisters opened Saint Joseph's Hospital for Consumptives at Parramatta and three years later erected a new 50-bed facility next door. Saint Joseph's moved to Auburn in 1892. At its opening in 1889, the Sacred Heart Hospice at Darlinghurst admitted people who were dying of TB. Whereas Saint Joseph's was for patients who were able to be rehabilitated, the Home for Consumptives, founded in 1877 by philanthropist John Hay Goodlet at Picton outside Sydney, was a hospice for incurable cases. Between 1886 and 1893 the home admitted 960 people, of whom 226 died. To celebrate Queen Victoria's jubilee, the Queen Victoria Homes for Consumptives Fund was established in 1897. In 1898 the fund assumed control of the home and in 1903 opened another one in the Blue Mountains, west of Sydney.

The Tasmanian sanatorium was opened in 1905 as a charitable institution. By 1935, artificial pneumothorax was the standard treatment for appropriate cases. By the early twentieth century, Queensland had sanatoria at Dalby, South Brisbane, Westwood (near Rockhampton), and, in 1923, Stanthorpe. In Western Australia, where tuberculosis among miners was, as in Victoria, a serious problem, a sanatorium was opened in 1906 in Coolgardie, one of the gold-mining centers. In 1915 the patients were transferred to the new 200-bed sanatorium at Wooroloo, near Perth. In the 1920s, active treatment began with the use of tuberculin, then pneumothorax, and, after that, thoracoplasty. In South Australia, the James Brown Memorial Trust decided in 1893 to build a sanatorium at Kalyra. It avoided becoming a dumping ground for advanced cases, as was the Hobart or Perth sanatorium. The first large sanatorium in Victoria was Heatherton. Gresswell was not established until 1933. While some thoracic surgery was done, the great majority of patients had the "rest cure" until chemotherapy was applied about 1950, and most were rehabilitated (Proust, 1991, 148–51; Layland and Proust, 1991, 27–29; Abrahams, 1991, 47; Edwards and Johnson, 1991, 52).

In 1872 (when national statistics first became available) New Zealand had a tuberculosis mortality of 126 per 100,000 population, which was substantial but well below the mortality rate in England and Wales, where it was about 300 per 100,000. Among white settlers, the mortality from TB fell almost 30 percent in the last two decades of the nineteenth century. In the early 1900s, health authorities mounted the first campaign against TB. In 1903 the New Zealand Department of Public Health established the first sanatorium, Te Waikato, as a model for hospital boards elsewhere to emulate. Te Waikato offered the latest in sanatorium treatment: good food, fresh air, rest, and labor appropriate to the fitness level of the patient. In 1904 Dr. T. H. A. Valintine raised funds for a small sanatorium near New Plymouth. Near Christchurch, Sybil Maude, a nurse, did the same for a camp for the poor, which became Cashmere Hills Sanatorium in 1909. The Wellington Hospital Board established Otaki Sanatorium in 1906. The Auckland Hospital Board placed patients in the Costley Home for the Aged Poor (later Green Lane Hospital) in 1908, and in 1910 the Otago Hospital Board established Pleasant Valley Sanatorium near Dunedin.

By 1910, health authorities believed that, while provision for early cases was satisfactory, care for advanced cases was not, primarily because hospitals would not readily admit them. In the interwar period, the number of beds increased only slightly. In the early 1930s, a survey of all sanatoria, 25 hospitals, and 74 medical practitioners revealed that 18 patients had had thoracoplasty and 256 had had artificial pneumothorax (Bryder in Proust, 1991, 79–83; Smith, 1988, 7–10).

The standardized death rate from TB in England and Wales declined from about 330 per 100,000 population in 1860 to about 180 in 1900 and to about 95 in 1930. The standardized death rate for pulmonary TB from 1930 to 1932 ranged from 61 per 100,000 for upper- and middle-class males to 125 for unskilled males (Bryder, 1988, 4–7).

In the early 1900s there were four specialist hospitals in London, two at Bournemouth, the National Hospital at Ventnor, and special wards in Liverpool, Manchester, and Newcastle. Except in Edinburgh, there were no hospital beds in either Scotland or Ireland. By 1910 there were 61 public and 29 private sanatoria. Poorer workers could not obtain access and thus used outpatient facilities or dispensaries or remained at home. When chronic or terminal, they often ended up in the Poor Law infirmaries. Indeed, about 60 percent of the 11,000 people admitted each year to these infirmaries had TB. Most of the sanatoria would admit only early cases, partly because they required much less nursing assistance.

The National Insurance Act of 1911 allowed local government to fund 60 percent of the capital costs of sanatoria. In 1911 about 2 percent of sufferers were resident in sanatoria in Britain and Ireland. In 1935, 11 percent were in residential institutions. Those with advanced TB who had the means went to private nursing homes, and a tiny number of indigent patients entered a charitable hospice like the Friedenheim in London. Thousands of the disadvantaged were accommodated in the Poor Law infirmaries, but most of the sufferers spent their last days at home (Smith, 1988, 97–130).

In 1870, Philadelphia, with 674,000 people, was the second largest city in the United States. As in other parts of the country, the municipal government was responsible for caring for the destitute. Outdoor medical care was supplemented by the Philadelphia Hospital and Almshouse. While most TB deaths occurred at home, 7 percent of the city's deaths from consumption occurred at the poorhouse, the U.S. version of the British workhouse. In 1876 the Protestant Episcopal Mission established the Home for Poor Consumptives as a new department that provided mainly home care, with a few indigents with advanced TB admitted to the House of Mercy. In 1886 it opened the new Chestnut Hill Home, where early cases were helped to recover. A conflict began developing between the traditional Christian care approach and a more confident medicine, whose goal was to cure. By 1898 the mission was listing the institution as the Hospital for Diseases of the Lungs at Chestnut Hill.

In the mid-1890s the Catholic-backed Free Hospital for Poor Consumptives was created to assist advanced cases among the poor. The hospital did not care directly for patients but paid for their care at other institutions: at first, at Rush Hospital and Saint Mary's Hospital, one of three Catholic hospitals. Later on, Saint Agnes Hospital, University Hospital, and the German Hospital also took consumptives. In 1901, just as the City Mission had, the Free Hospital stated that it considered TB to be a curable condition, and a camp with a sanatorium-like regime was opened in the east Pennsylvania mountains. By the early twentieth century, more affluent patients were also entering sanatoria, which were privately run and more comfortable. However, with the Depression's adverse impact on incomes, by the mid-1930s such private sanatoria had virtually disappeared (Bates, 1992, 42–58).

The institutional care of consumptives had been initiated by those with spiritual and moral goals—primarily, saving the souls of the terminally ill. But by the 1890s these goals were becoming secular and medical—segregation to prevent the spread of infection and, next, cure, became objectives. The urge to cure by focusing on early cases competed with the care of chronic cases. In the medical model, the latter was justified not in terms of saving their immortal souls but preventing the spread of the disease. With the advent of effective chemotherapy in the 1940s, expansion of the state system of sanatorium beds ceased. The White Haven Sanatorium was donated to the Jefferson Medical College in 1946 to improve the training of doctors and nurses, and ten years later it was closed down. State sanatoria at Hamburg, Gresson, and Mont Alto were closed in 1959, 1963, and 1968 respectively. The Home for Consumptives at Chestnut Hill changed its focus first to chronic diseases and then to rehabilitation. The Philadelphia Jewish Sanatorium for Consumptives changed its disease focus to alcoholism and other drug addiction (Bates, 1992, 329–39).

By 1910 the United States had about 400 sanatoria, about one-third of which were run by local or state authorities. Overwhelmingly, these concentrated on early cases, and 50 percent of beds were intended for poorer patients.

Both Canada and the United States experienced a decline in TB mortality in the first half of the twentieth century, but in both countries it continued to be an important disease among immigrants and Native Americans. Yet, 20 years before the United States developed a policy on the use of the bacillus Calmette-Guérin (BCG) vaccine, the National Research Council of Canada had approved its use in 1925. Apart from teaching personal hygiene, Canadian sanatoria appear to have focused on the usual physical rehabilitation of patients through good diet, rest, and heliotherapy. The high cost of sanatorium care and a shortage of beds encouraged the spread of collapse therapy in the 1930s (McCuaig, 1982, 299–302; Feldberg, 1995, 8, 92–93, 102; Lerner, 1998, 56).

By the 1890s the term *incurable* was considered unacceptable in Australia (and other Anglo-Saxon countries). Indeed, in 1891 members of a Victorian Royal Commission inquiring into charitable institutions said they would seek a legislative change of the name of the Austin Hospital for Incurables to the more positive-sounding Austin Hospital for Chronic Diseases, but nothing came of this. In 1911 a proposal was made to change the name, but again, nothing happened. Finally, in 1927 "incurable" was removed from the name, and the institution at last became the Austin Hospital for Chronic Diseases.

The new medical superintendent, Rupert Willis, encouraged a curative approach, promoting initiatives such as laboratory work and the surgical treatment of pulmonary TB. In 1929 David Rosenthal was appointed resident radiologist. Deep X-ray and radium treatment of cancers was introduced. A new wing for 100 cancer patients was opened in 1931, and in 1933 the name of the hospital became the Austin Hospital for Cancer and Chronic Diseases. In his 1935 report, the medical superintendent said the Austin was now the largest cancer hospital in Australia.

In 1948 Kaye Scott brought back new treatments from the United States:

chemotherapy using nitrogen mustard to attack cancer cells was introduced, and radioactive isotopes were used in suitable cases. For the first time in the history of the Austin, people who had earlier been considered terminal had recovered enough to return home. In 1958 a cancer unit was formed where cancer specialists—physicians, surgeons, and radiotherapists—could consult with one another on the optimal therapy. At weekly case reviews, up to 12 specialists might discuss a patient's case.

These developments in cancer care in the first few postwar decades were part of a larger transition of the Austin to the status of a major general hospital. In 1958 the admission of chronic cases was suspended. An outpatient and casualty wing was opened in 1960, and in 1965 an agreement was signed with the University of Melbourne under which the Austin became one of its teaching hospitals (Gault and Lucas, 1982, 102–5, 116–19, 131–38, 243–53).

The Development of the Hospital

The Premodern World

In early Greece, patients might be treated at the shrines of Asclepius or in a physician's own house, but hospitals were unknown. In ancient Rome, sick slaves and soldiers might be treated in institutions called *valetudinaria,* but no hospitals served the general population. Care of others in Greece had been based on a principle of reciprocal hospitality and in Rome on family-based responsibilities. However, in Christianity, charity was the basis of care of others. The Church of Antioch, as early as the 340s, established *xenones* or *xenodocheia* (hospices) to house the poor. Aetius began to treat diseased and injured hospice inmates in the 340s, and from this developed the *nosokomeion,* the specialist facility for the sick, although the line between hostel and hospital was not always clear.

In the Western Roman Empire, the first *xenon* was established in Rome by Fabiola, a wealthy Christian convert. In the early ninth century, church synods linked established xenodocheia or *hospitalia* to cathedral chapters. However, it was the monasteries that became increasingly significant as centers of care. Indeed, from the fifth to the tenth century, monastic medicine was in the ascendant (Porter, 1996a, 208–9; Risse, 1999, 70–97).

In the sixth century, new xenones were established with imperial aid to house the poor and the sick in Constantinople and other important cities. Under the Emperor Hereclius (610–641), the first institution that was primarily medical (nosokomeion) was established. In the twelfth century Emperor John II Comnenus and his wife, Irene, endowed a monastery to honor Christ the Healer—the Pantocrator (supreme ruler). Within the Pantocrator was the traditional *triclinon* (infirmary) for monks in need of care, and outside the walls was a large xenon for sick pilgrims and the sick among the local poor. The first notable Arab hospital was opened about 707 in Damascus, where the bulk of the people were Christian. It was modeled on the xenones and nosokomeia of the Byzantine Empire. A royal *bi-*

maristan (place for the sick) was opened in Baghdad in the 790s. Muslim rulers established large bimaristans in a few major cities: Cairo (874), western Baghdad (918), eastern Baghdad (981), Damascus (1156), Cairo (1284), and Granada (1366). These were impressive imperial institutions, and physicians loomed large in their activities, including clinical teaching and therapeutic innovation (Risse, 1999, 120–30).

In medieval England, the word "hospital" might be applied to four types of institution—leper houses, poorhouses, hospices for poor travelers, and institutions that housed the nonleprous, sick poor. Of 1,103 hospitals identified in medieval England and Wales, 345 were establishments for people with leprosy. There were 742 poorhouses, and in both poorhouses and leper hospitals, lay brothers and sisters cared for the ill. Hospices for travelers did not provide medical care as such. Hospitals for the sick poor—12 altogether—used the services of lay brothers and sisters and only rarely those of physicians or surgeons. Over time, corruption and poor administration led to the closing of many hospitals. Of the 112 in medieval times, by 1535, 24 had disappeared (Carlin, 1989, 21–36).

During the English Reformation the crown seized church property, including the hospitals. After being petitioned by citizens, Henry VIII in 1544 gave London Saint Bartholomew's and, two years later, the Greyfriars. His son, Edward VI, gave Bridewell and also the endowments (but not the buildings) of the Savoy. The five institutions were funded by donations (later taxes) from city parishes and were intended to form a centralized system of welfare for the poor. Each had its own target population: Saint Bartholomew's, the sick; Saint Thomas's, the aged; Christ's Hospital within Greyfriars, orphans and foundlings; Bethlehem (Bedlam), lunatics; and Bridewell, the idle poor, who were given employment in useful trades.

The growth of London from 100,000 people in the mid-sixteenth century to more than 350,000 by 1640 meant the five royal hospitals could not cope with the needs of the sick and the poor. The Great Fire of London in 1666 led to the reconstruction of two of the royal hospitals—Bridewell and Christ's. Then in 1676, a new Bedlam was built. The example of Les Invalides, the military hospital of Louis XIV, inspired the building of Chelsea Hospital. The royal naval establishment, the Greenwich Hospital, and Chelsea in turn inspired the rebuilding of Saint Thomas's in the 1690s and 1700s. The rebuilding of the rival Saint Bartholomew's began in the 1720s. After Thomas Guy provided funds for the purpose in 1724, a new hospital for the incurable sick and infirm, Guy's Hospital, was erected next door to Saint Thomas's.

Britain in the Eighteenth Century

In 1720, members of the Anglican Society for Promoting Christian Knowledge (SPCK), founded in 1699, helped establish the first public hospital, the Westminster Hospital. The founders were members of the Charitable Society, established in 1716 to carry out traditional acts of mercy such as visiting the sick. The society was in part inspired by the work of the Daughters and the Ladies of Charity in Counter-Reformation France.

The founding of Westminster Hospital and other public hospitals represents the redirection of charitable effort toward the provision of medical care. The development prefigured the modern hospital, but it also harkened back to the sixteenth-century models of institutional support for the poor. Guy's Hospital was originally to house incurables and in this respect was the same as Saint Thomas's. However, the parish-based relief system provided most of the support for the sick poor in this and the following century. Moreover, the new hospitals were for the working poor. Members of the pauper class were the responsibility of the workhouse.

By 1760 there were 16 public hospitals in provincial England, and by 1800, 38. The hospitals excluded a range of classes of patients—parturient women, children, people with mental illness, those with smallpox, VD, and TB, and the dying (Hart, 1980, 448–53; Porter, 1989b, 150; Granshaw, 1992, 201; Slack, 1997, 234–48).

Specialist hospitals began to appear in the mid-eighteenth century and came in a flood in the nineteenth. Lying-in hospitals for unmarried mothers and poor women with nowhere else to go began to be established: the British, 1749; the City, 1750; the General, 1752, and the Westminster, 1765.

By the 1860s, at least 66 specialist institutions were functioning in London. Usually set up by doctors seeking to take advantage of the expanding market for medical services created by middle-class prosperity, these institutions were to provide for classes of patients excluded from general hospitals and allow doctors to practice specialized skills. Indeed, specialization fitted well with the movement in medical theory away from a holistic, humoral conception of sickness to one of localized disease. In 1804 John Cunningham Saunders opened an eye hospital, subsequently known as Moorfields. During the next 20 years, at least 18 eye hospitals were opened across Britain. General hospitals responded by establishing eye departments in the 1850s and ear departments in the 1860s.

Hospitals were becoming more integral to medicine as the growing importance of clinical experience mandated student attendance in hospital wards. The Royal College of Surgeons in England required one year on the wards for licensing, while a licentiate of the Society of Apothecaries was required to have spent six months. By the 1860s hospital medical schools had become central to the education of medical students, and the requirements of the Medical Act of 1858 helped lock this into place (Granshaw, 1992, 201–8; Porter, 1996a, 213).

By the late nineteenth century, community attitudes toward hospitals, especially among the middle classes, were becoming more positive partly because the professionalization of nursing on the Nightingale model had produced a clean, disciplined, and trained nurse. The sanitary movement encouraged cleanliness not only in the home and the civic environment but also in the hospital, and in 1876 compulsory elementary education meant that lower-class women were a literate group ripe for recruitment into nursing. The multiplication of hospitals and the growth of medical interventions increased the demand for nurses. The more complicated surgery now performed required a hospital rather than a domestic environment for its effective practice.

Socioeconomic changes also affected the hospitals. The expansion of white-collar work saw members of the urban lower middle class seeking hospital care, and late in the century public hospitals began to take paying patients. Hospital insurance funds provided contributors with admission tickets, as did friendly societies and unions.

The Great War—World War I—saw all ranks treated in hospitals according to need. In 1920 Lord Dawson of Penn recommended a national network of primary health centers for lesser problems and secondary health centers staffed by specialists and based in major hospitals. Financial restrictions, among other factors, led to the shelving of the report. During the interwar period, the public hospitals struggled continuously with financial problems.

In 1948 the Labor government set up the National Health Service, in which the hospitals enjoyed a preeminent place. The high status of the public hospitals and their consultant staffs was now underwritten by the central government. Early in the new century, organizations such as the Imperial Cancer Research Fund and the Medical Research Council encouraged the development of a research culture. Even the new district hospitals were expected to promote research (Granshaw, 1992, 209–16; Lewis, 2003a, 209).

The public hospitals admitted operable cancer cases, but they banned inoperable ones because they increased the mortality rate. Most of the respectable poor with advanced cancers died at home, and paupers met their end in the workhouse infirmary. Among the specialist hospitals that proliferated in the nineteenth century was the cancer hospital. When his wife died of ovarian cancer in 1852, Dr. William Marsden, who had founded the Royal Free Hospital in London, established a small cancer facility, the London Cancer Hospital (later the Royal Marsden). From 1857 to 1886 imitators established cancer hospitals in Leeds, Liverpool, Manchester, and Glasgow. None of these survived into the interwar period of the twentieth century.

By the late nineteenth century, radical surgery for cancer (e.g., Halsted's radical mastectomy) was becoming standard treatment. The growing demand for space fueled by the promise of cure partly explains why the cancer hospitals of London, Manchester, and Glasgow decided to create separate facilities for the dying—Friedenheims—on the model of the homes for those dying of TB established in Germany in the 1880s. However, such facilities were never opened as commitment to curing was bolstered by surgical progress and the growth of research laboratories (Murphy, 1989, 222–38).

In the 1860s, 11,000 patients were accommodated in public charitable hospitals, and 50,000 sick paupers were being cared for by workhouse medical officers. In 1871 the workhouse infirmaries emerged as the first public-sector hospitals.

The Metropolitan Poor Act of 1867 marked the beginning of a modern state medical service. Whereas in 1866 only 111 paid nurses worked in the system (nursing was largely done by fitter patients), in 1888 there were more than 1,000. While the medical officer had been a private practitioner who attended the workhouse for a set period each day, now medical officers and assistants were resident. Except in large urban centers that had special public institutions, the Poor Law infirmary was the only institution that would accept the chronically ill.

By 1911 public hospitals had about 43,000 beds, but the public-sector hospitals increased their bed numbers from 83,000 in 1891 to about 154,000 in 1911. By 1911 there were 40 additional TB hospitals and 35 additional chronic-disease hospitals. Because conditions in the Poor Law infirmaries had improved, an increasing number of nonpaupers sought admission (Abel-Smith, 1964, 202–383; Hodgkinson, 1967, 498–545).

The United States

Philadelphia was home to the first general hospital, which was established in 1751. New York Hospital was founded two decades later, and the Massachusetts General Hospital in Boston in 1811. Hospitals were either municipal institutions for the poor or charities that often became business oriented. Insurance developed on a wider basis than in Britain, and this underpinned the business nature of many U.S. hospitals (Granshaw, 1992, 217; Porter, 1996a, 214).

By the late eighteenth century, poorhouses for paupers had become in effect municipal hospitals for the sick poor. Little had changed by the Civil War. Indeed, the first national survey of hospitals in 1873 listed as few as 178 hospitals, including mental institutions, and the county and municipal institutions still accommodated the bulk of inpatients. Doctors used the charitable hospitals, although they did not control them. Lay trustees or, in the case of the Catholic hospitals, nursing nuns ran them.

By the end of the first decade of the twentieth century, great changes had occurred. There were now more than 4,300 hospitals located across the country, and the well-to-do, the respectable, and the poor all used them. By 1920 the criticisms of hospitals familiar at the end of the twentieth century were being voiced, especially the impersonality and absence of a caring environment and the lack of concern for the needs of the chronically ill and the aged. Professional administrators and physicians now ran the hospitals, which had become the site for the most advanced practice of medicine. From 1870 to 1920, as Charles Rosenberg notes, the basic shape of the modern hospital had been established. Antiseptic surgery, the clinical laboratory, and X-rays stood for a medicine that was not only scientific but also effective. In 1870, bacteriology, diagnostic procedures and therapeutic progress based on immunology, serology, and X-rays advanced the bias toward acute care. Only the county poorhouse would take chronic and incurable cases.

No longer could educated people understand medicine, and medical knowledge and practices were now monopolized by those who were certified. Costs continued to rise as medical technology and professionalization progressed. Thus, even not-for-profit hospitals had to focus more on increasing income from private patients. The presence of trained nurses and nursing schools transformed the ward environments, which had hitherto reflected the lifestyle of working-class patients and their attendants, who came from the same background. Efficiency and profit maximization rather than Christian benevolence and stewardship became central, but the idea of the public good never quite disappeared (Rosenberg, 1987, 4–9, 339–48).

By 1900, depersonalizing practices were in place. Admission then involved a standard physical examination, compulsory bath, and often delousing. It was common to refer to the patient by bed number, in part to prevent any overly familiar relations with nurses. Deaths no longer occurred in the wards because the dying were removed to special rooms. The chronically ill and the aged were mostly placed in public institutions. Even in the 1900s, except for the Almshouse Hospital, all of the general hospitals in New York refused to take cancer patients, and most of them would not admit TB cases.

As early as 1910 there was a chorus of complaints about the modern hospital: the environment was impersonal and bureaucratic; specialists focused on their area of expertise, and no one took responsibility for the whole person; there was excessive concern with acute conditions that lent themselves to a technical response, while chronic cases and convalescents were of little interest. In 1906 S. S. Goldwater, administrator of New York's Mount Sinai Hospital, lamented the fact that treatment might not be decided by the patients' needs but by the practice of the department in which they were located.

By the early twentieth century, even some of the municipal hospitals were becoming technically sophisticated. By World War I, Philadelphia General Hospital was similar to the nearby public hospital, the Hospital of the University of Pennsylvania. Radiology and clinical pathology were a routine part of care, wards were organized according to diagnosis, a nursing school was in place, and a dozen or more medical specialties were represented. Yet it continued to function as a repository for the chronically ill, whom the city's public hospitals did not want to house. Only in the 1920s were an "insane hospital" and a "home for the indigent" established as separate institutions (Rosenberg, 1987, 311–27).

Even at the beginning of the twentieth century, leading members of the medical profession clearly recognized the need for good general hospitals to serve the purposes of medical education and research. In his influential 1910 report on medical schools in the United States and Canada, Abraham Flexner proposed that training in wards, dispensaries, and clinical laboratories be provided for students. Both private and public hospitals began to appreciate the advantages of a university-appointed medical staff and costly laboratory equipment. Many teaching hospitals used philanthropic funding such as that offered by the Rockefeller Foundation to improve facilities.

University hospitals quickly took the lead in training interns and residents in specialties, as well as in providing basic medical education. Specialization encouraged the admission of referrals rather than community-based general care. Many patients were enrolled in controlled clinical trials carried out by researchers. The development of teaching hospitals and updating of their equipment were underwritten by extensive federal funding, first in the 1940s under the Hill-Burton Act and then under National Institutes of Health research and training grants in the 1950s and 1960s. While the gross national product grew 5–9 percent a year in these two decades, institutional budgets grew 15–18 percent, and there was a 624-fold increase in funds at the National Institutes of Health. A whole generation of full-time academics was funded by the federal government.

Even in the 1960s warnings were being voiced about biomedicine's isolation from social and economic issues relating to health care. The teaching hospitals were not addressing the social problems of their communities, but with their finances boosted by Medicare and Medicaid reimbursements, they established a range of specialist services—cancer management, coronary and intensive care, trauma and microvascular surgery, diagnostic imaging, neonatal units, neurosurgery, and organ transplantation. Medical students were presented with a hospital-based paradigm based on a select patient population with complex diseases as the primary model of medical practice. They learned aggressive therapies, and the use of medical technologies to keep death at bay was the epitome of practice. Very demanding working commitments and extended specialty training, combined with an emphasis on academic ability rather than a caring capacity in the selection of trainees, made for a dehumanizing environment.

The late 1970s saw multiple challenges emerge: increased student numbers ceased to attract capitation payments; federal research funding could not so easily be used to underwrite educational work; and clinical income regardless of cost became more important as these established forms of funding became relatively less significant. Yet, the teaching hospitals remained the acme of the biomedical system, and intervening to extend life in what were disease states that could not be reversed remained the primary aim of the system. A disinclination to accept any limits and an open-ended commitment to prolong life became locked in place when fundamental changes in disease patterns and life expectancy were occurring. Since the early twentieth century, the United States (and other Anglo-Saxon countries) had been involved in an epidemiological transition from acute to chronic disease and even earlier in a demographic transition from high fertility and mortality to low fertility and mortality, with resultant increased life expectancy and growth in the proportion of the aged (Risse, 1999, 576–79, 608–9).

Canada

In England and Wales in the mid-nineteenth century there were 900 institutions for the ill (inclusive of workhouses), and by 1920, 5,000 such institutions. In the United States, there were 3 hospitals in the first years of the nineteenth century but 6,000 by the early twentieth century. The same notable increase took place in Canada: from a single hospital in Ontario in 1829 (the York General Hospital), the number increased to about 70 by 1929. In Canada as a whole in 1933, there were 589 public hospitals, of which 486 had a radiology department, 209 a clinical laboratory, 230 a physical therapy department, and 119 an outpatient department (Agnew, 1974, 5; Connor, 2000, 6).

As S. E. D. Shortt has noted, the nineteenth-century Canadian hospital was as much a moral reformatory for the sick poor as a health-restoring institution. Only late in the century, as middle-class patients began to use its services (attracted by advances in medical technology and propelled by demographic changes affecting the family's capacity to care for its own) and doctors began to dominate the administration, did hospitals begin to assume their modern guise as centers of medical science and nursing expertise. By 1875 Toronto General Hospital had as medical superintendent a physician who enjoyed both administrative and medical authority. Kingston General Hospital took the same path just over a decade later. In 1875 the doctors at Toronto General collectively advised on patient classification, preparation of a pharmacopoeia, and student education. By 1894 Kingston General had likewise instituted a medical board. Even in 1847, Montreal General Hospital had some paying patients. Kingston followed a decade later, and by 1893 about 20 percent of its income came from this source. At Montreal General, 29 percent of income came from patients in 1907, and, 14 years later, more than 70 percent (Shortt, 1983–1984, 6–9).

The emergence of the modern hospital may be viewed in more detail in the history of Toronto General, one of two nondenominational hospitals—Montreal General is the other—that functioned during the period when, through union, Canada evolved from a collection of colonies to the status of a leading industrialized democracy. Conceived of in the 1790s, built in 1819, and opened to indigent patients in 1829, Toronto General was first known as York General Hospital. It was renamed Toronto General Hospital in 1834. In the second part of the century, it cared for skilled workers, as well as the destitute. By the close of the century, middle-class patients were being admitted. Indeed, by about 1897, income from paying patients was equal to that provided by the provincial government. In the 1940s the availability of insurance plans removed much of the difference between public and private patients. The hospital's patients came not only from Toronto but also from a good deal of the rest of the province. Reflecting its emergence as an acute-care hospital, by the end of the nineteenth century the average stay of a patient was one month, and by the close of the twentieth century it was a week. In 1874 the intake of chronic cases and incurables decreased because of government financial pressure. This contributed to the growth of a more respectable image.

Between 1904 and 1930, the institution emerged as a significant academic hospital because of its links with the newly created Faculty of Medicine at the University of Toronto. Even before the first medical school had opened, the hospital had educated students because the sick poor had no choice but to act as clinical material. Late in the nineteenth century, not only were more students accommodated but training for nurses was also introduced, and the program eventually became Canada's largest. By 1930 the hospital was quite medicalized. The scientific side of the hospital had been growing, with the progressive introduction from the mid-nineteenth century of general anaesthesia, antisepsis, asepsis, X-ray technology, and laboratory medicine.

In the 1930s technological advances continued with the provincial government's endorsement of the war on cancer and its provision of funds for hospital-based institutes of radiotherapy. Toronto General's Ontario Institute of Radiotherapy was the most prestigious of these. Between 1930 and 1990 Toronto General came to occupy a leading position nationally in research and academic medicine (Connor, 2000, 9–11, 258–68).

Australia

In the nineteenth and early twentieth centuries, the large general hospitals in Australia were intended for the sick poor, although working-class people above the indigent level could be admitted if they paid a portion of the costs. Honoraries provided free care and in return gained clinical experience, prestige, and no doubt also personal satisfaction from their altruism.

The Australian colonies had foresworn Britain's Poor Law in dealing with the issue of the health and welfare of the poor, relying on a mixture of private charity and state support instead. Many private, for-profit hospitals, some of them quite small, existed, and even people of modest means used them. The larger private ones, usually established by religious bodies such as the Sisters of Charity or the Little Company of Mary, were not-for-profit and well run. The advances in medical science noted in other Anglo-Saxon countries also meant that the quality of medicine in the large public hospitals was outstancing what could be provided in the home or in small private hospitals.

In the smaller states, the large general hospitals were funded by the government, but in the more populous states—New South Wales and Victoria—they evolved as government-subsidized charities. The Launceston General Hospital in Tasmania's second oldest city was a government hospital. It decided in 1916 to admit all classes of patients, who were to pay according to their means. The following year, all public hospitals in Tasmania became committed to this policy. Angry, the medical profession boycotted the voluntary system. Not until 1930 did doctors again take honorary appointments at Hobart General Hospital.

The Adelaide Hospital in South Australia experienced a similarly inspired doctors' strike before the twentieth century, and patients were required to pay for their stay according to their income. The state government ran seven hospitals in extrametropolitan areas and paid subsidies to a number of small institutions. In Western Australia, in the face of the inadequacy of public contributions, the government had since colonial times provided most of the hospital funding. Means-tested maintenance fees were levied on patients in the 1920s.

Queensland hospitals likewise depended heavily on public funds. In 1920 all of the public hospitals in Brisbane and the South Coast region, the heavily populated part of the state, came under a government-appointed board. Country hospitals depended on the support of local people plus government subsidies. In the early 1920s, patients paid means-tested fees for their care (Thame, 1974, 259–66).

A more complex state of affairs existed in New South Wales and Victoria, where nongovernment funds were a much greater proportion of total income. Public hospitals enjoyed much more independence. In 1922 Victorian legislation established a board that was authorized to direct government funds more according to needs. It encouraged the levying of patients' fees for maintenance but suffered from the ongoing failure of government to provide adequate funding. Similar NSW legislation was passed in 1929, establishing a commission that was to distribute annual government grants on the basis of need. However, inadequate government subsidies limited the impact of the new body.

Patient contributory plans were operating in most rural areas of the states, but the practice could not be adopted by individual metropolitan hospitals because these lacked defined districts where contributors resided. In Sydney, the Metropolitan Hospitals Contribution Fund (1932) quickly came to cover about half a million people. In Victoria, a similar mutual fund, the Hospital Benefits Association, was formed in 1935 (ibid., 267–84).

The Melbourne Hospital (359 beds) was established in 1848, and the Alfred Hospital in 1871. Saint Vincent's Hospital, run by the Sisters of Charity, did not open until the 1890s. In 1884 the Alfred Hospital decided to open wards for paying patients, and these quickly became an important source of income. However, in 1891 the hospital was told to abolish its pay wards if it were to continue to receive government grants. In the Depression-ridden early 1890s, Melbourne Hospital saw its government grant decline from £15,000 to £12,000. It finally introduced a contributions plan for inpatients in 1899.

Even in the face of its financial problems, Melbourne Hospital increased its services. In the mid-1890s, the annual reports discussed the provisions for outpatients of the specialties of women's diseases and diseases of the ear and throat. Radiology was one of the first specialist technologies to emerge. In 1896 F. J. Clendinnen was appointed honorary skiagraphist, the first such position in an Australian hospital. An honorary anesthetist was also appointed. From 1898 to 1906 the number of patients having surgery rose markedly in part because many could pay part of their expenses at a time when the hospital was deep in debt.

The Alfred Hospital could not afford to purchase X-ray equipment until 1898, although G. L. Laycock had been appointed medical electrician in 1889. The position of medical electrician and skiagraphist became that of radiologist in 1920. There had been eight specialist posts created before that of skiagraphist in 1898: dispenser (always salaried) in 1871; dentist, 1884; pathologist, 1885; galvanist, 1885 (called medical electrician beginning in 1889); throat and ear, 1886; eye, 1886 (called ophthalmology beginning in 1920); skin, 1886; and chloroformist, 1888 (called anesthetist beginning in 1899). The number of medical specialties and paramedical services introduced between 1901 and World War II escalated notably: children's department, 1901 (called pediatrics beginning in 1948); masseurs, 1903 (absorbed by the medical culture department); clinical pathologist, 1904; venereal disease clinic, 1911; psychiatry, 1923; gynecology, 1923; biochemistry (always salaried), 1924; asthma clinic, 1925; antenatal clinic, 1925; medical culture department, 1925 (always salaried; became the physiotherapy department in 1928); diabetic clinic, 1926 (but interest in diabetes predates the clinic); Baker Medical Research Institute, 1926; radiology, which was divided into diagnostic and therapeutic, 1929; dietetics, 1930; orthoptics, 1930; neurological clinic, 1931 (full honorary status from 1934); general clinic, 1932 (to relieve minor conditions); oral surgery, 1934; almoner (social service worker), 1934; and clinical photography, 1936 (formerly undertaken by the pathology staff) (Mitchell, 1977, 155–56, 212–14; Walker, 1998, 31–33).

Driven by the same forces of demographic and epidemiological change, the advance of medical science, and the advent of new technologies, Sydney Hospital, the first hospital in Australia, developed the same specialist departments as the Alfred at about the same time. In 1898 X-rays began to be used. The old massage department under the control of a masseur became the Department of Special Therapeutics in 1909 (Watson, 1911, 180–81).

When the University of Sydney opened its medical school in 1883, Sydney had three general hospitals—Sydney Hospital (1811), Prince Alfred Hospital (1882), and Saint Vincent's Hospital (1857). All medical students went to Prince Alfred until 1909, when Sydney Hospital's clinical school opened. In 1923 the superior general of the Sisters of Charity successfully applied for Saint Vincent's to be accepted as a clinical school, pointing out that Saint Vincent's in Melbourne had been a teaching hospital of the University of Melbourne for 14 years. Beginning with 100 beds in 1883, by 1923 Saint Vincent's in Sydney had 313 beds. A relatively new honorary medical staff was appointed in the 1920s: the senior physicians included D. A. Diethelm, S. A. Smith, H. H. Bullmore, and J. P. Tansey. The honorary surgeons to inpatients were a formidable group, including Sir Alexander MacCormick, John (later Sir John) McKelvey, and H. M. Moran; a gynecology department was opened with the distinguished Dame Constance D'Arcy as a member of the staff; in addition, there were honorary ophthalmic surgeons; honorary surgeons for diseases of the ear, nose, and throat; honorary dermatologists; an honorary orthopedic surgeon; honorary radiologists; an honorary pathologist; and an honorary bacteriologist.

In 1924 a new pathology department was established, reflecting the wider uses of pathology, as in biochemical tests for blood sugar after the discovery of insulin. The Department of Radiotherapy and the Victor Deep Therapy Unit passed from the control of the university to the hospital in 1934. A social service department was opened in 1936, and in 1938 a diabetic clinic was established (Watson, 1911, 180; Hickie, 2001b, 91–92; Hickie, 2001a. 128–32).

In the colonial era many of the chronically sick poor ended their days in government asylums. Some categories of incurables were heavily stigmatized. End-stage syphilitics were considered both dirty and difficult to manage. The matron of the Liverpool Asylum in the early 1870s had cancer cases moved away from near the entry to the main building because they produced unpleasant odors. At the Adelaide Destitute Asylum in the 1890s, the same offensive smell made people with cancer less acceptable than even the popularly feared cases of tuberculosis.

Very little effort was made to provide religious consolation for the dying. In the mid-1880s, the authorities of Adelaide Asylum said that if a person was thought to be dying, relatives were notified where possible, and a member of the clergy was summoned if the patient wished. The superintendent of the notorious Dunwich Asylum outside Brisbane told an official inquiry in 1884 that nobody there administered religious rites to dying patients. A Catholic priest, who visited the asylum when possible, said he did not attend the burials of paupers.

South Australia and Victoria had the more decent asylum systems. While Melbourne had the largest such institution, asylums also operated in Ballarat, Beechworth, Castlemaine, and Sandhurst in 1868. In contrast, in New South Wales, the asylum system was located in and around Sydney. The total inmate population at the Melbourne asylum was 32 in 1851 and in the Depression years of the 1890s climbed to a peak of 680. From about 1870 to 1912, the average age at death of males in the asylum rose to 75 years. The demand for medical care increased as the inmate population became older, and, by 1880, 383 of 625 were classed as incurable.

In 1852, the South Australian system was centralized around the Adelaide Destitute Asylum. The asylum from the outset was officially seen more as a hospital for the infirm aged than as a workhouse; thus. terminal cases were brought there from general hospitals. Catherine Helen Spence, a social reformer who had observed conditions in England, claimed that Adelaide inmates lived in a less degrading environment than inmates of workhouses there. The medical officer, W. T. Clindening, noted in 1889 that the institution was largely a hospital for the terminally ill. Medical and nursing care was of a higher standard in the Adelaide institution than in the asylums of the other colonies. By the mid-1890s, a medical officer attended patients each morning. The nursing staff consisted of a matron, five trained nurses, and five male attendants (recruited from among the fitter inmates).

In Tasmania and Queensland, the colonial governments applied a punitive approach to infirm paupers similar to that applied to convicts. The 1871 Royal Commission on Charitable Institutions was critical of the poor conditions at Hobart's male invalid institution and even more critical of those in the female institution. In 1889 an official inquiry noted that unpaid inmates, not trained nurses, cared for the most of the patients. As late as 1888, it was estimated that more than 80 percent of inmates were ex-convicts. Believing over time that death would solve all of their problems, the governments steadfastly refused to spend money.

In Queensland, people who suffered from tuberculosis, cancer, paralysis, senility, and blindness were sent from public hospitals throughout the colony to Dunwich Asylum, a former convict outstation. Care came from less debilitated inmates, and doctors visited only occasionally. Thomas Stanley, an aged inmate bold enough to complain to authorities, told an 1884 inquiry that he heard a dying man begging, to no effect, for water; at night no one attended to hospital patients. In 1885 a single doctor was appointed to care for 400 inmates, and untrained attendants continued to be used. More than 30 years later, Dunwich was still notorious for its deplorable conditions.

The NSW government housed the infirm and aged poor in very large asylums—males at Liverpool (1862), Rookwood (1894), George Street in Parramatta (1862), and Macquarie Street in Parramatta (1894), and females at Hyde Park Barracks (1862) and Newington Asylum (1884). No professional nurses were employed until 1887, and the asylums were in effect dumping grounds for incurable paupers, from whose care the general hospitals wished to distance themselves. In the early 1870s a bed in an asylum cost only £12 per year, whereas one in a hospital cost £41.

In 1886 and 1887 a board of inquiry concluded that the medical superintendents and the matrons of the Parramatta and Newington asylums had been negligent, brutal, and mendacious. At Newington the terminally ill were so neglected that they sometimes died of starvation. In the cancer ward a bottle containing a morphine solution was readily accessible. The solution was often diluted, so the pain of cancer patients was probably not well controlled. Deaths from the misuse of drugs or physical abuse could easily be disguised because the doctor provided a supply of blank death certificates already rubber-stamped with his signature. The only result of the inquiry was the dismissal of the dreadful medical superintendent and the appointment of a few trained nurses.

The factor that finally pushed the government into reforming the system was the fear that tuberculosis sufferers in asylums would be a potent source of infection for the community as a whole. The government finally built a public sanatorium at Waterfall, south of Sydney. In recognition of their new functions, Rookwood, Liverpool, and Newington were redesignated as state hospitals. Rookwood, with a population of 1,300 males in 1911 and 1912, had two resident medical officers and six honorary specialists. Newington (for females) also experienced an upgrading of medical facilities. In a time of growing medical concern with cancer, a special cancer ward was established at Liverpool to house postoperative and inoperable cases (Jalland, 2002, 199–239).

New Zealand

Government hospitals, the first facilities in New Zealand, had opened in Auckland, Wellington, Wanganui, and New Plymouth by 1851. They served destitute Europeans and Maori. By 1910, 56 hospitals served a population of more than a million, but more than 70 percent of these had fewer than 50 beds. A number on the west coast, where gold mining had developed in the 1860s, had by the turn of the century become refuges for aged and infirm miners.

Like British public hospitals, New Zealand hospitals were supposed not to admit incurable cases, but exceptions were made in cases that involved great hardship. In his 1887 report, the inspector general of hospitals, Duncan MacGregor, proposed that hospital aid boards build local refuges for the aged, and he and his successor, T. H. A. Valintine, requested that homes for terminally ill patients be opened to assist urban hospitals. Unlike in Britain, the funding of hospitals from public contributions was relatively modest: in 1882, the government contributed about 70 percent of the income of all hospitals and slightly more than 36 percent in 1910.

As in Australia, doctors repeatedly complained of "hospital abuse," that is, the admission of patients who were able to pay for medical care, which they received free of charge. In the same period, specialties began to develop in hospitals in areas such as ophthalmology, otolaryngology, and gynecology. Duncan MacGregor, one of Lister's students, had introduced antisepsis to New Zealand in 1872. New Zealand's practitioners then quickly advanced abdominal surgery. Just as doctors in Australia kept abreast of the latest advances in knowledge and techniques from the medical journals and personal contacts in Britain, the United States, and Europe, so did New Zealand practitioners. The transfer of information was made easier after the establishment of the *New Zealand Medical Journal* in 1887. Moreover, early radiologists such as P. C. Fenwick of Christchurch Hospital were training in London around the time that Roentgen discovered X-rays (Dow, 1991, 46–63). The therapeutic application of X-rays began at the hospital as early as 1909. In 1915 Fenwick left on active military service. After his departure, his supply of radium was little used because no one else was trained in how to use the dangerous material, although P. D. Cameron of Dunedin had been employing it since 1911.

In the early 1920s the public became more aware of the therapeutic capacity of radium. Public funds were raised in Wellington, Auckland, and Dunedin. Christchurch Hospital decided to purchase radium and also to install a deep therapy plant. In 1934, the existence of a consultation clinic meant that radiotherapists, dermatologists, surgeons, and sometimes pathologists cooperated in developing cancer treatment plans (Bennett, 1962, 199–205).

The early hospital honoraries rarely had postgraduate specialist training. After 1910, most hospital doctors had a background as general practitioner or military surgeon and had then spent a period overseas when postgraduate qualifications were acquired. They came back as general physicians or surgeons with a focus on pediatrics, orthopedics, or some other specialty. After 1950, the pattern changed: many spent four years or more as residents and then obtained a postgraduate degree from one of the Australasian Colleges. They then acquired more experience in specialist positions overseas and returned as specialists in subspecialties. Thus, while some still practiced as general surgeons, many now were ENT (ear, nose, and throat), ophthalmic, orthopedic, plastic, thoracic, cardiac, peripheral vascular, pediatric, urological, renal transplant, neuro-, or gynecological surgeons. The old-fashioned general pathologist was now a morbid histologist, microbiologist, virologist, immunologist, clinical biochemist, hematologist, cytologist, forensic, or neuro-pathologist (Henley and Henley, 1977, 40).

OBSERVATIONS

The fact that the societies and cultures of these Anglo-Saxon countries were incompletely secularized underlies the problem of postulating a neat symmetry between the rise of modern science (including scientific medicine) and the decline of religion. Rather, we seem even in this late-modern era to be in the complicated situation of having a science-dominated culture and an associated human-centered worldview, which, for many people, offers insufficiently comforting metaphysical answers to the great existential questions that confront us. Nowhere is that seen more clearly than in the area of death and dying. Even many who have long abandoned the doctrines and rituals of organized religion seem to need some notion of spiritual matters or of personal transcendence in the face of death.

This larger dilemma of how to accommodate the spiritual realm in a culture deeply influenced by a materialist and reductionist science (and in societies and economies driven as never before by belief in a technological solution to every human problem) is reflected in modern medicine's quandary of how to reconcile its reductionist objectification of the patient with the call to care for the whole person in a compassionate way.

2 THE RISE OF MODERN MEDICINE

Western medicine is situated in a social, cultural, demographic, economic, and political context, and its development may be viewed from both an internal and an external perspective. In this chapter I approach the evolution of medical theories and practices from both standpoints.

Modern medicine evolved within a culture and a society whose fundamental values were set by the Christian church. The fall from grace that took place in the Garden of Eden not only brought sin into the world of humanity but also introduced bodily suffering and death. Yet, the doctrine of the Trinity—the nature of the Godhead and the incarnation and sacrifice of Christ on the cross—signified the immanent sanctity of the flesh. Thus there is some ambiguity about the body, just as there is about pain and suffering. Pain was punishment for original sin, whereas suffering was to be welcomed by Christians because it could bring their spirit closer to God. However, illness was also to be relieved by medicine and charity.

After all, Christ himself carried out a number of miraculous cures, and the church has always offered rituals of healing through holy relics, pilgrimages, holy water, and shrines of saints. As late as the mid-nineteenth century, the religious visions of a French village girl turned Lourdes into a place of healing for millions of supplicant sufferers.

However, Greco-Roman medicine, which continued as the learned medicine of the Middle Ages and the Renaissance, was naturalistic. The Hippocratic corpus saw the body alone as the source of illness; in turn, the body was part of nature *(physis);* neither supernatural entities nor sorcery were the cause of illness.

Greco-Roman medicine was also holistic. Greek medical writers developed the doctrine of the humors (fluids such as bile, phlegm, blood, and black bile), which, when in equilibrium, produced a healthy body and mind. Animal spirits (very fine fluids) linked body and mind, while different souls directed different functions. The doctrine was concerned with the whole person in two ways: illness normally arose from inner, constitutional developments, not pathogenic attacks from the outside, and body and mind interacted so that emotions might produce illness (Nutton, 1992, 22–23; Porter, 1996c, 83–92).

Reliable anatomical and physiological knowledge, so fundamental to scientific medicine, was denied to Greek and medieval medicine by cultural opposition to dissection as desecration of the body. The decisive break with Galenic anatomy was made by Andreas Vesalius (1514–1564). He and the pioneers of the new anatomy who followed him based their work on observation of the dissected human body, even if they knew more about structure than function.

THE BEGINNING OF SCIENTIFIC MEDICINE

The scientific revolution of the seventeenth century, epitomized by Isaac Newton's gravitational physics of the solar system, deeply influenced medicine because, if nature were truly made up of matter and subject to the universal laws of mechanics, it was best conceptualized as a machine, and therefore humans were machines. Thus, London physician William Harvey (1578–1657) offered an explanation of the circulation of the blood that relied on the conceptualization of the heart as a mechanical pump. The iatromechanists sought to apply the laws of physics to the body. Giovanni Borelli (1608–1679) explored the mechanics of breathing and the contraction of muscles. The iatrochemists for their part applied chemistry. Johannes Baptiste van Helmont (1577–1644) argued that bodily "spirits" were not mystical entities but chemical ferments that transformed food into flesh. Iatrochemistry did not enjoy as much credibility because chemistry was at this time much less developed than physics, but both ultimately failed to contribute much to clinical medicine because the basic scientific data were lacking (Ackerknecht, 1982, 112–27; Porter, 1996b, 154–62).

In the eighteenth century, while biological knowledge progressed as a result of the attempt to apply the new science to medicine, in their practice doctors continued to apply the traditional, qualitative assessments of the patient's condition based on input from the doctor's natural senses—the "feel" of the pulse (not the beats per minute), the taste of urine, the sound of difficult breathing, the smell of necrotic flesh, and the appearance of the skin and eyes.

Some diagnostic and etiological progress was made. Notable was Leopold Auenbrugger's method of percussing the body (especially the chest) with the fingers to establish by sound the health of the internal organs. He was clear about his wish to enhance the physician's diagnostic capacity by reducing the traditional reliance on the patients' subjective account of their illness and on external appearance. However, he did little to publicize it or to relate the percussive tones to postmortem lesions and to symptoms in the living.

Like Auenbrugger, Giovanni Battista Morgagni wanted to establish objective evidence of disease. In 1761 he published *The Seats and Causes of Diseases Investigated by Anatomy*. Morgagni's work created certain principles that informed the education of physicians and the practice of medicine from then on: disease usually imprints itself on the tissues, and these imprints, observable postmortem, can be used to diagnose disease in the living (Reiser, 1978, 16–22; Ackerknecht, 1982, 122–23). In the course of the nineteenth century, the relationship between physician and patient changed— from the use of verbal exchanges to discover the patient's experience of illness, to direct contact with the patient's body using physical examination, to indirect contact with sickness in the body by the use of machines and technical expertise. Earlier in the century, physicians relied upon their personal judgment and sensory impressions from manual examination and quite simple instruments. The patient's own assessment was now seen as unreliable. Eventually the individual physician's impressions also came to be seen as unreliable. Evidence had to be reproducible and standardized— reproducible so that a finding might be exactly transcribed, and standardized so that different expert observers would make the same finding. The doctor's sensory impressions were replaced by numerical data and visual depictions. If the new science of the seventeenth century had encouraged the first steps toward a scientific medicine and Enlightenment rationalism had created a cultural climate receptive to the idea of a scientific medicine, it was nineteenth-century hospitals, laboratories, and universities that finally produced modern medical science.

HOSPITAL MEDICINE: THE FRENCH MODEL

The revolution in France swept away the traditional institutions associated with medicine, making it easier for new developments to occur in Paris. Medical education was reconstructed with an emphasis on clinical observation, and in this enterprise, the belief of Enlightenment philosopher Pierre Jean Georges Cabanis in the primacy of sense impressions as the source of information played a large role. The intellectual link between Morgagni's pathological anatomy and the clinical science of the Paris hospitals was Marie François Xavier Bichat (1771–1802). However, whereas Morgagni's pathology was based on the organs, for Bichat it was based on the tissues. Consequently, one now thought, for example, not simply of inflammation of the heart but also of pericarditis, myocarditis, and endocarditis. Bichat's work, drawing on more than 600 postmortems, was to connect Morgagni's pathological anatomy with Rudolf Virchow's (1821–1902) cell pathology.

The large public hospitals with their myriads of patients offered marvelous conditions for clinical research, and a generation of distinguished clinicians availed themselves of these opportunities. The greatest was probably René Théophile Hyacinthe Laënnec (1781–1826). Chief physician at the Hôpital Necker in 1816, Laënnec introduced the monaural stethoscope—a wooden cylinder that fitted in one's pocket and amplified the sounds of breathing and the heartbeat. The binaural stethoscope was invented in 1852 by G. P. Cammann, an American. Laënnec was able to identify and follow the course of chest diseases by listening to breath sounds. Using clinical and pathological descriptions of phthisis, he subsumed the different forms of the disease under one pathological concept (Reiser, 1978, 228–29; Ackernecht, 1982, 147–51; Porter, 1996b, 173–74).

For Pierre Charles Alexandre Louis (1787–1872), only information based on very large numbers of cases could permit general laws of medicine to be formulated. Just as important was his argument that signs (what the physicians noted), not symptoms (what the patient reported), were (when correlated with organic lesions) the true keys to diagnosis, prognosis, and therapy. Significant new things happened to medicine under the leadership of the Paris School in the first half of the nineteenth century: medical training became a training of the four relevant senses to interpret the signs of disease; diagnosis became a reasonable explanation of the sense perceptions; and the carefully delineated diseases described by the French clinicians took on the guise of real entities.

The Paris School attracted students from throughout Europe and North America. In London, Guy's Hospital was the center of the new hospital medicine, but other hospitals, such as Saint Bartholomew's, and the new medical faculties of University College and King's College greatly expanded their teaching capacity. As in Paris, surgery flourished alongside the new medicine, with luminaries such as Sir Astley Cooper, Benjamin Collins Brodie, and James Syme (James Lister's teacher) contributing to its reputation.

Even in the United States, where first-rate medical schools developed at a slower pace than in Europe, French medicine, at least in the East, had considerable impact. Between 1820 and 1860, about 700 U.S. physicians went to study in France, including leaders such as Jacob Bigelow and Oliver Wendell Holmes (Duffy, 1976, 100–1; Ackerknecht, 1982, 147–56; Porter, 1996b, 173–77).

THE NINETEENTH CENTURY: THE GERMAN MODEL

After midcentury, the foundation of scientific medicine became the laboratory. Although both the laboratory and the experimental method—the hospital model relied on observation—had been in use since the seventeenth century, they came to assume an unprecedented importance (and level of public funding) in this era. And out of this union emerged organic chemistry and physiology as basic disciplines of scientific medicine, as morbid anatomy had been earlier.

Chemist Justus von Liebig (1803–1873) instilled in his students a physiochemical conception of living organisms, classifying foodstuffs into carbohydrates, proteins, and fats and constructing the discipline that would later be called biochemistry. Driving this work was a reductionist faith that the physical sciences could fruitfully be used to understand biological entities. The progenitor of experimental physiology was Johannes Mueller (1801–1858), who taught some of the greatest of the next generation of experimentalists, including histologists Theodore Schwann and Jacob Henle, pathologist Rudolf Virchow, and physiologists Emil du Bois-Reymond and Hermann Helmholtz. In 1847 du Bois-Reymond (1818–1896), Helmholtz, (1828–1894), Karl Ludwig (1816–1895), and Ernst Brücke (1819–1892) jointly stated that physiology must endeavor to explain the living world by reducing it to physiochemical laws. Moreover, technology was becoming integral to that task. The kymograph, which translated changes in bodily functions into a line on a graph, was introduced by Ludwig. The microscope, much improved in design, was the means by which histology (the study of the minute structures of the tissues) linked anatomy and physiology. The new laboratory medicine attracted able German and other European students. Among those trained by Ludwig were Americans such as W. H. Welch, who helped promote the new research outlook through the new John Hopkins Medical School beginning in the early 1890s.

In 1838 Theodor Schwann (1809–1885) proposed that tissues of animals, like those of plants, were made up of cells. This cell theory, which was clearly reductionist, was to become a basic doctrine of modern biology. Rudolf Virchow (1821–1902) took cell theory further: first, he rejected Swann's idea that cells emerged from the blastema, an organic matrix, and maintained instead that each cell came from another cell; second, he showed that the cell was the basic unit in pathology, as well as in normal life. Cellular theory was established at the same time as atomic theory in physics (Ackerknecht, 1982, 157–66; Porter, 1996b, 177–80).

Britain and the United States were slower to develop this new medical science. Whereas in Germany in the second half of the nineteenth century, full-time professional physiologists and institutes were devoted to physiology, in Britain work in physiology was to a large extent done by medical practitioners. An emphasis on practical, fee-for-service medicine, the lowly status afforded research in universities, lack of government support, and a vigorous opposition to vivisection all conspired to retard development. The emphasis was on the art of medicine sensitively practiced at the bedside by a scholarly physician. Even so, by the 1880s, some developments were taking place. Michael Foster established a physiology department at Cambridge, and he, with his students John Newport Langley and Walter Holbrook Gaskell, helped create Cambridge's image as the most modern school of medicine in the United Kingdom (Ackerknecht, 1982, 164–65; Lawrence, 1985, 509–12; Porter, 1996b, 181–83).

For various reasons, including the destruction of medical schools in the South during the Civil War and the negative effect of the speedy settlement of the Western frontier on the regulation of medical education, poor-quality, short courses in proprietary medical schools mushroomed in the United States, pushing standards of practice to a low level. Only late in the century, under the influence of those who had been exposed to the German model, did educational standards begin to rise. A general solution, however, was not achieved till the Rockefeller Foundation and the American Medical Association achieved success in the reform and regulation of medical education.

BACTERIOLOGY AND COMMUNICABLE DISEASE

Nowhere more than in the field of microbiology did reductionist science transform nineteenth-century medicine. In the long history of interaction between human populations and pathogens, the "causes" of infections were at last revealed. Neither miasmas nor chemical agents but parasitical microorganisms produced communicable diseases. Indeed, the power of this explanation was so beguiling that it took some time for medicine to accept a multifactorial explanation, one that involved causes in addition to the mechanical interaction of pathogen and host.

In 1857 chemist Louis Pasteur (1822–1895) had begun investigating fermentation. Against the established view that it was simply a chemical process, he showed that it resulted from the activities of microorganisms. Having identified the anthrax and chicken cholera pathogens and developed preventive vaccines, in 1885 he developed a vaccination against rabies. In the next decade, other researchers developed vaccinations against diphtheria, typhoid, cholera, and plague. Robert Koch (1843–1910) was a German figure of substance. Having worked on the anthrax bacillus and the pathogens involved in wound infections in the 1870s, he identified the bacillus of tuberculosis (1882) and that of cholera (1883). Koch drew up his well-known postulates to aid in reliably establishing the identity of the pathogen in any particular infectious disease: (1) it should be found in each case of the disease, (2) it should not be found in other diseases, (3) it should be isolated, (4) it should be cultured, (5) when inoculated, it should produce the same disease, and (6) it should be recovered from the inoculated animal.

In a remarkable burst of activity, the pathogens of gonorrhea, typhoid, leprosy, malaria, TB, glanders, erysipelas, cholera, diphtheria, tetanus, pneumonia, epidemic meningitis, Malta fever, and soft chancre were identified in the decade beginning in the late 1870s. The United States and Japan, newcomers to medical science, now also contributed to bacteriology's advance (Ackerknecht, 1982, 177–84, 222–24; Gelfand, 1993, 1140).

SURGERY: CONTROL OF SEPSIS AND PAIN

The traditional surgeon specialized in the setting of fractures, therapy for venereal diseases and wounds, and amputation of limbs injured in battle or accidents. Indeed, surgery and pharmacy, not academic medicine, in Britain prior to the Napoleonic Wars had for social as much as scientific reasons provided the practitioners who carried out most of the community's medical care. Unlike the university-trained physicians, who served the upper classes, they received their training as apprentices. The affluent middle classes were now looking for all-round practitioners who could meet the medical needs of the whole family, and in 1815 legislation recognized the surgeon-apothecaries as general practitioners.

The new focus on pathological anatomy encouraged surgical interventions; for example, from a humoral perspective, the removal of internal tumors made no sense. Even so, the problems of wound infection and pain remained formidable. In 1847 Ignaz Semmelweis (1818–1865) greatly reduced the high mortality from puerperal fever by proposing routine hand washing in a disinfecting solution. He understood that puerperal and wound fever had the same cause, but his colleagues resisted this conclusion. In 1843 Oliver Wendell Holmes (1809–1894) had also made the connection between contaminated hands and the initiation of puerperal fever. He, too, was ignored. Twenty years later Joseph Lister (1827–1912) became concerned about the comparatively high death rate from compound fractures as opposed to that from simple fractures. Because the former were in contact with the air and with bacteria known to be in the air, Lister decided to protect such fractures with germ-killing carbolic acid. He applied antisepsis through the use of a carbolic acid spray generally in surgical procedures. A decade later, asepsis (using steam disinfection of instruments and other means of disinfecting hands and the area of operation) replaced antisepsis. As a result, the traditional high risk of wound infection in surgery was much reduced.

The problem of pain was also confronted in the mid-1840s, when American dentist Horace Wells began employing the anesthetic nitrous oxide. In 1846 dentist William Thomas Green Morton substituted sulfuric ether and arranged a surgical trial. In Edinburgh in 1847, James Young Simpson (1811–1870) began to employ chloroform, and it virtually replaced ether as the main source of general anesthesia. Chloroform was easy to use, whereas ether caused irritation to the lungs and vomiting. Other technical innovations such as rubber gloves and artery clamps promoted a more adventurous surgery. By the 1880s, areas of the body hitherto out of consideration were being operated upon—the joints, the abdomen, the head, and the vertebral column (Ackerknecht, 1982, 187–92; Shorter, 1996, 141; Porter, 1997, 367).

On the other side of the world, William Gilbee, surgeon at Melbourne Hospital, having read of Lister's method in the *Lancet* of March 16, 1867, carried out a successful trial. However, it was another 15 years before Lister's approach was used by most Melbourne Hospital surgeons. By 1900, so comparatively safe had surgery become that Melbourne Hospital reported, for the first time, a waiting list for operations (Walker, n.d., 17; Inglis, 1958, 52–56).

In the United States, the practice of anesthesia had, by the close of the Civil War, become widely accepted. Antiseptic surgery was another matter, however. In 1875 Moritz Schuppert brought the antiseptic method back from Germany to New Orleans. His retirement soon afterward saw the practice abandoned until 1887, when Frederick W Parham reintroduced it. Only in the 1890s did Listerian practices become popular, and the later acceptance meant the German-developed practice of asepsis quickly replaced antisepsis (Duffy, 1976, 247–56).

In Canada, ether was used in January 1847 during an operation to remove a tumor from a man's arm. Chloroform was first employed in January 1848. Lister's original paper appeared in March 1867, and within months articles were reprinted from British journals. In February 1868, S. E. Bain, a regimental surgeon, made the first report of the use of carbolic acid. Within a short time it was being used as a dressing by surgeons in major hospitals in the east. Two surgeons who did much to publicize antisepsis in Canada were Archibald Edward Malloch, one of Lister's house surgeons at Glasgow, and Thomas Roddick, who was also trained by Lister. Neither at first used the diluted carbolic acid spray during operations. Malloch first employed the steam spray in 1873, while Roddick used it four years later. Both engaged in the slow process of persuading the majority of Canadian doctors to apply Listerism (Roland, 1981, 238–50; Shephard, 1993, 2–4).

DUALISM AND MODERN MEDICINE

Over the last five decades, a powerful critique has emerged of modern medicine's reductionism and dualism. These characteristics have been blamed for its lack of humanity in the care of the dying, its focus on the cure of bodies rather than the cure of people, and its failure to provide compassionate care and proper palliation when cure is no longer possible. The dualism has been attributed to the influence of philosopher René Descartes at the beginning of the modern scientific era. René Dubos in the 1960s, Eric Cassell in the 1970s, Howard Brody in the 1980s, and Miles Little in the 1990s all make Descartes responsible for the heritage of dualism.

Descartes received his education at a Jesuit school in Anjou, which exposed him to Thomist theology and Aristotelian logic, ethics, metaphysics, and natural philosophy. Doubting the metaphysics of scholastic philosophy and influenced by Galileo's new observational and experimental approach to the natural world, he sought to ground his reform of ontological philosophy in the experience of thinking: "je pense, donc je suis" or "cogito ergo sum." This subjective certainty led to reliable science by combining with the existence of a benevolent God who guaranteed the truth of sense experience. Mathematics was the means by which to proceed from this ontological base.

In his discourse on the rules of reasoning, Descartes makes clear his adherence to reductionism: divide each of the difficulties into as many parts as possible and as may be required to resolve them; begin with the simplest objects in order to ascend gradually to knowledge of the most complex.

Descartes pictured the physical sciences as a tree with metaphysics as the roots, physics as the trunk, and medicine and other applied sciences as the branches. Matter was whatever has extension, *res extensa,* that which can be fully described in terms of size, shape, and the motion of its particles. Although he began by deduction from metaphysics, he valued observation and experiment, maintaining that the further knowledge progresses, the more significant empirical evidence becomes.

Descartes said the soul was that which ultimately moved the body. Where the body is material, extended, spatial, and divisible, the soul is incorporeal, unextended, nonspatial, and indivisible. While he located the central motive power of the body in the brain's pineal gland, the movements of which agitated the fluids of a hydraulic nervous system, the problem of the connection between the incorporeal soul—the final cause—and the body was not clearly resolved.

He set out to banish all Aristotelian speculative forces and ideal forms and to destroy the humoral conception of humans; thus he would mechanize the functions traditionally associated with the vegetative and sensitive souls. Where the vegetative soul was seen as controlling growth, nutrition, and reproduction, the sensitive soul was seen as controlling sensation, appetites, and movement, and the rational soul, the intellect and will.

His heritage of dualism is still potent. In health, there is the definition set forth by the World Health Organization—health as complete physical, mental, and social well-being—which expresses a black-or-white thinking when the idea of better health would be more realistic. The other legacy is reductionism. In medical practice and research, it is displayed ontologically in adherence to a structural explanation of disease and methodologically in the need to explain at the molecular and genetic levels. The lowest level of physical structure (level 1) is assumed to be the realm of ultimate causes in a hierarchy of levels:

6. social groups
5. multicellular living things
4. cells
3. molecules
2. atoms
1. elementary particles

One cost of reductionism is the inadequate way modern medicine has dealt with patient suffering. Cartesian medicine endeavored to cure the body (which is seen to cause suffering because of a structural or functional defect) but does not comprehend the need to cure the suffering of the soul—in modern terms, the person. Those with cancer or AIDS, when beyond cure, have too often been left unaided to deal with the loss of autonomy and the imminent loss of self (Little, 1998, 76–92).

Beginning with Vesalius, I have traced the evolution of medicine's naturalistic concern in the nineteenth century with the body and its development of a reductionist hierarchy of levels of knowledge from organs down to cells. In the twentieth century, reductionism progressed to the molecular and genetic levels.

Thus, it seems the heritage of Cartesian dualism and reductionism as the philosophical path of modern medicine has been a source not only of strength but also of weakness. However, according to Mark Sullivan, the true source of the dualism lies in the work of Marie François Xavier Bichat, two centuries after Descartes: his location of disease in the body's lesions found at autopsy is the real beginning of medicine as a natural science. The physician's eyes, by focusing on the interior of the body, became the tools of diagnosis, not the patients' words conveying their subjective experience. Prior to Bichat, symptoms were both the appearance and the reality of disease. Now symptoms were the appearance and lesions the reality. The patients' reports were merely another object to be known.

To provide a firmer base for knowledge of the natural world, Descartes relied on evidence of his consciousness, the cogito, and a nondeceptive God, the source of all truth. Bichat likewise wanted to make medicine, or at least diagnosis, an exact science, a natural science of the individual. But he had a more modern conception of knowledge. Disease categories emerge from the object; they are not God's but come from the everyday interaction of knower and known. The doctors' perception had to be objective, untrammeled by any contribution by them as knowers.

For Descartes, the mental and physical are different substances; he eliminated the mind from the body as he came to know the body as a mechanism. His dualism is an ontological dualism. For Bichat, however, it is an epistemological dualism that entails both knower and known, but no ontological difference is involved. Once the patient's experience becomes irrelevant, other advantages of the objective evidence are identified, in particular, the capacity for standardization and reproducibility. Only after the model of the visible lesion—after the lesion became both the necessary and the sufficient condition of disease—was treated as primary medical evidence could techniques such as auscultation and X-rays become intellectually coherent tools of diagnosis (Sullivan, 1986, 334–45). The increasingly technologized medicine of the nineteenth and twentieth centuries buried the sub-jectivity of the patient deeper and deeper beneath a pile of objective evidence. However, at various times countermovements within medicine have challenged the marginalization of the patient.

PATIENT AS PERSON

A number of developments worked to produce a rediscovery of the patient as a per-son. The interwar growth of concern with mental hygiene in Britain forced psychi-atry to deal with neuroses and depressive illness that were located at least in part out-side the body—in the patient's mind or familial relationships. In the same period but with greater force in the 1950s, in Britain and the United States, epidemiology and social medicine identified specific at-risk populations and thereby encouraged medical sociologists concerned with illness to focus on the patient's attitudes, beliefs, and behavior. The patient's world was at the center of their inquiries.

Interwar holism in the United Kingdom has its roots in the late Victorian and Edwardian eras. William Osler, regius professor of medicine at Oxford in 1904, is representative of this earlier view, which preferred the generalist physician to the specialist and a broad cultural outlook with regard to technical training. His suc-cessors of the 1920s and 1930s believed that health was essentially balance, and, as Oxford physician Alexander Gibson observed, the vis medicatrix naturae of Hip-pocrates will naturally restore that balance. John Ryle told a medical audience in 1931 that the physician was not an applied scientist but a naturalist, the whole pa-tient was to be treated, and medicine was the general biology of people in disease, not a collection of loosely linked sciences and fields of specialization.

In the United States between 1920 and 1945, an even more explicit holism was influential. In 1922 Lewellys Barker, who succeeded Osler at Johns Hopkins, de-clared that the scientific study of the human constitution was at last coming into its own. A group of distinguished physicians and biological scientists such as in-ternist Walter C. Alvarez and biologist Raymond Pearl saw this constitutional ap-proach as a concern with the idiosyncratic response of the individual patient to disease and with the connection between the mind and the body. Constitutional medicine (for its exponents, a new clinical science of people) was one contempo-rary face of antireductionism. Others were psychosomatic medicine, social medi-cine, and the movement to integrate social services within the clinical area. A number of factors have been identified as responsible for the decline in interest in constitutional medicine by 1950: all of its main exponents were retired or dead by then, the effects of World War II were becoming apparent, and specialization was increasing. The military directly encouraged specialization by offering better pay and higher rank to specialists, and higher incomes were then available in civilian life. Further, GI education benefits allowed veterans to obtain specialist training. Whereas in 1940, 24 percent of doctors were specialists, in 1955 the figure was 44 percent. The conditions of postwar medical practice and medical schools were not conducive to seeing the patient as a whole person.

In the 1970s something of a crisis developed in medicine as the costs of health care, driven very much by the greater use of high technology in diagnoses and treatment and by the epidemiological shift to chronic diseases, induced governments and economists in the Western world to question the benefits of the unchecked growth of biomedicine. At the same time, powerful intellectual critiques were being made of biomedicine and its relation to health—by Ivan Illich about physician-induced illness and medicalization of what were problems of living; by Vicente Navarro about capitalism's unending search for profit and thus the promotion of health-care markets in the growth of technological medicine; and by Thomas McKeown's minimization of the role of curative medicine in the great mortality decline that began in the second half of the nineteenth century in Europe (compared with the role of better living conditions, sanitary reform, and a favorable trend in the relationship between some pathogens and human hosts). Nonmedical factors had a much greater impact on the health of populations, McKeown concluded.

In North America, medical educators reacted to some of the criticisms by expanding instruction in behavioral sciences to counter the reductionist and biologically sourced orientation of biomedicine. The theoretical framework that informed this approach was that of George Engel's influential biopsychosocial model of disease, publicly articulated in 1977. Engel's model maintains that illness results from the interaction of environmental, social, psychological, and biological variables and thus explains why the severity and course of a disease can vary among patients. But, as Margaret Lock has persuasively argued, the model does not get us much beyond that of biomedicine because it does not address the fundamental issue of values in medicine and in particular in the patient-doctor relationship (Lock, 1995, 102–5; Lawrence and Weisz, 1998, 11; Lawrence, 1998, 94, 102–4; Tracy, 1998, 161–65, 180–81).

Anthropology has been particularly significant in raising the issue of values in medicine and in putting medical knowledge and practice into the larger cultural context that influences medicine. Indeed, the idea of a more or less separate medical system, distinguishable from other social institutions, is something constructed by Western culture and not found in all cultures at all times.

Out of anthropology has come the meaning-centered approach to clinical care, especially associated with the work of Arthur Kleinman and his colleagues. This method holds that the healing of illness (including the alleviation of suffering) is at least as necessary as the curing of disease. The patient's subjective experience of illness has to be included in clinical care, and Kleinman offers the explanatory model as a means by which to do this. The virtue of the model is that it brings into play both order and meaning and is part of the effort to rehabilitate the patient. The physician's explanatory model results from fairly uniform and extensively shared knowledge believed to be based in science. The patient's comes from lay knowledge as interpreted by families and individuals and contains ideas about causation, fears, and hopes about outcomes. The patient's needs must be part of the treatment process; disability is both a natural *and* a cultural phenomenon. The body inhabits both the physical and the symbolic world and is located at a particular point in historical time.

Although the structured inequality of the doctor-patient relationship makes it difficult, especially in hospital settings, negotiation must occur to accommodate both the patient's and the physician's models of the illness. The patient's report ceases to be just more information enabling the doctor to locate the lesion as the true cause of disease. There is no longer known and knower, as in Bichatian epistemological dualism, but rather two knowers, with the patient's self-knowledge regaining some of the standing it lost after the late eighteenth century and becoming integral to medical knowledge. Medicine must devise better methods of inquiry into patient explanatory models and attend more carefully to the diversity and complexity of the host of disease-producing factors. In doing so, medicine will cease to be a purely natural science. It will need to use insights from the social sciences and humanities to complete its work.

To establish a sense of existential control, humans seem to require explanations to make some sense of illness and suffering and to give order to their individual worlds. Such explanations are of a different type from those of modern science; they cannot be drained of their emotional and social content and be reduced to the materialism of science, where the suffering body is merely a malfunctioning machine or victim of fortuitous, natural events. In the clinical encounter, the presence of values needs to be openly acknowledged, and the virtues of objectivity and subjectivity equally recognized (Sullivan, 1986, 345–49; Lock, 1995, 102–25).

The analysis so far has looked to biomedicine as the active partner that must change its ways in relation to a passive patient whose voice needs to be heard in order to humanize medical encounters. However, there is evidence that laypeople are not simply passive. They are both active and passive; they exercise discrimination in their use of medical knowledge and expertise. Sociologist Anthony Giddens argues that ours is not a postmodern era but an age of late modernity in which the effects of modernity are becoming more radical. Like other social institutions, medicine is becoming more and more reflexive whether viewed from its knowledge base, its social organization, or the manner in which it is practiced. It is becoming more fragmented; some areas of high technology exist alongside more biographical (or holistic) medicine, seen mostly in general practice, where the patient's subjectivity and the psychosocial context of the illness are emphasized.

Where traditional society once fixed lifestyles, late modern society requires individuals and groups to decide how to live, and this involves conflict and struggle in a politics of lifestyles. Modern abstract systems of knowledge and expertise expropriate knowledge about and skills for living from laypeople. But laypersons reskill themselves by reappropriating technical knowledge and routinely applying it to their everyday activities; this reskilling is made much easier by access to personal computers and the Internet. In areas where medicine does not have much to offer or treatments are experimental, patients and lay groups have been critical of medicine. Self-help groups in health and medicine have pitted experiential knowledge against the instrumental rationality of medicine.

Alternative and complementary therapies are no longer patronized only by small numbers of the unorthodox and unconventional. They receive widespread patronage from mainstream citizens who evince a determination to attain control over their bodies and their environments. This reskilling or reappropriation of knowledge and expertise by laypersons applies to areas of late modern life other than health and illness, but this may be a more salient issue in the area of health, which seems to have become the symbolic site for conflicts about wider social issues of control. Conversely, doctors have historically enjoyed a certain status that comes from dealing with matters of life and death, and in late modern society they have come to occupy some of the space thereby enjoyed by the clergy in traditional society; they have also come to represent a source of security in an increasingly uncertain world. Certainly, the paradox exists that, on the one hand, doctors are criticized for abusing medical power and for their financial greed; on the other hand, access to mainstream health care is seen as an inalienable right (Williams and Calnan, 1996, 1611–18).

TWENTIETH-CENTURY MEDICINE

In the twentieth century, medicine achieved an unprecedented understanding of the structure and functioning of the human body and its pathologies. With some exceptions such as diphtheria antitoxin, diabetic insulin, and nicotinic acid for pellagra, the revolution in knowledge was until the late 1930s unparalleled by a revolution in therapy. In that period the first of the true magic bullets, sulphanilamide, became available. In the 1930s the hospitals were full of patients dying from pneumococcal pneumonia or congestive heart failure due to syphilis or rheumatic fever, staying in bed because of pulmonary tuberculosis, or suffering from peritonsillar abscesses, mastoiditis, or bacterial endocarditis. By the 1950s, because of antibiotics, the disease pattern in hospitals was vastly different.

Around 1900, from the growth of nineteenth-century microbiology came immunology. Louis Pasteur had proposed that, in the process of the host's resistance to a pathogen, success was marked by the pathogen's loss of the capacity to reproduce. However, he was committed to the development of new vaccines rather than to elucidation of the process of immunity. It fell to Elie Metchnikoff in the 1880s to identify phagocytosis and to show that white blood cells ingested pathogens. His cellular theory of immunity, popular in France, did not impress the Germans. In 1890 Emil von Behring and Shibanuro Kitasato proposed that serum or blood that was made immune to tetanus or diphtheria by administering the toxin concerned would be useful in treating someone afflicted with either infection. Use of serum therapy (passive immunization) for a range of infections received some endorsement, but the development of vaccines (active immunization) was considered a more rewarding path to follow.

Paul Ehrlich developed a chemical view of immunity that, in its focus on the molecular level, foresaw the development of drugs and the new chemotherapy of infections. His side-chain theory explained how antigens and antibodies interacted and demonstrated a chemical affinity between some drugs and some cells; a specific drug might then be developed to bind and destroy a specific pathogen, as Ehrlich did in 1910 with Salvarsan (arsphenamine) and *Treponema pallidum,* the spirochete of syphilis (Ackerknecht, 1982, 181–82; Porter, 1996b, 189–92).

In Germany, von Liebig and his students investigated the way in which food produces energy for the body. Wilhelm Kühne, a Heidelberg physiologist, proved that substances called enzymes produce chemical changes. At the beginning of the twentieth century, the notion of a disease caused by a chemical deficiency began to be formulated. Christiaan Eijkman, working on the dietary deficiency disease beriberi, showed that what became known as vitamin B1, contained in the husks of rice grains, was missing from polished rice; the absence of the vitamin was responsible for the disease. At the same time, Frederick Gowland Hopkins demonstrated that such "accessory food factors" were essential for turning protein and energy into growth. Researchers in the United States soon came to take the lead in nutrition research. The work of Elmer V. McCollum, Harry Steenbock, T. B. Osborn, and L. B. Mendel led to the identification of vitamin A in 1913 and vitamin B in 1916. In 1914 Joseph Goldberger proved that pellagra was not an infectious but a vitamin B–deficiency disease. In 1922 McCollum and Steenbock identified vitamin D, the deficiency of which produces rickets. Rickets involves deformities of bony structures including the female pelvis, the prevention of which reduced mortality associated with childbirth. Later, the elements of the vitamin B complex came to be understood, and other vitamins (C, K, E) were identified. However, with bacteriology dominant, it took some time for the importance of dietary deficiencies as causes of disease to be accepted.

The identification of serums, hormones, vitamins, and anticoagulants, together with radiotherapy, surgical advances, and especially chemotherapy made the capacity to cure and rehabilitate the mark of twentieth-century medicine, just as progress in pathology and prevention had marked nineteenth-century scientific medicine.

Endocrinology (study of internal secretions) became a full-fledged field of inquiry in the twentieth century. William Bayliss and Ernest Starling constructed the idea of the hormone (from the Greek for "to arouse") from work on proteins and enzymes. The first hormone so named was secretin in 1902. Secretin stimulates the pancreas to produce digestive fluids. Endocrine (ductless) glands send chemical messengers via the blood supply all over the body, and the pancreas, ovaries, thyroid, and adrenals were shown to be endocrine glands. Imbalances in secretions were recognized as the cause of some diseases; diabetes was thus a hormone-deficiency disease and resulted from the pancreas's failure to release insulin and thus modulate blood sugar levels. The isolation of insulin in 1921 by F. G. Banting and Charles Best made possible the rational management of diabetes. In 1912 American surgeon Harvey Cushing demonstrated that a disordered pituitary gland (secretes growth hormone) produced obesity. Surgeons could remove the adrenal glands or pituitary tumors to cure thyroidism and pituitary disorder, respectively. Estrone (the female sex hormone) and testosterone (the male sex hormone) were recognized in the 1930s. Two decades later this research led to the oral contraceptive pill for women.

Until the twentieth century, few drugs were specific cures for particular diseases; quinine was a rare example. Moreover, their curative effects had been established only empirically. Paul Ehrlich's biochemical research created the field of chemotherapy, while also making clear the underlying mode of action. There were no new antibacterials until 1935, when Gerhard Domagk produced the first of the sulfa drugs. In the 1940s these were superseded by penicillin (Ackerknecht, 1982, 232–33; Porter, 1996b, 193; Porter, 1997, 456–57).

The development of the electron microscope made possible the growth of virology. Poliomyelitis was first clinically identified at the close of the eighteenth century. Outbreaks of poliomyelitis (sometimes leading to paralysis) were experienced in Europe, North America, and Australasia in the nineteenth century but grew more severe in the twentieth. In the 1900s Simon Flexner proved that it is an infectious disease. Albert B. Sabin and Peter K. Olitsky were able to culture the virus in human brain cells in the 1930s. In 1953 Jonas Salk reported success in testing a killed virus, and a nationwide campaign of vaccination was undertaken in the United States. However, Sabin had been developing an attenuated, live-virus vaccine that had the advantage of conferring long-term immunity and being able to be given orally. In 1961 and 1962, Sabin's vaccine replaced Salk's in the United States and, soon after, in the other Anglo-Saxon countries (Duffy, 1976, 244; Porter, 1997, 695; Lewis, 2003b, 35–42).

Surgery advanced into new areas of the body—chest, brain, heart—and organ transplants. Neurosurgery was but one of the new specializations as specialist clinics were established for urological, thoracic, orthopedic, and pediatric surgery. Innovations in diagnostic technology assisted greatly in advancing clinical knowledge of heart disease. Opening the heart became much less risky after antibiotics were available. A frequently encountered defect of the heart was mitral stenosis. Leading surgeons in the 1920s attempted without success to widen the narrowed valve, but success did not come until 1948, when Dwight Harken was able to open the valve with his finger and then cut away the calcified ring. Since the late nineteenth century, babies with congenital heart defects have been well known to medicine, but only in 1944 was a successful surgical intervention developed. The next great advance was open-heart surgery. Before this could take place, a technological alternative to the heart's function had to be developed. John Gibbon of Philadelphia constructed a heart-lung machine and used it in operations in 1952 and 1953. In the 1950s surgeons were replacing failed arteries in the limbs. Then, in 1967, René Favaloro of Cleveland carried out the first coronary artery bypass. This has now become a well-established procedure.

Plastic surgeons in Britain had worked on facial reconstructions during World War I, and they were called upon to do reconstructive surgery again during World War II. Organ transplants failed because of host immunological rejection. However, when this rejection process was clarified by Peter Medawar's work in the 1940s, immunosuppressive drugs began to be used in the 1950s to deal with the problem, although substantial gains were made only in the late 1970s (Ackerknecht, 1982, 237; Porter, 1997, 611–26).

Nineteenth-century experimental neurophysiology greatly advanced understanding of the nervous system. Charles Sherrington showed that electrical impulses pass from one neuron to another. However, it soon became known that chemical agents were also involved. In the 1920s Henry Dale demonstrated experimentally that, after electrical stimulation of motor nerve fibers, acetylcholine was secreted at nerve endings. Otto Loewi showed experimentally that, after stimulation, a frog's heart secreted the enzyme cholinesterase. This chemical in-hibitor stopped the acetylcholine stimulator, and thus the transmitter–inhibitor pattern was emerging. Walter Cannon found that, when stimulated, the sympa-thetic nerves release a chemical substance that was later identified as noradrenaline. The main transmitters were noradrenaline at sympathetic endings and acetyl-choline at most other locations. Once chemical transmission was understood, the possibility of treating neurological diseases such as Parkinson's disease emerged. In 1967 a new therapy was introduced using L-dopa, a chemical analogue of dopamine, to enhance the production of dopamine and thus to enable patients to overcome muscle stiffness and to walk again (Porter, 1996b, 193–95; Porter, 1997, 570–73).

In the second half of the twentieth century, basic science, clinical inquiry, and medical practice came together notably in the field of genetics. Darwin himself of-fered no convincing explanation of inheritance, and Gregor Mendel's 1865 report of his experiments in hybridization, which became the basis of modern genetics, remained little known. Exploration of the etiology of two diseases—sickle cell anemia and Down's syndrome—promoted the case for heredity. Thus, in 1867 John Langdon Down proposed that a European person with Down's syndrome (a form of intellectual disability accompanied by a specific set of physical traits) might be a throwback to an earlier, "inferior," Mongol race type. Only in 1959 was it shown such a person had an extra chromosome—chromosome 21.

However, a fundamental breakthrough in molecular biology was required be-fore medicine could advance in the area of genetic diseases. Nucleic acid had been discovered at the core of all cells, and by the 1920s, it was known that two types of nucleic acid—DNA (deoxyribonucleic acid) and RNA (ribonucleic acid)—exist. Then, in 1953, Francis Crick and James Watson destroyed the existing idea that DNA simply acted to hold the protein together in chromosomes and showed that DNA's double helical structure indicates a genetic code. By the 1980s, the code could be "read," and genes could be isolated and duplicated. By the 1990s genes had been identified that were behind a number of diseases, including muscular dystrophy and cystic fibrosis. Treatment could be provided, at least in principle, for diseases due to a defective gene or the lack of a particular gene. The gene encoding the desired protein could be isolated, and the protein produced in adequate amounts (Porter, 1996b, 195; Porter, 1997, 586–88).

MEDICAL RESEARCH: THE RISE OF AMERICAN PREEMINENCE

The winning of the Nobel prize in physiology or medicine may be treated as a rough indicator of the quality of a nation's medical research. Between 1901 and 1995, the smaller medical research powers among our five Anglo-Saxon countries fared as follows: F. G. Banting and J. J. R. MacLeod of Canada won in 1923 for the discovery of insulin; Howard Florey of Australia shared the prize in 1945 for his work on penicillin (although it was carried out in Britain); F. M. Burnet of Australia shared the prize in 1960 for research on acquired immunological tolerance; and J. C. Eccles of Australia shared it in 1963 for research on the biophysics of nerve transmission.

There were prizewinners from Britain on five occasions between 1901 and 1939, and, except for Canada in 1923 and the United States in 1933 and 1934, the other prizes were distributed among Germany (8), France (4), Austria (4), Russia (2), Sweden (1), Italy (1), Spain (1), Denmark (3), the Netherlands (2), Switzerland (1), Belgium (2), and Hungary (1). In 1943 the pattern changed. The key difference is the preeminence of the United States. On at least 39 occasions between 1943 and 1995, the prize went to or was shared with someone from the United States (Porter, 1996b, 198–99).

This grand U.S. achievement was built on growing support for medical research. As French medical science based in the Paris hospitals had led the world in the early nineteenth century and German medical science based in the laboratory did later in the century, so U.S. clinical and basic medical science became the setting of advances in medical knowledge from the 1940s on, when the United States far outstripped the rest of the developed world in the size of financial and institutional resources devoted to the task. Between 1945 and 1965 the annual research expenditure at the celebrated Massachusetts General Hospital increased 17-fold, while that at the federally funded National Institutes of Health increased a massive 624-fold. University hospitals were the bases for a new type of full-time researcher whose training and ongoing work were funded by federal grants. Their research, whether clinical or laboratory, was the source of their status, income, and professional identity (Risse, 1999, 578).

In the 1870s in the United States, the populist idea that all worthwhile knowledge was within the grasp of ordinary citizens was being replaced by one of respect for specialized knowledge and professionalism, particularly among the expanding middle classes. The shift in attitude is evident in the increased number of higher education institutions, as well as professional associations across a range of fields.

This faith in expert elites was reinforced in the Progressive era, when the community accepted scientific knowledge as carrying its own authority. The use of laboratory science raised the prestige of the medical profession, and laboratory training became a sine qua non of a first-rate medical school. Philanthropic foundations and the government played a vital part in the emergence of a medical research infrastructure, and none more than the Rockefeller Foundation. Abraham Flexner's famous 1910 report on medical education in the United States and Canada detailed the shortcomings of medical schools in the former. Only three universities besides Harvard and Johns Hopkins could claim to be proper medical research centers: the universities of Pennsylvania, Chicago, and Michigan. The Rockefeller Foundation introduced the idea of full-time clinical chairs in specialties such as cardiology and provided funds for Johns Hopkins. With much support from Rockefeller, the idea took hold in other parts of the country. By the mid-1920s the United States could boast of 20 research institutions as good as any in Europe.

Government was also a large funder of research. The National Institute of Health became the National Institutes of Health (NIH) in 1948 and quickly became a major promoter of medical research. In 1945 the National Institute of Health had received research funds of $180,000. In 1950 the NIH received $46 million, of which a substantial proportion was used to fund extramural research. Its budget grew from $81 million in 1955 to $1.4 billion in 1967 (Warner, 1992, 134–39; Porter, 1996b, 196; Lewis, 2003a, 271–72).

The organization and adequate funding of medical research was slower to develop in Britain. Until World War I, the medical schools in London did little to foster research, but things began to change as a result of Lord Haldane's inquiry into university education. In 1913 he proposed that modern departments doing research be established in the medical schools. By the mid-1920s the 12 London schools had five chairs of medicine among them. A school of postgraduate medicine was opened at Hammersmith Hospital in 1935. This West London institution was an important source of education for clinical researchers. Research funding came mainly from the Medical Research Council (MRC) and from medical charities such as the Imperial Cancer Research Fund, the British Heart Foundation, and the Wellcome Trust. The Rockefeller Foundation also provided very considerable funds for research projects, buildings, and positions in Britain (and in other parts of Europe and Australia).

In the 1940s the MRC supported two significant projects: one was the carrying out of the first randomized, controlled trial involving human subjects to be reported; the other, the use of epidemiology in a clinical matter—the likely cause of lung cancer mortality. In this development of medical statistics and clinical epidemiology, medicine's search for understanding of disease had moved beyond the hospital and laboratory to the randomized control trial and the social survey (Porter, 1996b, 200–1).

SCIENTIFIC MEDICINE OR VALUES-BASED MEDICINE?

In the 1970s the estrangement of biomedicine from humane traditions was considered to be so great that there was a call for a conscious enrichment of medicine through the teaching of the humanities. In the Society for Health and Human Values, the Institute on Human Values in Medicine, and the *Journal of Medicine and Philosophy* (first issue in 1976), Edmund Pellegrino helped create academic vehicles for a wider discussion of issues in the medical humanities, bioethics, and philosophy of medicine. Others such as André Hellegers, who established the Kennedy Institute in 1971, and Daniel Callahan, who, with Willard Gaylin, established the Hastings Center in 1969, also contributed to this process (Engelhardt, 1986, 3–5; Engelhardt, 1990, 238–39).

In the United Kingdom, the intellectual and professional response to the crisis in the humanity of medicine that was associated with the increasing use of expensive high technology was somewhat different. More and more, epidemiologists questioned whether clinicians could justify by statistical analysis a good many of their treatments. The most outspoken critic was Archibald Cochrane, who argued that a disproportionate share of the resources of the National Health Service

(NHS) was going to cure rather than to care sectors. Only the applications of randomized controlled trials could reduce the growing gap between the sectors and promote the effectiveness and efficiency of the health services. Thomas McKeown's critique of high-cost, high-technology medicine was based on an analysis of the contribution of medical interventions to the historical decline in mortality in Europe. Moreover, McKeown, as much as Cochrane, was concerned with what he saw as a lopsided NHS dominated by hospital-based specialist services that inevitably failed to deal with the key health problems, which were those of the infirm aged and people with mental illness. It was a health care system with acute separated from chronic patients, home care from hospital care, and preventive measures from curative services. Both McKeown and Cochrane emphasized the caring function of medicine to balance the high-technology, highly specialized, hospital-based medicine that received funds that might be better spent on other services. They wanted greater policy emphasis on what they saw as a neglected medical tradition, the physician's caring function (Kunitz, 1991, 256–60).

In the United States Daniel Callahan and Eric Cassell were also calling for medicine to rediscover the lost art of caring. Callahan, on the grounds of humanity and economic sustainability, claimed the health system had to cease giving primacy to a high-technology medicine that aimed to cure all diseases and, in a godlike way, forestall death itself. The primary task should be caring, which provides solidarity in the face of the disintegrative threat to the self and the body that illness presents and empathy in the face of suffering. Caring binds the sick to the community in the face of the alienation produced by illness and overcomes deep fears of abandonment. For most of our biological history, human existence has been precarious in view of the fact that illness and death, famine, war, and social violence have been inescapable threats. Mutual caring, physically, psychologically, and spiritually, was essential to survival. But the vulnerability is never transcended; at best, it can be kept at bay; misadventure or as yet uncontrolled diseases can still strike us down.

Caring is required at the general and particular levels. At the general level there are four aspects: caring for patients' feelings that are evoked by their condition; meeting the patients' need for others to understand how their mind works; responding to what they value in life; and finally, trying to understand how they relate to others. The individuality of a patient requires caring at the particular level. This is captured nicely by sociologist Arthur Frank (who himself survived two life-threatening illnesses), when he says that treatment commonly makes a compromise between efficiency and care by creating an illusion of involvement. However, particulars are what make an experience real, and using the same common name for the anger or grief of two different persons only obscures what is happening for each of them (Callahan, 1990, 135–37; Callahan, 1998, 270–74; Callahan, 2001, 12–24).

Miles Little has pointed out that medicine and health care more generally in first-world countries are exhibiting signs of crisis:

1. Medical litigation is growing by leaps and bounds. In Australia, the largest insurer against litigation recently went into voluntary litigation because it was unable to fund an increasing number of claims.

2. Costs of technology and services are approaching an unsustainable level, and rationing of services, de facto or otherwise, is standard.
3. There is an uneven distribution of human, physical, and technological resources across healthcare systems.
4. The huge investment in technology is resulting in diminishing returns in terms of population health.
5. More and more citizens are using practitioners of alternative (or complementary) medicine in part at least because they listen to and care for them better than biomedicine practitioners.
6. Healthcare workers endure high rates of mental and stress-related illness.

While great success in the sense of measurable outcomes is enjoyed by scientific medicine, the crisis indicates an underlying problem. That problem, according to Little, is reductionism. By focusing on a reductionist approach, medicine privileges one strength, cure of disease, while dehumanizing suffering; it suggests that material explanations are sufficient to underpin our decisions in health and medicine. Thus, once a genetic account of colon cancer is established, present suffering, fear, and effort may be ignored in favor of a vision of the future in which colon cancer has been eliminated because someone will have found a genetic cure or method of prevention.

Little says that values-based medicine is the paradigm that is best able to deal with the current crisis because values and beliefs ultimately strengthen the whole enterprise. The fact is that we consider suffering and untimely death bad because we intrinsically value individual human life from both a quantitative and a qualitative perspective and because we understand that its flourishing requires supportive social conditions. The well-known principles-based ethics of medicine—respect for the autonomy of others, beneficence, nonmaleficence, and justice—themselves rest on the bedrock of such values and beliefs.

The new paradigm encourages us to consult our values and to avoid reducing medicine to one of its parts, whether that be care or evidence. We can have science and evidence as well as compassion and concern. Science and evidence in a values-based model take on value just because they vitally assist us to promote human autonomy, security, and flourishing (Little, 2002, 319–21; Little, 2003, 177–78).

MODERN SOCIETY

Scientific medicine has been shaped by internal factors such as the growth of knowledge in the modern hospital and laboratory. It has also been shaped by demographic and epidemiologic changes that have accompanied the growth of modern society and a culture of modernity.

The demographic transition has seen a shift from high mortality and high fertility (which characterize traditional society) to low, and the epidemiological transition, a movement from a cause-of-death profile dominated by communicable diseases to one dominated by chronic, degenerative diseases. Connected with these transitions has been a historically unprecedented growth in average life expectancy at birth and an unprecedented rise in the proportion of aged people in the population. This is the new world of mortality and morbidity that emerged in parallel with scientific medicine and to which scientific medicine was required to respond.

In the Greco-Roman world, the average duration of life was 20–30 years, and in medieval and Renaissance Europe, 25–30 years (although it is known to have varied by socioeconomic status). Since the eighteenth century, average life expectancy has risen quickly in Western Europe, North America, and Australasia. In the United States, for example, it was 33 years in 1800, 49.7 in 1900, and 68.7 in 1950. Since the mid-nineteenth century, the proportion of older people in the United States and the United Kingdom has increased markedly: in the former, 4.1 percent in 1850, 6.4 percent in 1900, and 12.6 percent in 1955; and in the latter, 7.2, 7.5, and 16.5 percent respectively (Grmek, 1958, 86–90).

Premodern societies in Western Europe had high death rates, intermittently driven even higher by ferocious epidemics of infectious disease such as plague. More efficient interventions by the central governments of nation-states (themselves a key feature of modern society) during the eighteenth century helped banish these crises of mortality. Endemic infectious diseases such as tuberculosis now became more significant as causes of death. The upward movement of life expectancy slowed. Only in the later nineteenth century did a substantial decline in mortality begin again, and much of this decline resulted from falling child and, subsequently, infant mortality.

The new Anglo-Saxon countries—the United States, Canada, Australia, and New Zealand—also experienced this long-term decline in mortality. In the early twentieth century, the epidemiological transition to chronic, degenerative diseases saw cardiovascular disease and cancer dominate. Like Western Europe, they experienced the great fertility decline of the later nineteenth century. Australia's fertility decline was similar to those in northern Europe and the United States, so it can serve as an example: the decline was from 43.3 births per 1,000 population in 1862 to 35 in 1877. By 1900 it was down to 27.3 per 1,000. All of these countries then passed through the final phase of the demographic transition to a modern regime of low mortality and low fertility. The third period of the long-term secular decline in mortality occurred after World War II and was fueled by the antibiotics, although other factors were also involved (Quiggan, 1988, 1, 19; Schofield and Reher, 1991, 1; Riley, 2001, 22–23.)

In premodern society, more than half of the population was dead before they became adults. In the Anglo-Saxon countries by the second half of the twentieth century, dying as a baby, child, or adolescent was unusual. The modal age of death was no longer infancy but old age. The accompanying change in the leading causes of death from communicable diseases (and associated conditions) to chronic, degenerative diseases (of the aging) can be seen if the leading causes of death in the London bills of mortality (1701–1776) and in Britain in 1992 are compared: in the London bills, they were convulsions (babies; mostly the result of infection), 28.3 percent of the total mortality; tuberculosis, 16.6 percent; and fevers, 14.7 percent; and in 1992 Britain, diseases of the circulatory system, 46 percent; cancers, 26 percent; and respiratory disease, 11 percent (Riley, 2001, 17). The change in the modal age of death and in the cause of death in the late twentieth century made possible the exercise of greater control over, and personal autonomy concerning, the process of dying. The epidemiological transition in England involved not only a shift in the leading causes of death from acute infections to chronic diseases; it also involved a decrease in the risk of death while ill and an increase in the duration of episodes of illness. Diseases that had quick resolutions were replaced by ones that had slow resolutions as causes of death (Riley, 1987, 587–88).

AGING AND PREPARATION FOR DEATH

In the Greco-Roman world, Hippocratic medicine identified heat as the basis of life. Over the course of life, the finite quantum of heat each person possessed declined. Galen elaborated on this theory by postulating a drying process that began when the embryo was formed from the drying of blood and semen. To these ideas Christianity added a spiritual and moral factor, original sin; aging and death came into the world when Adam and Eve were expelled from Eden.

In medieval Christian thinking, aging was a preparation for death and eternal life—a pilgrimage to God. In an agrarian society the natural rhythms of daily life and the cycles of the seasons marked the passage of time. Salvation and eternity, not longevity, were the goals of life.

The Reformation brought time and work into a new alignment. Faith, not works (pious acts), justified one and brought hope of salvation, said Luther. Before the Reformation, the manner of one's dying decided the fate of one's soul; now how one lived one's entire life was what was important. Concern about time and death became focused on health and control of the body.

By the late seventeenth century, the personal anxieties and social upheavals of the Reformation era had abated. A bourgeois ideal of life could come to fruition, along with the emergence of the scientific revolution itself. The Puritans took Protestant conceptions of aging to America; aging was seen as a sacred pilgrimage to God's final judgment. They also took a patriarchal ideal of family life in which the husband's and father's authority prevailed.

Demographic historians talk of a northwest European demographic regime, seen most clearly in England from the sixteenth to the mid-eighteenth century, which was different from that occurring elsewhere in the world at this time: comparatively low fertility, late marriage, considerable individual freedom of choice in marriage, comparatively low mortality, high geographical mobility, a tendency for children to leave home well before marriage, weak kinship connections, and the small size of coresident groups.

In addition to the establishment of independent households by the newly married, another consequence of this arrangement was that at least half of all elderly people in England are thought to have lacked children living nearby; thus the community had to underwrite the security of individual aged people who were unable to provide for themselves. It is no accident that the Elizabethan Poor Law was a public welfare system unique in early modern, northern Europe, nor that for two centuries a large body of English literature discussed the individual's right to community assistance. The idea of rights is seen in John Locke's constitutional theories, in the rural reports of Arthur Young and William Cobbett, and in the testimony of laborers given to inquiries into the Poor Law (Thomson, 1991, 210–12; Cole, 1992, 9–49).

Social hierarchy and patriarchy within the family were increasingly challenged in the eighteenth century as a market economy spread, economic individualism advanced, and the value of the ordinary, rational person was extolled by Enlightenment thinkers. For Thomas Paine, the equality of generations was implied by the equality of people, and Thomas Jefferson said the Creator made the earth for the living, not for the dead. The prestige enjoyed by age declined with the growing challenge to traditional authority. Until the end of the eighteenth century most Americans continued to be Calvinists, but the patriarchal authority of the Calvinist God was also challenged. Thus by the 1820s a more benevolent God had for many replaced the omnipotent ruler. The Calvinist ideal of old age was one of active pious example to the rest of the community; piety was required of the old, but it also advanced their possibilities of salvation and enabled them to overcome the frailties of body and mind (Cole, 1992, 52–70).

In the 1840s, the Victorian moral code, developed by middle-class moralists but purporting to speak for all society, emphasized self-control and personal responsibility. In the United States, it grew out of the Protestant religious culture of the North and sought to guide the individual through the emerging democratic, competitive, and increasingly urban society that had supplanted the Puritan nexus of piety and politics in an organic and stable community. At the same time as Puritanism collapsed, poorhouses, asylums, and penitentiaries were being erected to deal institutionally with what had traditionally been the community's informal responsibility (Stannard, 1977, 170).

While Catholics and Protestants in the sixteenth and first half of the seventeenth century differed in how they dealt with imminent death—the former's anointing, giving of the sacraments, and taking of confessions were rejected by the latter as superstitious—both were quite clear that the priest or minister was the key figure, not the doctor. Indeed, both the Catholic and the Protestant churches were preoccupied with the craft of dying as part of living a fuller Christian life. Rationality, calmness, moral strength, and faith in the face of death together promoted expectations that the dying person would be received in heaven and were indicators of the "good death." However, in the late seventeenth century, the religious aspect declined, at least for some members of the elite, as the Enlightenment's emphasis on the primacy of this world grew. The secularization of death went hand in hand with the growth of the medical management of death (McManners, 1985, 457; Wear, 1985, 55–66; Houlbrooke, 1989, 41; Wear, 1992, 120–25).

Changes were afoot without and within medicine. Georgian Anglicans began to see illness not in providentialist but in naturalistic terms, and the idea of a gentle, "natural death" faced rationally and with stoicism took root among the elite. At the same time, the attendance of the family at the deathbed became central, with the stress on an atmosphere of intimacy and peace.

Because of his reputation for managing the dying process well for members of the upper class, Sir Henry Halford (1766–1844) was perhaps the most successful physician of the early nineteenth century. Halford approached his task by stages: the first, where he refrained from telling the patient the truth and promoted optimism; the second, where he told the truth, leaving time for the patient to deal with any unfinished business; and the third and most challenging, where he managed the pain and fear of dying, generously using his own opium-based medicines. If death were to be made as easy as falling asleep, resorting to liberal doses of alcohol and opium to sedate the patient was necessary. If in the mid-seventeenth century a good death required courage and faith as the final test of the Christian, 150 years later the good death was being medically managed, as an extension of the doctor's therapeutic role, to be as smooth as the transition to sleep. Death was being medicalized, at least for the elite (Porter, 1989a, 84–94; Porter, 1995, 474–75).

As Americans turned away from the absolute sovereignty of the Calvinist God in the first half of the nineteenth century, health reformers preached the pursuit of longevity and promised that moral and physical hygiene would bring a long life. A number of distinguished English and other European physicians produced books on longevity and hygiene, including George Cheyne, *An Essay on Health and Long Life* (1724); Samuel Tissot, *Advice to the People in General, with regard to Their Health* (translated, 1781); and C. W. Hufeland, *Macrobiotics, or the Art to Prolong One's Life* (1796).

Health reformers in the United States commonly conceived of people's vital energy as their physical capital. Like financial capital, it had to be used to yield both good health and long life. All unnatural stimulants like tobacco, coffee, tea, alcohol, and excessive sexual activity brought premature death. The reformers proposed that dwellings be properly ventilated, bathing be regular, and clothing be frequently changed. Long life and healthy old age were attainable through sensible self-control; infirmity and dependency were the results, then, of the individual's moral failure. The health reformers capped the idea of a long healthy life with a painless, natural death, leading to heavenly salvation.

In sixteenth- and seventeenth-century northern Europe, the urban middle classes became devoted to the idea of an orderly progression through the stages of the individual life, commonly represented iconographically by a rising and falling staircase, with each age having appropriate virtues and vices. In the seventeenth century, this widespread iconography referred to a fearsome death and God's judgment. In the eighteenth century, a tamer death was represented. By the mid-nineteenth century, the iconography spoke of a life course in which self-help brought health, and material advantage as concern with a Christian eternity was replaced with progress in historical time, health, social usefulness, and success in this world.

By the mid-nineteenth century, evangelical Protestantism had a Romantic flavor that included the idealization of children, women, the family, old age, and death. Americans Theodore Parker and Henry Ward Beecher saw the reward of not dissipating vital capital as a high life expectancy, health and independence in old age, and a natural, pain-free death. They did not address the question of the social usefulness of the aged, assuming that preparation for old age was the same as preparation for death. Of course, self-control and natural health had their opposites in sin and bodily ills.

A literature of self-help manuals, usually authored by women, advised readers on how to live a civilized old age. This involved healthy, productive, and useful independence for as long a time as possible—the darkness of evening would come at 70 years—and the cultivation of a spiritual life to assist with the losses of old age.

Around the 1870s the Victorian dualistic conception of old age produced a struggle between those opinion makers who saw old age as a sort of barrier to progress and those who promoted the view that a long life and healthy old age were indeed possible. The late nineteenth century saw a number of factors accumulate to reinforce a pessimistic view of old age—aging of the young immigrants of yesteryear in North American cities; the beginning of the epidemiologic transition as the dominance of infectious disease was replaced by chronic, degenerative conditions, with the result that older people were often ill for long periods before death; and medicine's identification of old age as a clinically distinct period. It was also a time when state and professional management of health was taking over from the tradition of self-responsibility. Perhaps no one publicized the pessimistic viewpoint more than William Osler, the eminent physician. In his valedictory speech at the Johns Hopkins Medical School, Osler talked of men's creative years as extending from 25 to 40 and of the uselessness of men over the age of 60. Although the tone was humorous, the dismissal of older men—he spared older women from euthanasia—evoked much public interest. One notable feature of Osler's argument was the use of a secular, utilitarian criterion—the capacity to work (Cole, 1992, 96–174).

During the nineteenth century, then, the long-established Christian conception of life as a spiritual voyage was overtaken by a scientific worldview, and at the beginning of the twentieth century, the criteria of productivity and efficiency were being applied to the aged. In the first four decades of the new century, those seeking greater collective responsibility for the marginalized aged—the sick and the poor—inadvertently reinforced the negative side of the Victorian dualistic approach by painting the aged as inevitably dependent, sick, and poor. The price was a tendency to stereotype the aged as unable to contribute in a meaningful way—through their labor—to society and requiring much professional, especially medical, assistance.

Like the other Anglo-Saxon countries, Canada experienced the aging of its population in the second half of the nineteenth century. Of the population in West Canada (Ontario) in 1851, 3 percent were over 60 years of age; in 1871, 4.6 percent; and in 1901, 8.4 percent. A declining birthrate combined with still substantial child mortality meant that a large proportion of old people had no surviving children with whom to live. However, the poverty, ill health, and dependency of the aged were much exaggerated by the government. It was true during the 1890s that the elderly became a large proportion of the institutionalized population, but for each institutionalized, aged person, 33 aged people were living with family or on their own.

A similar situation prevailed in the United States and England. Indeed, only 3–5 percent of those over 60 years of age in North America during the nineteenth century lived in institutions. As in Australia in the 1890s, economic depression in Ontario forced many elderly, working-class people into dependency just as it pushed governments into fiscal restraint. The Ontario government, like those in the United States, Britain, and the Australian colonies, sought to reduce spending on social welfare by having families assume more responsibility for the dependent aged (Montigny, 1997, 34, 47–49, 82, 99–103).

Waves of young immigrants kept colonial Australia a young and vigorous society, a fact that made the colonials feel proud and which they contrasted with the situation of "old" Europe. At the peak of immigration to eastern Australia in the 1850s, those 65 years of age and older constituted just 1 percent of the population. The populations of the original convict colonies, New South Wales and Van Diemen's Land (Tasmania), aged more gradually than those of the newer colonies, Victoria and South Australia. The latter suddenly aged in the 1880s and 1890s as the large, free immigrant populations of the 1850s became old. The elderly were a comparatively small proportion in colonial Australia—about 4 percent in 1901 (compared with 11 percent in 1986)—but the speed of aging (compared with Britain) and the fact of serious economic depression in the 1890s heightened the sense of crisis. At the same time, the onset of declining fertility reinforced the anxiety, as did the fact of the high masculinity of the aged portion of the population, which meant an excess of single or widowed males: in 1891, 143 males per 100 females among those 65 years of age and older, compared with 73 per 100 females in 1986.

The apparent increase in the numbers of the dependent aged was especially unwelcome because Australians believed theirs was a prosperous society where the great majority who were industrious could reasonably anticipate a financially independent old age. Indeed, they had long resisted the mother country's stigmatized workhouses for the poor. As elsewhere in the Anglo-Saxon world, evangelical Protestantism spread widely the notion that a virtuous life would bring a healthy and independent old age. A vicious youth would bring a miserable old age.

Australia was second (NSW and Victoria, 1900) in the world to New Zealand (1898) in introducing noncontributory old-age pensions provided by the government, first at the state level, then federally (1908). The pension programs brought greater financial security but also something of the stigma that withdrawal from paid work carried.

By the early 1900s, ideas of national efficiency and national fitness, fueled by social Darwinian concern about interpersonal, international, and interracial struggles for survival, were to adversely influence attitudes about old age.

New York physician George Miller Beard, who published *American Nervousness* in 1881, substantially influenced debates in Australia and the United States. Beard, claiming to have sifted through the biographies of almost all of the greatest names in history, established the mean age at which they had carried out their original work. He showed that work peaked at age 40 and achievement went downhill thereafter. There was undue reverence for the aged, and old men did not deserve to control, as they did, most of the world's wealth and prestige. His graph resembles the traditional iconography of the ages of life. However, there are some differences. Not only is the peak reached at 40 instead of 50 years, but the fall from that point is sharper and longer. Gone are the images of early modern iconography that have to do with seasons, salvation, and eternity. Productive capacity is the only index of value.

Like Beard's, William Ostler's views on old age were widely reported in Australia. Vitalist ideas on old age were reflected by Philip Muskett, an Australian doctor who wrote *The Attainment of Health* (1909). Muskett, who published a number of books on health for the layperson, saw a steady decline in physical, mental, and sexual power in men beginning in the mid-forties. Although old men (those 55–70 years of age) contributed "peaceful reasoning" to the goods of the world, in all other ways the old were simply unfit for a competitive society. Some women writers rejected the ageism of mainstream thinking. Feminist Louisa Lawson believed the status of older people was governed by attitude, not physical fitness, and old women, if elected to parliament, would spread altruism and justice in affairs of state (Cole, 1992, 163–68; Davison, 1995, 43–58).

English novelist Anthony Trollope (who visited the Australian colonies in the 1870s) in his futuristic satire, *The Fixed Period* (1882), offers a solution to the problem of the burdensome old. In the progressive republic of Brittanula, the Fixed Period law requires all citizens at the age of 67 to enter a special college called Necropolis, where they are to live comfortably for a year, reflecting on life in an educational process intended to be of value to the young, as well as the old. They are then to be euthanized with chloroform and cremated. However, the first person due to be "deposited" in the college protests against the law. Even so, President Neverbend proceeds to implement it, but a British warship arrives to prevent the opening of Necropolis. Neverbend is to return to England and be jailed. Beard and Trollope, each in his own way, highlight the irrelevance of the aged to a capitalist, secular, rationalist society in its high industrial phase (Cole, 1992, 168–69).

In the United States in the early twentieth century, the idea of old age as a period of healthy self-reliance was replaced by the assumption that the majority of the aged were noncontributors to the real world, which was that of work. In the 1960s, in an environment of minority movements seeking social justice, older people also organized to combat ageism; in this they were supported by a growing number of health and social service professionals, as well as sympathetic people in the media, labor unions, and business, who promoted the view that the aged could be healthy, socially involved, and sexually active. For the middle-class aged at least, this cultural and political facelift brought increased lifestyle choices. Almost at the same time, there began to emerge the possibility of intergenerational conflict. By the 1980s, welfare liberalism had delivered to the retired aged substantial public benefits. However, facing the rising medical costs of an aging population, the expanding life expectancy of older people, and in the future a smaller labor force to provide for their own retirement, younger citizens began calling for generational equity.

As Thomas Cole insightfully points out, old age in the United States in the late nineteenth century came to be devalued because it seemed a barrier to the individual right, inspired by the Enlightenment promise of material progress and that of liberal capitalism, to accumulate health and wealth. Of course, the masses of the aged poor, whether immigrants or native born, urban working class, could not be part of this middle-class dream.

Elsewhere in the Anglo-Saxon world there was concern about the economic and social implications of an aging population. Thus, in Britain in the 1930s and

1940s, pessimistic projections forecast a 1980 population of only 29 million, of whom about 30 percent would be 65 years of age and older. What actually happened was that the birthrate increased, and in the 1950s large numbers of young immigrants came from the Caribbean and the Indian subcontinent. The total population in 1981 was 60 million.

Modern liberal capitalist society's faith in material progress has, as Christianity's hold on our hearts and minds receded, turned health into a form of secular salvation and the physical (and mental) decline that aging brings into something culturally unacceptable.

The modern idea of the journey through the ages of life was developed among the urban middle classes of the Renaissance and Reformation era to help individuals establish a sense of life as a meaningful progression ending in transition to an afterlife. By the second half of the twentieth century, a secularized and rationalized version of this progression was expressed in Anglo-Saxon countries in age-oriented institutions: educational institutions to prepare the young for their career paths; jobs organized to maximize the productivity of young and middle-aged adults; and government-financed benefit programs for the retired aged (who were unable to provide for themselves) whose productivity was considered too low to keep them in full-time work.

Members of the modern hospice and palliative care movement have criticized the social and spiritual inadequacy of the dying process that has accompanied this twentieth-century organization of the stages of life devoted to the maximizing of human performance and material productivity. As well as criticism, there have been attempts to substitute for the traditional Christian goal of salvation (for those for whom it no longer has meaning) a focus on exploration of the complexity of the inner life in a search for self-transcendence that goes beyond contemporary society's strong valuation of healthy physical functioning, status advancement, and material success. In effect they pursue the very difficult goal of reconciling the ancient advice to submit to natural limits with the contemporary emphasis on individual development for all. In such a quest the interpersonal and social-relational dimensions are critical because individual fulfillment seems to lie with giving to others after we have accomplished self-stability at the middle stage of life; our death might then become our final act of giving (Cole, 1992, 233–251; Thane, 2000, 13).

DEATH AND DYING

The material and sentimental extravagance of funerary and mourning rituals in Victorian Britain and other parts of the Anglo-Saxon world reached a peak in the later nineteenth century, just when reformers advocating cremation began to gain some support. Reformers wanted to promote a more sanitary disposal of remains, especially in crowded cities, and to simplify funeral rituals. They also sought to change basic attitudes toward death. Victorian doctors now played a larger role in the patient's dying, at least in the upper and middle classes. The world of the dead and the world of the living became disconnected, yet it was not a simple movement toward secularism. The religious created new roles in the drama of death and dying, specifically caring for the dying in special hospices. These were the forerunners of the institutions created by the larger, modern hospice and palliative care movement.

Until the 1870s, the evangelical model of a good death was widely influential. Central to it was the doctrine of Christ's dying for human sins. Death was very important because it was the last chance for experiencing conversion and thus salvation. For evangelicals, a triumphant death meant victory over the devil, in which they believed. All nineteenth-century Christians agreed on the need for family support during the dying process. A long illness was to be preferred because it permitted time for finalizing worldly matters and for spiritual preparation for death. Evangelical Anglicans and Nonconformists put more weight on faith than on the giving of the last rites by a member of the clergy. Prayers and Bible reading by the family sustained the faith of the dying person, but for Catholics, the priest's presence was essential for the administration of the last rites (Jalland, 1996, 19–21, 26–31).

In the late seventeenth century, the taste for extravagant funerals began to spread from the aristocracy to the middle classes. The process culminated in the first half of the nineteenth century as the middle class became more prosperous in an industrializing economy. Nevertheless, an awareness was growing of the public health risks from the overcrowded graveyards of London and other European capitals, particularly the pollution of drinking water and of the air by the dangerous miasmas, then mistakenly thought to cause fevers and other disease. In 1850 the Metropolitan Interments Act put an end to interments in churchyards. It closed old interment grounds and provided for a fixed charge for funerals in cemeteries. The provisions of the act were applied to all of England and Wales in 1853. Societies devoted to promoting moderation in funeral arrangements were created. By the 1870s, simple ceremonies were common.

The sanitary aspect of interment also came to the fore. Cremation, associated with Roman pagan practices, had not been carried out in Europe since early Christian times. Italian and French burial reformers had discussed it at length since the mid-eighteenth century, but this discourse had remained confined to the readers of scientific and medical journals. Indeed, until 1877 as few as 10 official cremations took place in Europe, but in the course of the 1870s, Italy, Germany, Holland, Belgium, and the United States acquired cremation societies.

Distinguished urologist and president of the British Cremation Society, Sir Henry Thompson became a cremationist after visiting the Great Exhibition in Vienna in 1873. He stated the case, based on sanitary and utilitarian grounds, in an article in the *Contemporary Review* in early 1874. His blunt economic arguments against burial, calculated to appeal to bourgeois economic computations, underestimated the continuing strength of religious and sentimental attitudes to disposal of the dead. Later cremationist works wisely appealed to rural nostalgia, as well as making arguments based on economics and hygiene. Sir Henry's deploring of the waste of good fertilizer to be made from human remains was just too outrageous.

For three decades, the multifaceted debate continued, covering religious, sentimental, legal, and even political grounds. Sir Frances Seymour Haden, an eminent physician, emerged as Thompson's main opponent when he established the Earth to Earth Society in 1875. Haden argued for more efficient decomposition of the body by the use of coffins constructed of easily biodegradable material such as wicker.

The Cremation Society built a crematorium at Woking in 1879 but stopped experiments when the home secretary, pushed by strong community feeling, threatened prosecution. In 1884 a judge, Sir James Stephen, declared that cremation was not a criminal act. Crematoria were brought into use in Woking in 1885, Manchester in 1892, and Scotland in 1891. In 1902 the Cremation Act regulated the practice. In 1889 only 53 cremations were carried out, and two decades later only 795 a year. It was not until the 1960s that cremations were carried out for 50 percent of deaths.

The slowness with which cremation became popular indicates the durability of religious and family traditions. Cremation was most strongly supported by the upper-middle and upper classes. However, even among them, continuing adherence to traditional Christian practice meant that support was not widespread (Leaney, 1989, 118–30; Jalland, 1996, 195–209).

Looking back over the nineteenth and earlier twentieth centuries, Pat Jalland, historian of death and dying, sees two major turning points in cultural attitudes. The first occurred around the 1870s and 1880s, when the decline in evangelicalism and in mortality combined to disconnect death and the Christian afterlife. Thereafter, Christianity became a more diluted, social creed. The second was the Great War, which speeded the slower-moving changes of the previous four decades or so.

For some of those moving away from Christianity in the late nineteenth century, spiritualism had appeal because it offered an alternate conception of one's postmortem state, in which one's identity survived. Spiritualism as a movement began in the United States in the 1840s. It came to Britain in the 1850s, when some middle- and upper-class individuals participated in small private séances as a form of leisure activity. Daniel Douglas Home, an English medium, made spiritualism so popular that a Convention of Progressive Spiritualists was convened in 1865. Nevertheless, the movement then lost momentum. In 1891, when the National Federation of Spiritualists (NFS) was established, it included 41 local societies. The NFS became the Spiritualists National Union in 1902. By 1913, the number of affiliated societies had increased to 141.

When the Society for Psychical Research was founded in 1881 by a handful of Cambridge philosophers and scientists, the spiritualist movement was put on notice that its claims would be subjected to rigorous investigation. The members included distinguished figures such as Henry Sidgwick, Frederick Myers, Leslie Stephen, Alfred Tennyson, W. E. Gladstone, Arthur Balfour, and John Ruskin. Whereas spiritualism on the Continent was deeply committed to scientific inquiry, in the United Kingdom many members were Christians, and a genuine religious yearning underlay the movement.

The great slaughter of World War I turned spiritualism into a mass movement as thousands refused to accept the finality of their personal losses. When dying was increasingly associated with old age and people believed the war would be over very quickly, the scale of death and disability was overwhelming. At the battle of the Somme, 20,000 soldiers were killed on the first day, the same number as the total losses in the Boer War. Somewhat fewer than 723,000 British citizens died— one in eight servicemen, and the British Empire's dead totaled more than one million. In addition, one and a half million were disabled.

Two prominent figures did much to popularize spiritualism, and both lost sons in the war. Sir Oliver Lodge, an eminent scientist, wrote a book about his psychic experiences concerning his dead son. In the three years after November 1916, the book went through twelve editions. Sir Arthur Conan Doyle produced his book in 1918, and until he died in 1930, he promoted the spiritualist cause ceaselessly. He went on a speaking tour of Australia and New Zealand in 1920 and 1921, the United States in 1922 and 1923, South Africa in 1928, and northern Europe in 1929. Where spiritualism had been a small movement before 1914, it went from strength to strength in the interwar period.

With funerary rites for most individual soldiers impossible and so many people not responsive to Christian ritual, new forms of public ritual had to be devised. Some developed from earlier Christian forms: thus, civic war memorials developed from traditional religious street shrines. The ritual of Armistice Day evolved gradually in response to public demand. The two minutes' silence observed at 11 AM on each Armistice Day was observed throughout the British Empire. London's Cenotaph, originally intended to be temporary, was replaced by a permanent structure, again because of popular pressure. The tomb of the Unknown Soldier in Westminster Abbey became another point of public ritual.

David Cannadine argues that if Armistice Day was the public recognition of bereavement, the spiritualist movement was the private denial of death. Pat Jalland has argued that World War I destroyed the final links with hundreds of years of Christian history that had fostered the hope of eternal life, with devastating cultural consequences for a population in mourning. Death became a major taboo and something standing in opposition to life, not life's culmination (Cannadine, 1981, 227; Jalland, 1996, 380–81).

Attitudes in World War II were different. British military deaths—270,000— were far fewer. Because Nazism was widely seen as evil, the ideological justification was strong. Civilians were not separated from the front so radically. Indeed, 60,000 civilian deaths were recorded by the end of hostilities. It was the "people's war."

The Anglican and dissenting churches, in the main, would not identify Christ with the nation's war effort. However, the Roman Catholic Church publicly endorsed the cause as forthrightly as it had in the Great War. Yet, where there had been a common Christian eschatology in World War I, it was now meaningful only to believers. Liberal theology and secularism had helped destroy the central role once taken by Christianity. Interestingly, even concern with spiritualism had eroded. A more diffuse and pantheistic attitude toward death was abroad. If the carnage of the Great War cast a dark shadow over the interwar years, the first few decades after World War II were darkened by the deaths of 50 million people in the war, the memory of the Holocaust, the dropping of the atomic bombs on Japan, and the real prospect of global destruction through nuclear war (Cannadine, 1981, 197–233; Jalland, 1996, 358–81; Wilkinson, 1997, 158–62).

By the beginning of the nineteenth century, the Puritan view of dying as a prelude to likely punishment for sin was disappearing from the United States, although it lingered in rural areas. The grimness of Calvinism was replaced by a sentimentalization of death. One material expression of this was the replacement of locked burial grounds by open cemeteries featuring an idealized pastoralism—Mount Auburn in Boston in 1831; Laurel Hill in Philadelphia in 1836; and Greenwood in Brooklyn in 1838. The graves were seen as perpetual homes from where the dead might be in communion with their deceased friends and family (Stannard, 1977, 167–85).

Postbellum, the lawn cemetery took over from the rural cemetery, and fences around individual graves were removed. To permit a level lawn, grave mounds were banned, and unobtrusive monuments were encouraged. Death was thus being hidden.

More optimistic about God and people than traditional evangelicalism, liberal Christianity played down the conception of death as punishment for sin. The attitude of the very influential clerical figure Henry Ward Beecher represented the change. Beecher disliked the image of the traditional, black-crepe funeral, and on his death in 1887, his family organized a flower funeral.

Funeral services also changed. Previously, the home was where the religious service took place. After a short graveside ceremony, the body was buried. Now for the urban middle class, caskets replaced the wooden coffin, and professional undertakers directed the funeral. Focus on this-worldly matters meant the body was now dressed in everyday clothes instead of a shroud. Embalming, widely used during the Civil War to preserve bodies of combatants sent home for burial, made the body appear as natural as possible.

Funeral directors offered their funeral parlor, where economies of scale allowed them to market an attractive funeral for a reasonable cost. They took full charge of the arrangements and, with the cooperation of more liberal-minded clergy, even influenced the content of the sermon, directing it away from theological lessons about sin toward psychological relief of grief.

This disguising of death is very close to the denying of death and at its core is the drive for control of self, society, and the natural environment. Alexis de Tocqueville had noted that, because Americans readily concluded that everything in the world could be explained, they resorted to denying what they could not comprehend. Remarking on the American way of death in the 1980s, in a culture that encouraged the avoidance of dirt and unpleasant odors, the preservation of appearances with cosmetics, and a turning to plastic surgery to help people feel young, James Farrell concluded that it was difficult to confront the reality of death and senile decay (Farrell, 1982, 120–21).

By 1900, the changes that had begun half a century earlier were easier to see. Among these was the professional control of death and dying that themselves had become more private. Although most people still died at home, some were dying in hospitals. By the mid-twentieth century, the great majority were dying in hospitals. However, in this environment, the feelings of the dying person and the family tended to come second to the convenience and desire for efficiency of the professionals in charge. Indeed, it was at this time that the hospice movement developed in Britain and soon after in North America and Australasia in order to provide a setting where the needs of the dying and their families were foremost and where death again became a natural part of the cycle of life (Wells, 2000, 273).

As in the other Anglo-Saxon countries, in Australia between about the 1840s and the end of World War I, demographic, social, and cultural changes profoundly altered attitudes toward, and practices concerning, death and dying, especially among the urban middle class and better-off working class. Immigrants from Britain and Ireland brought to the Australian colonies the idea of the good Christian death, an idea supported by Protestant evangelicalism and the spiritual revival in Catholicism. However, the Christian approach to death appears to have lost credibility more quickly in the Antipodes than at home in England and Ireland. Lack of clergy, thinness of population, and the absence of women (and the family structures they sustained) in the bush, as well as the fact that many immigrants were working-class people who had given up the habit of regular attendance at church, worked to undermine the traditional Christian way of death. The Catholic way remained vital longer than that of the Protestants because of the centrality of the priest's ministrations to the dying person and the fact that the individualism of Protestant Christianity rendered it less able to defend itself against biblical criticism, Darwinian theory, and scientific materialism.

In the 1820s and 1830s, the Church of England failed to win the struggle to become the established church in Australia. The Antipodes lacked a wealthy elite able to endow Anglican churches and livelihoods, and the Church of England was closely associated with the hated convict penal system. Moreover, the immigration of members of other churches reduced its numerical advantage. In 1836 it was decided that state financial support would be provided for all significant churches. The mixing of attitudes toward and beliefs about death at the community level was promoted by extensive cross-denominational marriage, and in commerce, denominational difference did not produce social division. Public conflict was most marked between leaders of denominations, not their flocks.

Patrick Godman argues that, from the late 1830s to the early 1850s, as the age and sex structure of the population rapidly moved toward a normal state due to the influx of free settlers, the traditional emphasis on postmortem judgment began to decline (Godman, 1995). No unique Australian expression of attitudes toward death emerged. Rather, a regional variant of a recognizable model came into being.

The state-sponsored collection of mortality and other vital statistics supported pioneering efforts by public health reformers to advance urban sanitation. Between 1870 and the outbreak of World War I, the advance of public health and medicine, especially progress in bacteriology's capacity to identify the causes of the infections that produced so much mortality, gave a new sense of control over disease and even death itself. As I have already observed, hospitals changed their function from charitable refuges for the sick to centers of laboratory-based medicine and new technologies. The spread of education, cheap books, and newspapers allowed philosophical secularism to begin to influence mass attitudes and beliefs.

The Catholic Church resisted the secular attack on the doctrine of immortality more successfully than the Protestant churches. The Australian Catholic Church had its intellectual and doctrinal roots in Ireland and Rome, not urban Scotland and southeastern England, where the secular challenge was strongest. In 1870 the doctrine of papal infallibility greatly strengthened the authority of the clergy. Methodists also resisted the growing materialist influences, but while their beliefs concerning death did not change, the expression of these beliefs became privatized. In the 1890s some Congregationalist ministers, such as W. R. Fletcher, defended traditional faith and revelation against the secularizing influences. More liberal ministers tended to adopt the position that death was a material event whose effect on the living had to be worked through by grieving.

In the Church of England, Low Church evangelicals and High Church tractarians both defended traditional belief against Broad Church higher biblical criticism. However, even evangelicals could question the full sovereignty of God. By the end of the nineteenth century, the Presbyterians had given up didacticism concerning the need for timely repentance in favor of a human emphasis on sympathy and loss. As they sought to make the best of earthly life rather than prepare for death in life, the Presbyterians were open to the influence of utilitarianism. In contrast, the Baptists used the occasion of death didactically. Yet, as a predominantly urban denomination, Baptists were much in contact with secularizing forces. Indeed, they, like other city-dwelling Australians, were subject to the industrialized mentality well before large-scale industry came to Australia. By 1900 Sydney and Melbourne were by international criteria large cities, and the problems of urban life there were essentially no different from those of Europe or North America (Godman, 1995, 87–128, 176–91).

The early appearance of a secular approach to death and burial in colonial Australia is related to the isolation of bushmen from family and church on the frontiers of settlement and to the often forbidding conditions of life in the bush. Death in the bush was very different from the domesticated Christian deaths of the mother country, the model for death management in the more settled areas of colonial Australia. The ideal bushman's death was masculine and heroic and not infrequently violent.

In the Victorian gold-mining areas of the early 1850s, funerals were minimalist affairs. A doctor's son recorded that, on peering into a miner's tent at Castlemaine, he saw what he thought was a log of wood on the ground, but it was in fact two sheets of bark tightly tied around the body of a man. The other miners had fashioned a rough cross and placed it on the man's chest. They were away searching for a clergyman to conduct the funeral service. Bark might be used where there was no money for a coffin or suitable wood was not available or the body had to be buried quickly because of the hot climate (Bowden, 1974, 90).

Not only were traditional burials impossible in remote locations, but in foregoing them the bushmen may have been expressing indifference to British cultural practices. The bush grave also came to represent a sense of being at home in the often harsh new land. Jalland has identified three significant factors in the bushmen's approach to death: first, the wish to express their respect for the dead even if, by the middle-class standards of the time, their rituals were casual; second, a pragmatic, even stoical, acceptance of death, supported by the fact that the costs of formal mourning and rituals were too great when one's personal survival might be at stake; and third, the often riotous and alcohol-fueled wake as a tribute to their companion.

The bush wake is an example of the adaptation of a popular custom of the poorer classes of Ireland, Wales, and Scotland. In 1902 John Flynn, a Presbyterian outback missionary, came upon some bushmen burying a companion at a place almost 2,000 miles inland from the South Australian capital, Adelaide. They knew no formal ritual, even hymns, but decided to show their respect by singing "For He's a Jolly Good Fellow."

In the later nineteenth century, the doctor's role in Australia, as elsewhere, was considered more critical. Doctors of this era were well aware of the limits of their curative capacity and thus did not see a patient's death as a failure on their part. They were also well aware of the importance of hope in the struggle with disease; moreover, as prognosis was a less reliable matter than in more recent times, they were unlikely to talk of imminent death until they were sure. Pain control was one area of palliative care where nineteenth-century doctors could be more confident of effect.

In 1845 Fanny Bussell, the daughter of an upper-middle-class family in western Australia, nursed her dying mother through the painful final stages of cancer. Her mother received opiates twice a day, but the pain could not be fully alleviated. When Fanny's husband, Henry Sutherland, was dying of throat and lung cancer a decade later, she begged him to take a larger dose of morphine. Fanny died in 1881, after having received large doses of laudanum for six months. In the case of another upper-middle-class patient, pastoralist Samuel Winter, in 1878, just before death he was given laudanum by his medical attendant to induce sleep. At the other end of the social ladder, laudanum was employed to ease the pain of paupers dying in colonial benevolent asylums (Jalland, 2002, 93–99, 243–62).

The British style of funeral was practiced by the urban middle class and those of the respectable working class who could pay into funeral benefit funds, although after the 1850s funerals were generally more modest affairs than at home in England and Ireland.

After mid-century, funeral reform developed in the Antipodes, and middle-class progressives joined funeral reform associations in the 1870s to support the simplification of rituals. Rev. Charles Badham, professor of classics at the University of Sydney, stated that he wanted no idle pomp at his funeral. The republican and radical activist Rev. Dr. John Dunmore Lang wanted a plain coffin and no eulogy.

Of the Australian colonies, South Australia in 1891 was the first to enact legislation allowing cremation and the first, in 1903, to establish a crematorium. In the 1880s the Adelaide press had discussed the merits of cremation. In the colony, the Catholic Church in 1886 labeled cremation a pagan practice and published the decree of Rome's Holy Office opposing cremation for Catholics. In 1890 Adelaide surgeon R. T. Wylde called a public meeting to form a cremation society. His cause was supported by some prominent political and business figures, and the Royal Society of South Australia voted unanimously in favor of legislation allowing cremation (Wylde, 1890, 3–16; Nicol, 1994, 173–82; Jalland, 2002, 117).

In 1873 James Edward Neild, lecturer in forensic medicine at the University of Melbourne Medical School, addressed the Royal Society of Victoria on the advantages of burning the dead. In 1892 the Royal Society produced a favorable report on cremation, and a Cremation Society was formed with leading professionals and academics as presiding officers. Attempts to get enabling legislation through parliament succeeded in 1903 (Rusden, 1890, 1–24; Cremation Society of Victoria Report, 1892; Nicol, 1994, 173–75). In 1886 J. M. Creed introduced a bill in the parliament of New South Wales to regulate cremation. Support was forthcoming from the lieutenant governor and the former chief justice, Sir Alfred Stephen, and other notables. In London during his medical training Creed had been a clinical clerk to Sir Henry Thompson. In 1890 he helped establish the Cremation Society of New South Wales.

Nonetheless, beyond the doctors and other members of the elite, cremation was rejected until well into the twentieth century. While support for institutional Christianity declined, residual sentiment sustained popular support for burial. Moreover, Catholics were totally opposed to cremation. In the decade after the opening of Adelaide's crematorium in 1903, a mere 50 people were cremated. Crematoria were not opened until 1925 in New South Wales, 1927 in Victoria, 1934 in Brisbane, 1936 in Hobart, and 1937 in Perth (Creed, 1890, 3–16; Creed, 1916, 133; Nicol, 1994, 175, 320; Jalland, 2002, 117–118).

I have mentioned that, in Britain, World War I accelerated the decline of concern with the Christian mourning rituals and the good death. The same was the case in Australia, where, proportional to the population, the numbers of troops—all volunteers—killed, died, or wounded were greater than in the mother country. In a national population of only 4.6 million (1911), 60,000 men were killed. Of every three men in uniform, two were killed or wounded. The Australian and New Zealand Army Corps (ANZAC) legend, born of the fierce fighting against the Turks at Gallipoli in 1915, celebrated the fact the war, like the bush, called forth the qualities of stoic acceptance and endurance.

As in Britain, spiritualism was a popular alternative to traditional religion as a means of coping with death in World War I. In the 1850s, British immigrants to gold-rich Victoria had brought spiritualism to the Antipodes, and Melbourne became a site of its continuing practice.

For many returned servicemen, ANZAC Day memorial ceremonies became associated with the presence of the spirits of their fellow soldiers. In the inner sanctuary of the Australian War Memorial in Canberra, a picture of the Menin Gate and unending columns of ghostly soldiers marching in support of their comrades was eventually mounted. Immensely popular when it toured the country, it was seen by a million people nationwide. So spiritually self-sufficient did ANZAC Day ceremonies become that Anglican Archbishop Frederick Head of Melbourne and some Methodist chaplains left the 1938 ANZAC march in protest against the way a Christian presence had disappeared from the ceremony. The traditional Christian approach to death appears to have survived the Great War better among Roman Catholics than among Protestants. Institutional Protestantism was already losing support before 1914. Catholic church membership held up better because the glue of Irish ethnic and working-class loyalties reinforced that of the faith (Godman, 1995, 240–43; Jalland, 2002, 304–15).

As with the British, Australian casualties in World War II were, relative to population, much lower, and this war appears not to have had the impact that the Great War had on civilians' attitudes toward death. Somewhat fewer than 8,600 Australians were killed in action in Europe between 1939 and 1945 (much of the warfare involving Australians took place in the Southwest Pacific and Southeast Asia, not Europe, in this war). This was about the same number that died in the seven months of the Gallipoli campaign in 1915. Secularization of war memorials was taken a step further when, in a utilitarian way, public buildings such as libraries rather than specific monuments were dedicated to the dead.

In the 1950s and 1960s, the possibility of nuclear war seems not to have greatly affected attitudes toward death in Australia. Even in the Cuban missile crisis in October and November 1962, the media focused on the chances of conflict breaking out rather than on the terrible destructiveness of the weapons. In Australia, reaction to the nuclear threat was different from that in Britain and the United States. In Britain, closer to Soviet Russia, the fear of becoming a victim sparked a formidable protest movement. In the United States, fear was expressed mainly as an aggressive stance, with strong popular backing for the doctrine of massive nuclear retaliation. Because Australians felt distant from the probable areas of conflict, a widespread protest movement really got under way only in 1971, when France carried out nuclear tests in the Southwest Pacific. These were seen to threaten Australians' health, not their existence (Godman, 1995, 257–76, 284–85).

For six to seven decades after World War I an attitude of denial of death prevailed in Australia as in other Anglo-Saxon countries. The secular, private, stoic model of death and grieving that developed in the bush in colonial times and was adopted in the cities as a result of World War I was very much a masculine model. Indeed, in 1918 laywomen, who had been the primary caretakers of the dying, were increasingly displaced by health and funeral professionals, while the family home as the site of deaths and dying was replaced by the hospital, nursing home, and the funeral parlor.

As I stated earlier, the growth of scientific medicine was accompanied by an objectification of the patient and the dominance of a reductionist and materialist worldview. Medicine's capacity to cure took a quantum leap in the late 1930s, when antibiotics encouraged doctors to believe that, if they could cure bacterial infections, they could come to cure most diseases. Later, technological developments enabled lives to be prolonged even where a cure was not possible. Doctors almost came to believe that death was a sort of professional failure at the same time as the process of removal of death and dying from the domestic sphere was completed.

In the 1970s in Australia (but earlier in Britain), the denial of death began to break down. Postwar migration to Australia from parts of Europe where the culture of uninhibited expression of grief survived began to challenge the primacy of the stoic model. The variety of death rituals that marked the new, multicultural society of postwar Australia made it easier to accept the argument of the thanatologists and the modern hospice movement that open expression of grief and open discussion of death and dying were healing (Godman, 1995, 298–300; Jalland, 2002, 326–28).

OBSERVATIONS

This account of the rise of scientific medicine reveals the power of a metaphysics based on materialism, dualism, and reductionism to create an unprecedentedly reliable knowledge of the pathologies of the human body and historically unmatched technologies of diagnosis and treatment. However, medicine is not just an applied health science pursuing the cure of disease. It is also a moral enterprise that highly values the individual human life and the relief of human suffering. The drive to understand and cure disease may come into conflict with these commitments, especially in the care of those with advanced disease who are progressing toward death. This conflict, which the following chapter outlines, is highlighted in medicine's approach to cancer in the last century.

3 Cancer and Medicine in Historical Perspective

Emerging in the twentieth century as one of the primary causes of death and disability in Anglo-Saxon countries, cancer became in the popular imagination the modern scourge. It replaced syphilis (the "red plague") and tuberculosis (the "white plague") as the paradigmatic disease of modern life, believed from at least the early twentieth century to be related to the personal habits, the economic organization, and the physical environment of urban-industrial society.

Central to the history of modern medicine's response to cancer is the great emphasis on basic research. Indeed, cancer is integral to the rise of laboratory-based and clinical biomedicine and to the alliance, vital to modern health care, between laboratory, hospital, and clinical trial. Whereas traditional control of infections primarily involved prevention and prophylaxis, cancer control involved treatments that in turn called for the development of research. Both anticancer organizations and governments became involved in research support. In the early twentieth century, when an upsurge of scientific, clinical, therapeutic, and social interest in cancer took place, no effective preventive policy was at hand, so two strategies were pursued: a scientific one focused on more effective therapies and better knowledge, as well as adequate treatment facilities, and a social and educational one to encourage early diagnosis since the cancer had to be localized for any chance of cure with existing treatments. With such an approach, provision for incurable cases tended to be neglected, and no special policy was developed to deal with their care (Pinell, 2000, 671–82).

Historical Understanding of Cancer

Although cancer became identified as preeminently a disease of modern society, it is in fact an ancient one. Evidence of tumors has been found in Egyptian skulls from the First Dynasty (3400 B.C.). The Hippocratic corpus (ca. 400 B.C.) called noninflammatory hard tumors and ulcers of the skin, female breast, and genitalia (culminating in death) carcinomas. Hippocrates said the cause of cancer was excessive production of black bile, a bodily humor; a humoral imbalance produced by improper diet and lack of exercise; or problems arising from climate, season, and age. The primary cure was a special diet—a cure prescribed for the next millennium and a half—to restore the humoral balance. Galen maintained that cancer resulted either from a flux of black bile producing a scirrhous that might then become a cancer or from black bile unmixed with blood, which directly produced cancer. Since this theory saw cancer as a local expression of a primary diathesis, it tended to encourage systematic treatments such as bleeding or dieting rather than surgical excision. Surgeons in medieval Europe showed the same reluctance to use surgery, while the fact that medicine and surgery became separate practices in this era further discouraged surgical intervention (Ackerknecht, 1958, 114–115; Cantor, 1993, 540; Proctor, 1995, 16).

Gasparro Arelli's discovery of the lymphatic system in 1622 moved the focus to abnormalities of the lymphatic structures. Georg Ernst Stahl (1660–1734), Friedrich Hoffmann (1660–1742), and John Hunter (1728–1793) all saw cancer as simply an unhappy consequence of inflammation, the body's healthy response to trauma. For Hermann Boerhaave (1668–1738), the greatest physician of his time, local irritation produced cancer.

The development of pathological anatomy in France in the early nineteenth century advanced the general understanding of cancer. Marie François Xavier Bichat saw all diseases as being located in 21 subtypes of tissues, with cancer being situated in cellular tissue. In the 1830s, cell theory enabled pathological anatomy to descend from the gross level. Rudolf Virchow (1821–1902) proposed that cancer cells arose from "embryonic" cells located throughout the body's connective tissue, a view later shown to be wrong. His strong support for the view that cancers were of local origin reinforced the emphasis on surgical treatment. By 1900, the basic outlines of modern knowledge of cancers had become clear. First, cancers have been differentiated from other tumors such as cysts and tubercles. Second, tumors grow by cell division and are fed by the host's blood supply. Third, they are malignant if they invade adjacent tissue or metastasize to other sites and benign if they are encapsulated. Whether malignant or benign, they may be described as epithelial or nonepithelial (the former include those composed of cells lining the blood and lymph vessels and those lining body cavities) (Ackerknecht, 1958, 116–18; Cantor, 1993, 541–44; Benedek and Kiple, 1993, 102–3).

WAS CANCER MORTALITY INCREASING?

In 1843 Stanislas Tanchou pointed out that cancer deaths in Paris had increased from 595 in 1830 to 779 in 1840 and suggested that cancer was, like insanity, more common in civilized nations. Domenico Rigoni-Stern showed in 1842 that cancer was more common in urban than rural areas, female deaths were about eight times those of males, and unmarried women, in particular nuns, were at higher risk of breast cancer. At the same time, John Le Conte noted a remarkable increase in cancer mortality in England and Wales, proposing that it resulted from the wretched condition of workers in manufacturing and mining, although he recognized that some of the increase could be explained by more careful documentation and better diagnosis and pathology. In the 1883 edition of his classic *Handbuch der historisch-geographischen Pathologie,* August Hirsch argued that the supposed rise in the incidence of cancer was an illusion due to improvement in the collection of mortality statistics. Sir Arthur Newsholme, a distinguished public health doctor, suggested in 1899 that most of the alleged increase in mortality in England could be explained by the fact that deaths from "old age" or "indefinite causes" were now being correctly attributed to cancer; deaths from "indefinite causes" had declined from 143,000 in 1867 to 69,000 in 1895. As late as 1937, statistician Louis I. Dublin suggested that mortality in the United States was probably not increasing, but his view was not the prevalent one. Although some of the growth might be explained by improved diagnosis and access to medical services, more reliable data sources, together with the fact that age-adjusted rates showed an upward trend, pointed to a real increase (Proctor, 1995, 18–26). In Canada, too, a debate raged as to whether mortality was increasing. An Ontario Health Department pamphlet of the early 1930s stated that the rising incidence was due to some extent to better diagnosis, made possible by the wider use of diagnostic aids such as X-rays. However, the dean of medicine at the University of Toronto believed that the increase was real.

The same claims that mortality was increasing were also made in Australia. G. L. Mullins, physician at the Hospice for the Dying in Darlinghurst, stated in 1896 that the increase in cancer death rates in New South Wales between 1857 and 1893 was genuine: mortality in males rose from 13.4 per 100,000 population (1857–1859) to 41.6 (1890–1893); females, from 12 to 40.5 in those same periods. Heredity was the chief cause, but chronic irritation was a precipitating factor, and tobacco smoking, like the consumption of meat, alcohol, or tea, was not a primary cause. In 1902, T. A. Coghlan, New South Wales state statistician, said the figures showed an unmistakable increase, even after allowing for better diagnosis and aging of the population, with male deaths per 100,000 population rising from 15.5 (1856–1860) to 57 (1896–1900) and female deaths rising from 15.7 to 54.4 in the same periods. However, H. B. Allen, a pathologist at Melbourne Hospital, stated that most of the increase in the last three decades of the nineteenth century was fictitious and was actually due in part to a change in the age distribution of the population and in part to improved diagnosis, more regular medical examinations, and more explicit documentation (Mullins, 1896, 1–8; Cumpston, 1989, 250–51; Clow, 2001, 41).

The matter of an increase continued to be debated. M. J. Holmes of the Commonwealth Health Department reported in 1925 that cancer mortality in Australia had increased from 26.1 deaths per 100,000 population in 1870 to 89.1 in 1923, when the all-cause death rate was falling (largely because of declining TB, post-neonatal, and early childhood death rates). He was certain that a very serious increase in cancer mortality had occurred (Holmes, 1925, 3; Cumpston, 1989, 251). Ten years later, the Commonwealth Director General of Health, J. H. L. Cumpston, reviewed the trend in Australian cancer mortality between 1881 and 1933, and stated that there was worldwide interest in the question of whether cancer death rates were increasing. He concluded that mortality in people up to the age of 69 had not increased and that the increase in those 70 years of age and older was probably largely the result of improved diagnosis and certification (Cumpston, 1936, 95–106).

Epidemiologist H. O. Lancaster pointed out that Holmes had not allowed for changes in the age distribution of the population. He standardized cancer death rates between 1908 and 1955 and concluded that, for females, mortality had been falling since around 1920, but for males it had been rising since the mid-1940s because of increasing deaths from lung cancer (Table 3.1).

In the 1930s, a study of a series of private patients revealed a five-year survival rate in operable cases of 64 percent and in borderline cases of 27 percent. In the 1940s, a Victorian study traced 98 percent of 395 women treated for breast cancer. There was a five-year survival rate of 54.6 percent where combined surgical and radiation therapy was used and 48.9 percent where surgery alone was employed. Studies of uterine cancer in the 1930s, as well as the 1950s, indicated the positive impact of treatment, whether surgery and/or radiotherapy. However, more general factors such as personal hygiene, marital status, and age at marriage also likely had an effect.

According to H. O. Lancaster's 1958 review, death rates for prostate cancer, which had been increasing, had now stabilized for those under 75 years of age while still increasing for those above that age Interestingly, Lancaster does not mention lung cancer, which had been rising markedly since about 1930. From 1.7 per 100,000 population between 1910 and 1914 (age standardized to the world population), it rose to 47.6 per 100,000 between 1975 and 1979. While lung can-

Table 3.1. Crude and Standardized Mortality from All Forms of Cancer in Australia*

Period	Crude Mortality	Standardized on Population of England/Wales, 1901	Standardized on Life Table Population of Australia 1939 Census	Equivalent Average Death Rate
Males				
1908–1910	72.4	71.3	154.0	82.6
1911–1920	80.8	74.4	162.6	87.3
1921–1930	95.0	77.5	175.4	83.8
1931–1940	112.3	78.6	182.5	77.5
1941–1945	118.0	75.5	177.7	71.6
1946–1950	125.6	77.5	180.1	76.0
1951–1955	122.7	79.1	184.2	78.1
Females				
1908–1910	71.5	83.4	171.1	96.2
1911–1920	77.1	82.9	173.3	93.9
1921–1930	90.7	84.9	181.3	92.6
1931–1940	107.4	83.1	181.3	87.0
1941–1945	121.5	83.5	183.3	84.8
1946–1950	123.5	80.4	176.6	82.6
1951–1955	117.0	75.9	167.4	76.5

Source: Lancaster, 1958, 353.

* Mortality per 100,000 population

cer mortality in women was rising during the twentieth century, it was not until the 1960s that the rate of increase became marked, and it was a counterweight to declines in mortality from stomach and uterine cancer; the first fell by 15.1 per 100,000 population in the five decades since about 1925, while the second fell by 12.3 in the same period. Male deaths from stomach cancer declined by 23.6 per 100,000 population in those same 50 years.

The declines in stomach cancer were linked to improvements in food preservation techniques. Greater exposure to risk factors (e.g., the increasing prevalence of smoking) and improvement in diagnosis and accuracy of death certification influenced these trends. Lung cancer mortality in males began to fall in the late 1980s. In some cancers, more effective therapy and thus better chances of survival produced some decline; for example, improved treatment of acute lymphoblastic leukemia in the 1970s promoted survival rates and thus produced the decline in death rates from this disease during this period. In turn, the decline in this leukemia was mainly responsible for the marked decline in overall leukemia mortality (Lancaster, 1950, 1–6; Lancaster, 1958, 350–56; Armstrong, 1985, 126–27; Taylor, Lewis, and Powles, 1998, 42).

In Canada, too, male mortality from lung cancer rose around 1930, and between that date and the mid-1970s, most of the increase in the male cancer rate was attributable to lung cancer. The overall female cancer rate fell continuously beginning in the mid-1930s, but after the mid-1960s, a growing lung cancer rate slowed the overall decline. In the mid-1960s, mortality from cancer of the stomach and rectum in men and women, as well as cervical cancer, declined. Mortality from cervical cancer was falling before cervical cytology screening programs were created, but the rate of decline was more substantial in areas where screening was at a high level. Between 1991 and 2001, the male cancer incidence rate fell from 469 to 445 per 100,000 population, but the female rate rose from 337 to 344. Whereas in the same period the male lung cancer incidence rate declined from 91 to 77 per 100,000 population, the rate for females increased from 38 to 47 per 100,000. Both breast and prostate cancer incidence rates rose in that decade (Wigle, 1978, 119–20; Martin, 2002, 1,582).

RESEARCH

Effective therapy was considered central to cancer control; therefore, research was to be promoted on pathogenesis, the biological effect of radiation, the development of therapeutic protocols, and the production of more effective X-ray and radium therapy technology. While research on etiology and pathogenesis was deemed important, during the interwar years radiation medicine was more important. Furthermore, as efficacy in therapy was critical, the provision to hospitals, often by the government, of radium and penetrating X-ray equipment was treated as vital in the five Anglo-Saxon countries we are discussing. Thus, by the early 1930s, the United States had 12 cancer hospitals and 68 general hospitals that had cancer departments with specialist equipment. Britain had 18 hospitals or approved cancer centers.

In the heyday of bacteriology in the late nineteenth century, it was widely believed that, once the "cancer germ" was identified, the appropriate therapy would quickly be developed. Indeed, research on etiology during the twentieth century swung between two poles—the effect of exogenous factors, whether viruses, parasites, environmental chemicals, or radiation, and that of endogenous factors such as genetic mutation. A great deal of intellectual effort and money went into this research, which largely focused on such proximate causes or mechanisms. Comparatively little funding was provided for research at the macro or social level of causation. Moreover, the issue, especially in the United States, was politicized—the left emphasizing social causes; the right, research at the molecular level (Pinell, 2000, 676–78; Proctor, 1995, 14).

New laboratories were set up to accommodate the upsurge of experimental inquiries. In the first case of direct state support for cancer research, the New York Pathological Laboratory was inaugurated in 1898 to pursue research into the parasitic hypothesis. The following year the Harvard Medical School received an endowment, with which it established the Caroline Brewer Croft Cancer Commission. In 1902 the Memorial Hospital in New York used an endowment to set up the Collis P. Huntington Fund in partnership with the Loomis Laboratory at Cornell University Medical School. The American Cancer Research Society was set up in Chicago at the turn of the century. In England, at Middlesex Hospital, after three years of conflict between cancer surgeons over whether the institution should continue as a haven for incurable cases and innovators wishing to establish a program of systematic research, laboratories were opened in 1900. Public proposals were soon made for a national fund to support research. The Cancer Research Fund was formally established under the control of the Royal Colleges of Physicians and of Surgeons in 1902, and two years later it became the Imperial Cancer Research Fund (ICRF). In the interwar years, an argument was to rage between the Medical Research Council and the Royal Colleges about which side would exercise authority over the direction of research pursued by the fund. By World War I, most of the capital cities in Europe boasted a radium institute, and a sizeable number of national and international cancer organizations had been formed (Austoker, 1988, 13–26; Cantor, 1993, 548).

The first decade of the new century saw much concern about the infectious origin of cancer. In 1907 Amedee Borrel proposed a viral origin, while in 1908 Vilhelm Ellermann and Oluf Bang contended that chicken leukemia was caused by a virus. In 1911 Peyton Rous transmitted a chicken sarcoma by a cell-free filtrate. Then the focus shifted to host resistance and other endogenous factors. Theodor Boveri's somatic mutation theory of 1914 postulated that chromosomal abnormalities or factors producing such abnormalities were the causes of cancer. The endogenous emphasis was reinforced by H. J. Muller's demonstration in 1927 that radiation, in changing a cell's genetics, produced uncontrollable cell proliferation. The theory also called into question explanations that were couched in terms of chemical reactivity after chemists demonstrated that polycyclic aromatic hydrocarbons were the coal tar constituents that caused cancer. By the 1950s it was firmly established that mutations in bacteria and animals could be induced by exposure to carcinogenic chemicals. In the 1930s a number of tumor-producing viruses in animals were identified, and fresh attention was paid to the role of viruses. Both DNA and RNA-type viruses were found to be carcinogenic in animals.

With the identification of tumor transplantation antigens, concern with tumor immunity expanded again in the early 1960s. Virus research led to the identification of enzymes that were able to split molecules at particular sites. Retroviruses contained an enzyme called reverse transcriptase. A retrovirus (made of RNA, not DNA), having penetrated a cell, used the reverse transcriptase to transform its core of RNA into DNA. Howard Temin's protovirus theory hypothesized that the viral genome is incorporated into the cell's nucleic acid by virion-RNA-directed polymerase. The instability of the resulting protovirus means that any disruption may produce cancer. The viral oncogene theory of Robert Huebner and George Todaro posited a type of RNA virus located in the human genome as an ongoing legacy of human evolution. The normally suppressed oncogene may be awakened, they contended, by the impact of any of many environmental carcinogens (Cantor, 1993, 544–47).

BRITISH AND AMERICAN RESEARCH

Between 1860 and 1875 a movement for the "endorsement of research" developed in the United Kingdom. This set out to convince the government and the public that not only was basic scientific research needed for economic progress but also that it should be supported by state or private endowment. Endowment and an institutional infrastructure for experimental medicine eventually emerged: the British Institute of Preventive Medicine in 1891 (in 1903, the Lister Institute); the Wellcome Physiological Research Laboratories in 1894; the London School of Tropical Medicine in 1899; and the Cancer Research Fund in 1902. In the United States, facilities for medical research expanded notably with the creation of the Rockefeller Institute for Medical Research in 1901. This transition did not occur without tension, however. Many doctors were ill informed about research and saw the change of focus from the patient to laboratory experiment as threatening. Nevertheless, the need for reliable knowledge of the nature of cancer was manifest, and the failure of surgery to reduce death rates (which many believed were increasing alarmingly) was equally clear.

Ernest Bashford, the young researcher chosen as founding director of the Cancer Research Fund, had worked in Germany with Paul Ehrlich. His plan for research envisaged the pursuit of statistical inquiries, investigation into the ethnographical and zoological distribution of cancer, and studies on the comparative pathology of tumors, as well as experimental research into the etiology of cancer. Although statistical and comparative studies were carried out—a large study of the geographical distribution, type, and site prevalence, as well as the effect of lifestyle on incidence, concluded that cancer was to be found among all races and in all climates throughout the British Empire—the emphasis was on experimental research.

From 1907 to 1913, Bashford and colleagues carried out more than 211,000 experiments on animals to study resistance to transplanted tumors. By World War I the widely agreed position was that natural resistance was inherited, tumors could be propagated only in the same species, ease of tumor transplantation differed with different tumors, and the capacity of tumors to grow in foreign territory could not be predicted. It has been proposed that Bashford's work, that of American geneticist C. C. Little on the genetics of mammal tissue transplantation, J. B. Murphy's experiments on transplantability, and William Woglom's critical analysis of earlier studies provided the basis for Peter Gorer's key findings in the 1930s concerning the conditions under which tumor transplants were accepted or rejected.

Indeed, in the interwar period, the speedy growth of new institutions and societies created a need for the international exchange of ideas and information. The American Cancer Society (ACS) arranged an international meeting of experts in New York in 1926, while in London in 1928, the British Empire Cancer Campaign (BECC) hosted the First International Conference on Cancer. The conference convened thereafter in different locations every four years, and in 1930 the BECC also hosted informal biannual meetings.

The cancer control movement in the United States had been established to promote lay education as envisaged by Charles Plumley Childe, who had failed to win support in the United Kingdom. By the late 1920s the American Cancer Society was pushing for cancer centers so that the efforts of researchers, clinicians, educators, and administrators could be coordinated. The federal government became involved in 1930, with the creation of the National Institute of Health, which among other things funded research on cancer. Congress strongly supported the National Cancer Institute Act of 1937. Government funding for clinical and basic research under the act was overseen by a National Advisory Cancer Council.

In Britain, no comparable commitment of public funds to cancer had been made. Not only were cancer services unevenly distributed, but doubts about treatment modalities were also growing. Although opinion was turning against the use of radical surgery, surgical intervention continued to be seen as the most effective treatment. It was not until the end of the 1920s that radiotherapy was widely endorsed. Chemotherapy or metallotherapy had been discredited by various failures. In the late 1890s, George Beatson's employment of ovariectomy in Glasgow had generated interest in hormone therapy. Although this diminished as the role of estrogen carcinogenesis in tumor formation was recognized, work on prostate cancer by Charles Huggins in 1941 resurrected concern with hormone therapy.

In 1929 the local authorities assumed responsibility for cancer services, but neither the quality nor the availability of these services improved. In the same year, the National Radium Trust and the Radium Commission came into being to supervise the provision of radium, which was used for intracavitary and interstitial therapy. From the outset, the commission restricted the use of radium to a small number of hospitals. However, it soon became clear that only a fraction of cases would be able to obtain treatment: in 1936, of an estimated 100,000 cases, 40 percent were considered treatable, but as few as 8,000 actually received treatment. Facing declining subscriptions, the public hospitals simply lacked the funds to extend quality services. When the government began to deal with the problem of better access under the Cancer Act of 1939, it ran into difficulties because of the rivalry between the public hospitals and the local authority hospital systems.

Further, the opportunity was lost to follow the United States in developing more integrated facilities by providing public funds for research under the Cancer Act. The concern of the Ministry of Health about opposition from clinicians meant that nothing was done, and the public organizations continued largely to fund basic research: £700,000 was to be spent on treatment facilities, but only £90,000 a year from the ICRF and BECC, plus something from the Medical Research Council (MRC), would be going to cancer research.

Under the National Health Service Act of 1946, diagnosis and treatment became the responsibility of the Regional Hospital Boards and the Boards of Governors of the English and Welsh teaching hospitals. However, the central advisory system was not an effective replacement for the Radium Commission. The shortcomings can be seen in the lack of promotion of cancer education because of reluctance to accept the link between smoking and lung cancer, as well as in the slow progress toward comprehensive cancer documentation. Even by the mid-1980s, the National Cancer Register had not established complete standardization between regions.

In the 1940s and early 1950s in the United Kingdom and the United States, chemotherapy became established as a treatment modality and an area of cancer research. Used first in warfare in 1915, sulfur mustard produced leukopenia aphasia of the bone marrow and dissolution of lymphoid tissue. Knowing the lymphocytolytic effect of mustard gases, Alfred Gilman carried out tests with nitrogen mustard in 1942, but because of wartime restrictions he was unable to describe the effects until 1946. Soon afterward, Sidney Farber used the antifolate aminopterin to effect temporary remissions for 10 of 16 children suffering from acute leukemia. Chemotherapy studies required cooperation between basic and clinical researchers. Cooperative programs in drug development were developed at institutions in the United States and Japan and at the Chester Beatty Research Institute and the Royal Cancer Hospital (now the Royal Marsden Hospital) in the United Kingdom. While the BECC and MRC supported research with chemotherapeutic relevance, the fund failed to pursue such inquiries (Austoker, 1988, 27–62, 162–98; Cantor, 1993, 557).

The MRC had largely failed to develop clinical research facilities in the period between the world wars, but, pushed by concern to bridge basic research and medical practice, it became more active in the 1930s, and the establishment of the National Health Service provided a further boost. Where in 1930 the MRC conducted one clinical research unit, in 1939 it ran three, and in 1948, eighteen. The Cancer Fund set up the Clinico-Pathological Research Unit in 1951. J. Stretton Young worked on the structure of human breast cancer and its mode of spread. L. M. Franks worked on prostate cancer, in particular the role of aging and hormones in the production of malignant and benign tumors. Modern endocrine therapy for breast cancer began in the 1950s. Identification of those likely to benefit became essential, and methods for measuring hormonal status were investigated. In 1954 Joseph Bamforth conducted a consultant service in exfoliative cytology, mainly providing early diagnosis of cervical cancer.

In 1957 the Cancer Fund cooperated in breast cancer research with the breast clinic at Guy's Hospital. During the 1960s, the number of clinical trials run by the clinic grew considerably. The most widely known of these trials was the study of therapy for early breast cancer (1961–1971), in which a comparison was made between wide excision plus modest-dose irradiation and radical mastectomy plus local irradiation.

In the postwar era, the ICRF and BECC (later the Cancer Research Campaign), private charities both, provided a growing proportion of funding for British cancer research: in 1952, 29 percent of total funding (£296,220), but in 1985, 79 percent (£46,270,660). Funding in the United States in this period was on a much greater scale. Not surprisingly, the leading edge of research in cancer became established there. Moreover, although opposition to "big government" was traditionally powerful in the United States, one of the most publicly supported research infrastructures in the world developed there.

In the mid-1940s, Mary Lasker, wife of a wealthy businessman, worked with C. C. Little, managing director of the American Society for the Control of Cancer (ASCC; later the ASC), to transform the voluntary body into a formidable funder of research. She then worked with Surgeon General Thomas Parran; James Shannon, head of the National Institutes of Health (1955–1968); Congressman Frank Keefe; and others to persuade Congress to substantially increase funding for the National Cancer Institute. From $1.75 million in 1946, funding rose to $14 million in 1947 and $100 million in 1961.

Lasker and her allies called for a "war" on cancer. During Pres. Richard Nixon's administration, the National Cancer Act of 1971 was passed, and public funding thereafter climbed astronomically: from $400 million in 1973 to $1 billion in the 1980s. Interest in the viral origins of cancer had revived, and the idea of a vaccine, just when vaccination against polio was proving so successful, had helped to build support for the increased public appropriations. Those who criticized the vast outlays for fundamental research vainly pointed out that viruses were implicated in only a small number of cancers. Many cases of cancer were preventable, the critics argued, if only the National Cancer Institute (NCI) would offer leadership in anti-smoking campaigns and promote cervical cancer screening.

Environmental theories of cancer etiology were not welcomed by the NCI and the ACS. Cold War conservatism pushed experts into denying the threat of atomic radiation, and it was not until the end of the 1950s that physicians began to address the issue seriously. There were also intellectually respectable reasons for questioning cultural and environmental explanations. First, with chemical carcinogens, since tests on animals in the main provided the evidence, would the effects on humans be the same? Second, most cancers were marked by long periods of latency, and their production was very likely multifactorial. Even when smoking was implicated, only some of those who were exposed to the carcinogen went on to develop cancer. Moreover, significant cultural values supported the orthodox emphasis on fundamental research into the cellular biology of the individual. The status and prestige of reductionist science, and medical science in particular, were very high at this time. Moreover, the free enterprise economy was again delivering prosperity. Most citizens did not want federal regulation of industry (and government intervention more generally), with the economic depression of the 1930s and World War II having safely receded into history. Only with the cultural and political revolt of the young against the Vietnam War and mainstream materialist lifestyles in the late 1960s and the economic dislocation following the end of cheap Middle Eastern oil in the 1970s did the environmentalist approach gain widespread credibility (Austoker, 1988, 212–17, 244–70; Cantor, 1993, 550–52; Patterson, 1987, 184–90).

Development of British and U.S. Cancer Services

The Middlesex Hospital in London had special cancer wards in 1792, while a Society for Investigating the Nature and Cure of Cancer came into being in Britain as early as 1802. In the second half of the nineteenth century, a number of cancer hospitals were established: the London Cancer Hospital (later the Royal Marsden) and institutions in Leeds, Liverpool, Manchester, and Glasgow.

In the United States, the process began with the establishment of the New York Cancer Hospital in 1884; then came the Saint Rose Free House for Incurable Cancer in 1899, followed by institutions in Buffalo in 1898, Philadelphia in 1904, and St. Louis in 1905. In the United States, some of the initiatives reflected a belief that research would soon produce cures so that hospitals would cease to be repositories for the incurable and dying. Around 1900 the same optimism in Britain saw the abandonment of planned Friedenheims, separate homes for those dying of cancer. The funds were spent instead on treatment and research. In 1887 a small cottage on the grounds of the London Cancer Hospital was converted to a facility for incurables. In 1911 it was demolished and replaced by an extension to the east wing. Two years earlier, a research institute (later the Chester Beatty Institute) was founded.

Along with the increasing support for laboratory research was growing support for X-ray and radium therapy, which were seen as alternatives to surgical treatment or at least as supplementary to such treatment. Concern about increasing cancer death rates fueled this development.

In 1919 the MRC looked into the medical uses of radium left over from World War I. In 1923 prominent clinicians, concerned about growing cancer mortality, set up the British Empire Cancer Campaign. The MRC saw the clinicians, facilely confident of speedily finding a cure, as likely to promote unrealistic public expectations of research. With requests for radium proliferating, in 1929 the British government set up the National Radium Trust and Commission. Using public and charity money, the trust bought radium for the commission. In turn, the commission, working with the King Edward's Hospital Fund for London, established a national network of radium treatment centers inspired by French and Swedish examples. The commission also worked to divorce the practice of X-ray therapy from X-ray diagnosis and, following the integration of the practice of radium and X-ray therapy, oversaw the training of radiotherapists. When the National Health Service was established in 1948, cancer hospitals were merged into general hospitals, and therapy was centralized in one location in each of the new health regions. The radium commission was closed down.

Provision of specialist care for the incurable and the dying was the aim of a new charitable organization, the Marie Curie Cancer Relief Fund, created in 1948. This organization offered home care for terminal patients. Pain associated with terminal cancer began to be investigated at St. Luke's Hospital in 1948. Physician Cicely Saunders expanded upon this work at St. Joseph's Hospice in Hackney from 1958 to 1965 (Cantor, 1993, 547–50). Her concept of "total pain" was to underpin the greatly improved pain control that she provided at St. Christopher's Hospice in the late 1960s.

So dreaded was cancer in the United States at the turn of the century that doctors in Philadelphia who established a cancer hospital in 1904 called it the American Oncological Hospital rather than the American Cancer Hospital. Fear of the contagiousness of cancer was so great that between the 1890s (when the New York Cancer Hospital allowed noncancer patients to enter) and 1913, cancer patients were housed separately from those suffering from other conditions. As early as 1899, only four years after their discovery, X-rays were being hailed as the source of a "cure." The problem of standardizing doses soon dampened medical enthusiasm, however. Radium was more favorably viewed because of its consistency in supplying rays, but radium did not bring respite, let alone cure, for most of the common cancers.

In 1913, in partnership with the Bureau of Mines, James Douglas, chair of the Phelps-Dodge Copper Mining Company, established the National Radium Institute. Cancer physicians were not enthusiastic about radiotherapy and wanted the earliest possible diagnosis followed by treatment through surgery. General practitioners remained poorly informed about cancer.

Founded in 1913, the American Society for the Control of Cancer was dominated by doctors. For more than 30 years, it preached early detection and surgery. While its primary activity was health education, it also pressed for the development of facilities for diagnosis and treatment. From fewer than 15 in the early 1920s, the number of special facilities grew to 345 in 1940. More than 500 hospitals were providing X-ray therapy by 1931. Nevertheless, the extent of therapeutic facilities was insufficient because most people resided quite a distance from a clinic. The opposition of private medical practitioners to the creation of publicly funded clinics and doubts about their efficacy meant that laboratory research rather than clinics continued to be the preferred route to cancer control. Many citizens remained poorly informed about cancer: a 1939 opinion poll revealed that 41 percent of respondents still believed cancer might be contagious.

The immediate postwar decades were economically prosperous, and the public was hopeful about progress in science. Philanthropy underwrote the expansion of major treatment and research facilities. In Philadelphia in 1945, the Lankenau Hospital Research Institute (created in 1927) became the Institute for Cancer Research, and from 1946 to 1957 its staff increased threefold. Similarly, the M. D. Anderson Hospital for Cancer Research in Houston received considerable funding. In 1945, a 300-bed facility, the James B. Ewing Hospital, was opened at New York's Memorial Hospital. At the same time, a gift of $4 million from the Sloan Foundation enabled the establishment of the Sloan-Kettering Institute for Cancer Research at Memorial (Royal Cancer Hospital, 1951, 7, 15; Patterson, 1987, 37–142).

Following the discovery of the structure of DNA in 1953, many researchers were confident that the advance of molecular biology would bring a speedy understanding of cancer. Pressure for greatly increased resources for cancer built up. R. Lee Clark, head of the M. D. Anderson Hospital, said that, with funding of $10 billion over a decade, cancer could be beaten. At the end of 1971 President Nixon, seeing political advantage in a war on cancer, signed into law the bill in support of the NCI.

By the late 1970s the war was not going all that well, and critics of the NCI were becoming more vociferous. Epidemiologists demonstrated the influence of diet: immigrants took on the eating habits of natives and also their pattern of cancer incidence. The new evidence about diet made possible the idea that prevention could be extended beyond the reduction of smoking prevalence. The orthodox medical emphasis on laboratory research and early treatment was subject to attack by those who blamed modern urban lifestyles for the high level of cancer. The link between emotions, immune system defenses, and various diseases, including cancer, interested those who were espousing unorthodox views of cancer etiology. Of alternative therapies, laetrile from apricot stones became the most notorious in the 1970s. Perhaps 70,000 people in the United States (20 percent of U.S. cancer deaths) were using laetrile in 1978.

By the early 1980s, as political conservatism increased in influence, the powerful tide of support for environmental controls was beginning to turn. The orthodox emphasis on fundamental molecular research remained well supported. Moreover, the treatment armamentarium was formidable, with new developments such as immunotherapy and the "natural drug" interferon in the offing. The subspecialty of medical oncology had 5,000 practitioners by the mid-1980s. However, the cost was substantial. In 1980 cancer therapy accounted for one-ninth of the total health expenditure. For most major cancers, five-year survival rates do not appear to have improved much since the 1950s. In the mid-1980s, two epidemiologists, arguing for more resources to be put into prevention, claimed that 35 years of effort against cancer, in the main involving treatment, had to be seen as a qualified failure (Patterson, 1987, 244–306).

CANADA

In early 1902 three papers on radiotherapy were published in Canada's *Dominion Medical Monthly;* one paper pointed out that the advantages included relief of pain, removal of fear of surgery and of the odor of cancer, and the painlessness of the treatment. At the 1902 Canadian Medical Association's annual meeting, a session on X-ray therapy included a presentation by Gilbert Girdwood of Montreal on the treatment of skin and breast cancer and one by Charles Dickson of Toronto on treating a range of conditions, including stomach and rectal cancer. Girdwood was the first radiologist at Royal Victoria Hospital in Montreal (Lewis, 1969, 155, 214; Hayter, 1998a, 663).

In North America, enthusiasm for radiotherapy grew as quickly as it did in Europe. In 1916 a group of physicians in Philadelphia formed the American Radium

Society and unanimously elected Canadian physician William Aikins as its first president. In 1907 Aikins, having visited the Laboratoire Biologique in Paris, opened the Radium Institute of Toronto as a private clinic. In the early years most radiotherapy treatments in North America were carried out by general practitioners and surgeons in their own offices. As editor of the *Canadian Medical Review,* Aikins compiled data on 133 patients, the published case reports of which painted a glowing picture of radium therapy.

That radiotherapy became part of medical practice despite the lack of a scientific basis for its use—clinical trials for new treatments in controlled conditions did not develop until the 1920s—had much to do with the power conferred on clinicians from having an effective technology for a disease that produced desperation in patients and often a sense of helplessness in doctors. In any case, though cure might not be possible, palliation often was.

In the 1920s the practice of radiotherapy became located in hospital departments or special clinics, and training programs were instituted. The new locations permitted follow-up and evaluation of large numbers of patients. Also, as laboratory investigation of its basic science took place, controlled trials more clearly established its role in cancer treatment (Hayter, 1998a, 663–88). Canadian provincial governments became involved in supporting cancer treatment in the interwar period. Quebec was the first in 1922.

In 1931, with the Ontario Medical Association (OMA) urging it to act, the provincial government established a royal commission on X-rays and radium. The commission was much influenced by radiologist Gordon Richards, who was eager to centralize all control activities. The commission proposed that Ontario purchase radium and create radiotherapy centers in the three cities that had medical schools. It took the government a decade to implement its recommendations in part because of the financial stringency imposed by the Depression, but by early 1934 clinics had been established in hospitals in Toronto, Kingston, and London.

However, the system of cure was fragmented from the outset. While the commission had recommended comprehensive clinics, the focus was on radiotherapy, with individual surgeons in the community responsible for surgical cases. Wary of the intrusion of government into treatment, the OMA was opposed to centralization. Moreover, the centralization of clinics in cities meant that sparsely populated areas were underserved. The commission had rejected the organization of care in Australia as a model although it was also beset by the problems presented by remote, low-density populations and great geographical size. The Australian system involved having the main centers in the capital cities and a few smaller regional centers treating simple cancers but passing complicated cases on to the main centers.

For six decades, the provision of comprehensive and accessible care proved beyond the reach of this centralized system, which was also characterized by conflict between surgeons and radiation oncologists, university and nonuniversity centers, and doctors and government. Furthermore, although the commission had recommended community education, the approach was overwhelmingly one of treatment. Prevention and screening were left far behind (Sellers, 1940, 72–73; Hayter, 1998b, 1,735–40).

By the 1990s there was a clear need for treatment centers to provide palliative care for the incurable. Standing in the way were the different background cultures of palliative medicine and oncology. The former developed from hospice care and focused on the emotional and physical needs of patients, not the disease. The latter developed from the biomedical model, wherein the disease is central and cure (or at least prolongation of life) is usually the goal. The interdisciplinary team is integral to palliative care, but in fact the great majority of terminal patients are under the care of family physicians.

As treatment became more complex, oncologists had to deal with interdisciplinarity, but the team approach was not universal. Too often the referral of patients from cancer centers to palliative care was delayed or simply did not occur. Equally, palliative care physicians sometimes failed to see how often oncology could be palliative—from 1985 to 1991, 46 percent of radiation therapy in British Columbia was for palliation. Yet, physicians were more likely than oncologists to treat pain and other symptoms properly. The recommendations of the Palliative Care Expert Panel to the Cancer 2000 Task Force have helped to bring palliative medicine and oncology closer together. Cancer centers now commonly have symptom control clinics, and some university departments of oncology include a division of palliative medicine. Cancer centers in British Columbia, Winnipeg, Ottawa, and Halifax have established cooperative relations with palliative care services. In 1995 palliative medicine physician Eduardo Bruera, as chair of the Clinical Trials Group Symptom Control Committee of the National Cancer Institute of Canada (NCIC), was charged with conducting clinical trials in the management of symptoms; in 1997 oncologists and palliative care physicians used an NCIC workshop to specify areas of symptom management in which basic science research might be fruitfully carried out (Mackenzie, 1998, 1702–3).

AUSTRALIAN RESEARCH

In 1914 a donation funded a research scholarship for work in cancer at Melbourne University. Thomas Cherry became John Grice Research Fellow in Cancer in 1921 and retained the post until 1934. He was struck by the apparent connection between trends in tuberculosis and cancer mortality. He also explored the relationship between TB and cancer in experimental work on mice. In 1933 he presented his conclusions: the rise in cancer resulted from the association of declining TB mortality with a continuance of opportunities for reinfection; cancer was not caused by the reigniting of an old form of infection but by a new invasion of the bacillus (*Australasian Medical Gazette,* 1914, 518; *Medical Journal of Australia,* 1914, 47; Cherry, 1933, 215–16; Russell, 1977, 101).

In Australia, the University of Sydney began establishing facilities for research on radiotherapy. In the 1920s private and public donations, as well as state and federal funds, were used to set up facilities. The Cancer Research Committee proposed that the main focus of research be on the effects of radiation on living tissue. Warnford Moppett, a Sydney medical graduate, carried out experiments on the behavior of the chorioallantoic membrane of fowls' eggs when exposed to "homogeneous" X-rays of different wavelengths. The work of Moppett and W. H. Love, a physicist, led to studies in which biological action was correlated with the content of lead, uranium, and molybdenum in tissues of incubated eggs. This work in turn led to the introduction at the university's teaching hospital, Royal Prince Alfred Hospital, of treatment of cancer with colloidal lead.

From 1925 to 1927 Moppett's work dominated the Sydney program. His novel hypothesis was that homogenous X-rays of certain frequencies could efficiently produce changes in cells, some of which caused cell death and others, proliferation. Rays of the two types inhibited each other; the novelty lay in the claim that there was selective action at specific places in the X-ray spectrum when the existing explanation of selective action posited differences in biological action of whole regions of the spectrum or a general effect on quality emerging as stronger radiation was employed. In the meantime, microchemical work on cell architecture offered a different explanation in terms of the standard physics of photon absorption. Further, experiments in the United Kingdom failed to find evidence for selective action or offered instead more plausible biological explanations for the Moppett effect. Eventually it was quietly discarded by Moppett himself. With the "failure" of Moppett's research, the Sydney program was in trouble.

The University of Melbourne should have been a significant center of radiotherapy research because physics professor T. H. Laby was an internationally known expert on ionizing radiation. However, the university advanced in this area only after the Commonwealth located its radium laboratory in Laby's department. In 1935 the Commonwealth laboratory became the keystone of a national system in which the physicists in the university of each state provided services related to standardizing radiation doses and to the quality of X-ray beams for local hospitals. Each state's anticancer committee funded this work, but none of them pursued an ambitious research program like the intellectually flawed one in Sydney (Hamersley, 1988, 199–216).

In 1926 Dr. Arthur Burrows of Manchester was consulted on the use of radium. The University of Sydney then installed a deep therapy X-ray machine at Royal Prince Alfred Hospital and another at the biophysical laboratory on campus. The Commonwealth government purchased ten grams of radium for distribution to the states for cancer treatment. A radium clinic was also set up at Royal Prince Alfred.

In 1928 F. P. Sandes, McCaughey Professor of Surgery at Sydney University, became director of cancer treatment for the cancer research committee. H. G. Chapman, professor of physiology, became director of cancer research. H. M. Moran, a prominent cancer specialist and member of the research committee, claimed that the science professors on the committee strongly opposed Chapman's appointment on the grounds that his research ability was doubtful. Unhappily, those who were concerned about this were proved correct. Chapman carried out no work and poorly supervised that of others. However, reporting to the Australasian Medical Congress in 1934, Chapman called for governments and individuals to provide more funds for research, pointing out that decreased income had forced Sydney University to discontinue the services of a number of researchers. Meanwhile, in the face of Chapman's continuing refusal to allow his accounts to be audited, the chancellor in early 1934 threatened to suspend him. Chapman suicided in May 1934. He had embezzled £3,360 from the Royal Society of New South Wales, of which he was treasurer, and more than £15,000 from the Australian National Research Council (the forerunner of the Australian Academy of Science), of which he was also treasurer. Although Chapman did not defraud the university of cancer funds, his behavior destroyed the high hopes of those who founded the research program, although some research work continued into the late 1930s. The program had supported the publication of the *Journal of the Sydney University Cancer Research Committee*. However, at the 1937 Australian Cancer Conference, it was decided that there was insufficient support for a special cancer journal, and the publication was allowed to expire (Chapman, 1934, 20; *Medical Journal of Australia*, 1937, 237; Young, Sefton, and Webb, 1984, 205–14, 423).

In 1957 Sir Macfarlane Burnet, distinguished director of the Walter and Eliza Hall Institute of Melbourne, talked pessimistically about the prospects for cancer control. Ten years later one expert commentator admitted that, in that decade, the outcomes of orthodox cancer treatments had improved but little (Starr, 1968, 733). Nevertheless, there were some notable developments in research and treatment infrastructure.

Following advice from Ralston Paterson of Manchester's Holt Radium Institution to centralize treatment and research facilities, the Victorian government appointed a committee (including Peter MacCallum, chair of the Victorian Anti-Cancer Council, 1946–1963) to implement the advice. In December 1948 an act was passed that established a cancer institute for research into and treatment of cancer for the benefit of the people of Victoria and Tasmania.

Twenty-five years after its establishment, research ranged from basic inquiries to clinical applications. The endocrine research unit was examining cancer-caused disturbances in hormone function; the hematology research unit, clinical research on RNA analyses of tumors; and the biological research unit, cell population dynamics and mechanisms controlling cell population and differentiation. Clinical trials were in progress for leukemia, non-Hodgkin's lymphoma, and cancer of the breast, lung, stomach, pancreas, and colon. Trials for ovarian cancer and melanoma were also being considered (MacKay, 1949, 729; Ilbery, 1978, 573–75).

In 1955 the New South Wales State Cancer Council Act to promote research and treatment was passed. The Hospitals Commission set aside 30 beds at the Prince of Wales Hospital in Randwick for cancer research. The clinical services of the unit were not intended to replace those routinely offered by metropolitan hospitals, nor was the unit to accommodate terminal and dying patients. By the mid-1960s the council was regularly providing research grants for fundamental and clinical research (*Medical Journal of Australia*, 1956, 1049–50; 1957b, 44; 1964, 202).

In 1976 Donald Metcalf, head of the cancer research unit at the Hall Institute in Melbourne, publicly argued that smaller nations such as Australia had both the capacity and the duty to carry out cancer research. Pointing out that it was known how to prevent only two of the common cancers (skin and lung), he stated that, in the treatment of childhood leukemia and Hodgkin's disease, great progress had been made, while management of breast and prostate cancer had usefully progressed. However, overall, in 30 years, cancer therapy had advanced but little. A national research plan would include the following elements based on the idea of consolidating existing efforts: units of 10–12 people would be the key, funded entity; as an interdisciplinary enterprise, cancer research could not be confined to one university department; specific cancer funding should not go to normal members of teaching departments; Australia, with its high rate of skin cancer, had a special responsibility to investigate that disease (Metcalf, 1976, 45–47).

In the early 1980s, to commemorate the centenary of Sydney University's Medical School and of Royal Prince Alfred Hospital and also to halt the drain of researchers from New South Wales, a group of medical academics proposed the establishment of a center of excellence like Victoria's Hall Institute. However, in 1984 a working party of the Australian Science and Technology Council criticized the proposal as too ambitious. In 1985 the institute was set up by state legislation. Tony Basten was appointed director in 1989, and his Clinical Immunology Research Center became the core unit of the institute. Preeminent immunologist Peter Doherty had, at the official opening of the new building in 1997, described the institute as the country's major research center in immunology. The institute aimed to combine cellular immunology with cancer-oriented molecular biology (Basten, 1999, 634–36).

Reviewing the future of cancer research at the close of the 1990s, two cancer control experts, R. C. Burton and B. K. Armstrong, declared that the critical point in cancer research had been passed. It was now known that cancer was due to mutated genes. The primary types of genes at work were proto-oncogenes, whose products are involved in signaling pathways to cell-cycling, tumor-suppressing genes, the products of which control the proto-oncogenes and DNA-repair genes. Research priorities needed to be set according to mortality burden, current etiological knowledge, and the availability of proven preventive and treatment options. Fundamental biological research offered the promise of great progress, but well-supported research covering environmental, epidemiological, behavioral, social, and cultural questions was also needed to underpin the edifice of contemporary, evidence-based cancer control (Burton and Armstrong, 1997, 180–81).

AUSTRALIAN TREATMENT SERVICES

Cleaver Woods of Albury, New South Wales, is reported to have used X-rays in 1896 to treat cancer of the larynx. In 1899 Herschel Harris became honorary skiagraphist to Sydney Hospital. An X-ray department opened at Royal Prince Alfred Hospital in 1904. With the appointment of E. H. Molesworth and Langloh Johnston as honorary dermatologists in 1910, radiotherapy began at Saint Vincent's Hospital in Sydney. In 1909 Harris and P. E. Bennett (dermatologist at Royal Prince Alfred Hospital) initiated radium treatment of rodent ulcers.

X-ray and radium therapies were also being tried in other states. In 1902 T. G. Beckett, honorary medical electrician at the Alfred Hospital in Melbourne, argued that, in easily accessible sites, cancers could be cured by this therapy, contrary to the views of many doctors; moreover, the therapy eradicated pain (Beckett, 1902, 450–57). Dermatologist at the Alfred Hospital in 1902, A. W. Finch Noyes is said to have initiated the use of radium in Melbourne. In a 1910 report to the Victorian government, a leading Melbourne specialist, Hermann Lawrence, proposed that it subsidize the cost for hospitals with a skin department. Two years later, radium valued at £1,500 was offered by the government to the Melbourne, Alfred, and Saint Vincent's hospitals on the condition that each meet a third of the cost. In 1913 a donation from Thomas Baker, who helped found Kodak (Australia), allowed the Alfred Hospital to accept the offer.

In 1914 Stanley Argyle, Beckett's successor in 1908, had a special electrical pavilion set up at the Alfred Hospital. The Felton Bequest purchased a deep X-ray therapy plant. In 1925 Argyle was able, through the bequest funds, to purchase radium valued at £4,500. In 1929, the last year of his directorship, Argyle's department dealt with 6,000 inpatients and 45,000 outpatients and carried out just under 20,000 X-ray examinations.

E. J. Roberts, senior resident surgeon and radiologist at Hobart Hospital, addressed the Tasmania branch of the British Medical Association (BMA) in 1913 on the therapeutic value of secondary rays produced from metal by the action of roentgen rays. In Launceston, when John Ramsay became interested in the potential of deep X-ray therapy, he visited Germany in 1919 to purchase equipment form Siemens. W. P. Holman, who became a radiologist at Launceston Hospital in 1925, had radium needles made in Brussels and used them to treat breast cancer.

In 1896 a Perth engineer, W. J. Hancock, ordered X-ray equipment from London and gave it to Perth Hospital in 1898. D. I. Smith became the first radiologist in 1920. In 1924 A. Johnson and J. Johnson, both doctors, treated hospital as well as private patients in their rooms until the hospital acquired a deep therapy unit.

In 1925 the Commonwealth provided funds for cancer research at the University of Queensland, after which a cancer campaign committee was established. The committee raised £52,000, and the Queensland Cancer Trust (part of the British Empire Cancer Campaign) administered the monies. The trust set up Queensland's first clinic at Brisbane's Mater Misericordiae Hospital at the end of 1928. The clinic used a deep X-ray therapy machine. In 1929 the Brisbane hospital arranged for patients to have radium therapy.

In 1927 Royal Adelaide Hospital possessed 80 milligrams of radium, a large part of the national total. When urged by public health expert Frank Hone in 1928, the University of Adelaide set up an anticancer campaign committee to work with the hospital to extend access to treatment. The Anti-Cancer Foundation financed the acquisition of equipment, staff salaries, and other initiatives, including a cancer registry. In the 1940s the state government funded the acquisition of further equipment, and the foundation subsidized a physics division (Ryan, Sutton, and Baigent, 1996, 219–21, 232–52).

The growth of radiotherapy in the first three decades of the twentieth century was not uncontroversial. Reviewing cancer treatment in 1913, the *Australasian Medical Gazette* pointed out that the only successful mode of therapy was surgery. Honorary radiologist to the Adelaide Hospital, H. Carew Nott observed in 1922 that the value of radiation was not sufficiently recognized (*Australasian Medical Gazette*, 1913, 149; *Medical Journal of Australia*, 1922, 342–43).

L. J. Clendinnen compared the results of surgery with those of radium therapy in cases of breast cancer treated in the five-year period ending June 1933 at the Melbourne Hospital Clinic (Table 3.2).

A history of radiotherapy in Australia (Ryan et al., 1996) claims that radiotherapy has historically suffered from a failure to commit adequate public funds to support it. The attitude has been that the cure (other than radiotherapy) was just around the corner—whether this was chemotherapy in the 1970s, immunotherapy in the 1980s, or gene therapy in the 1990s. A major advantage of radiotherapy, of course, is that the diseased organ is preserved relatively intact.

In the interwar years in Australia, as in Britain, injections of colloidal preparations of various heavy metals were used to treat inoperable cancer. J. L. Jona of the gynecological department of the Women's Hospital in Melbourne was a leading exponent of this approach. Using preparations of bismuth, lead, and copper, Jona injected 14 patients with cancer in various sites whose condition was rapidly deteriorating. All had had surgery, and many had also had deep X-ray or radium therapy, or both. Almost all showed some temporary improvement, and one woman, who was near death, lived for three months. One year later, in 1929, Jona reported further on the treatment of inoperable cancer with lead, copper, and bismuth. His therapy, he argued, was always useful as an adjunct to other modes of treatment. Surgery was often disappointing and sometimes involved the most awful mutilations; radiation failed with many forms of cancer; and metallic therapy could deal with metastases. In 1934 the *Medical Journal of Australia* said that the use of lead therapy would not only benefit hopeless cases but would also offer researchers a new field to explore. In 1936 it reported on 114 very advanced cases treated in Basel, Switzerland, by neurohormonal therapy; the journal was enthusiastic about the therapy, which had seen health restored in many patients and great improvement in many others (Jona, 1928, 587–89; Jona, 1929, 457; *Medical Journal of Australia*, 1934b, 519–20; 1936a, 191–92).

Table 3.2. Results of Treatment for Breast Cancer

Type of Case	Treatment	Number of Cases	Local or Adjacent Recurrences	Distant Recurrences (Bony or Visceral)
Operable and Borderline	Surgery	102	83%	34%
	Radium Therapy	17	6%	6%
Inoperable	Surgery	26	100%	58%
	Radium Therapy	30	13%	16%

Source: Clendinnen, 1934, 32.

GOVERNMENT ACTION IN AUSTRALIA

In 1925 the Commonwealth Royal Commission on Health had proposed that governments subsidize cancer research. At its first session, the Federal Health Council in 1927 urged the Commonwealth government to establish a radium bank (which would lend radium to the states for therapy purposes) and to subsidize deep therapy under controlled conditions so that the results might contribute to overall scientific knowledge of cancer. It also urged hospitals to keep records of cancer patients on a uniform basis.

We have seen how the cancer research committee was established at the University of Sydney. At that time the governments of New South Wales, Queensland, South Australia, and Western Australia each donated £5,000 to the work of the local cancer committees. The University of Sydney and the Queensland Cancer Trust unsuccessfully sought the assistance of the federal health department to create a national coordinating authority for cancer control. However, the department did sponsor national conferences on cancer in Canberra during the 1930s (*Medical Journal of Australia,* 1931c, 88).

The first Australian cancer conference was held in 1930, and the second, in 1931. The representatives included the following members of the Federal Health Council and cancer experts from the states: from New South Wales, Sir Alexander MacCormick, Prof. O. U. Vonwiller, and Doctors H. G. Chapman, F. P. Sandes, E. H. Molesworth, H. M. Moran, R. H. Kenny, A. T. Nisbet, L. Keatinge, A. Arnold, and T. Wilkins; from Victoria, Prof. T. H. Laby, Doctors W. Cuscaden, H. Flecker, N. T. Bull, R. Fowler, J. Clendinnen, J. O'Sullivan, T. F. Ryan, K. Scott, A. J. Trinca, and A. H. Turner; from Queensland, Doctors J.V. Duhig, L. M. McKillop, and Capt. E. R. B. Pike; from South Australia, Doctors F. S. Hone and B. S. Hanson; from Western Australia, Dr. M. Bromhall; and from Tasmania, Dr. V. R. Ratten.

M. J. Holmes of the Commonwealth Health Department reported that, over a period of two and a half years, 4,373 people had been treated with radium at the participating centers; of 1,699 treated for cancer (excluding rodent ulcer) over a two year period ending June 1930, 41 percent had had no recurrence of symptoms.

The conference made various recommendations, including the introduction of a degree in radiology; publication by the Commonwealth of periodic statistical studies on cancer morbidity and mortality; consultation in the different states concerning a national educational campaign to stress the importance of early diagnosis; and, in all X-ray treatments, the recording of dosages in ionometric units (*Medical Journal of Australia,* 1931a, 515–16; 1931b, 607–8).

At the third Australian Cancer Conference in 1932, M. J. Holmes reported that, while the work of the cancer committees in New South Wales and South Australia was progressing satisfactorily, clinical meetings at the Brisbane consultative clinic in Queensland were not well attended and in Victoria no proper clinics had been established (*Medical Journal of Australia,* 1932, 697). Reporting to the fourth conference in 1933, Holmes pointed to the problem of a national shortage of beds, especially since more patients with early cancer were seeking treatment. He proposed that those with advanced cancer not be allowed to occupy beds for long periods in order not to exclude those with a reasonable hope of recovery. In NSW, Commonwealth radium had now been supplied to the government's Coast Hospital, the Royal North Shore Hospital, and the Ryde Home for Incurables. In Victoria, although no progress in the creation of a state cancer organization had been made, patients who were treated with radium at the Austin Hospital in Melbourne had tripled in number, and Saint Vincent's in Melbourne was building a large new wing for radium therapy. The University of Sydney had begun offering a degree in radiology in the hope of helping to reduce the dangers of treatment to patients and staff alike. Unhappily, only Queensland and Tasmania were carrying out community education (*Medical Journal of Australia*, 1933, 79–80; 1934a, 302).

The Commonwealth X-ray and Radium Laboratory expanded its work considerably in 1935. The new physicist in charge, C. E. Eddy, reported that a total of 29,033 millicuries of radon had been issued that year. In 1930 the total had been only 11,380 millicuries. Eddy was now making periodic visits to different states to consult on X-ray and radium matters.

M. J. Holmes told the 1936 Australian cancer conference that one of the significant problems that had to be addressed was closer cooperation of specialists like surgeons, radiologists, pathologists, and others so that patients obtained the best care, especially when combined treatments were involved; too often, patients were lost to sight when transferred from a radiotherapy department to a general or surgical ward.

J. H. L. Cumpston addressed the issue of public and professional education to encourage early diagnosis and treatment, saying that much remained to be done to advance the cause. He counseled his colleagues in the delicate matter of relations with patients, urging clinicians to be compassionate doctors rather than cold judges. The importance of the educational issue led F. P. Sandes to reopen the question of a national organization. He proposed, and in this was supported by the conference, the creation of an Australian Cancer Commission composed of representatives of the federal health department, the BMA, the Royal Australasian College of Surgeons, the Australian and New Zealand Association of Radiology, and representatives of the general public, the universities, the hospitals, and other appropriate bodies nominated by the federal health minister.

Some of the long-standing objectives of the members of the Australian Cancer Conference were realized in 1936. With the creation of the Victorian Anti-Cancer Council, each state now had an organization to handle cancer control matters. With the establishment of the National Health and Medical Research Council (NHMRC), Australia at long last had a national research body with funds to encourage cancer research, and extrametropolitan centers for diagnosis and treatment were being developed, as was the case, for example, with Bendigo Base Hospital's consultative clinic (*Medical Journal of Australia*, 1936b, 238–39, 245; 1937, 234).

The tenth and last prewar conference on cancer was held in Wellington, New Zealand, in February 1939 as an Australasian meeting. While the conferences in the 1930s did much to build organizational infrastructure to extend access to treatment, attempt to standardize treatments, and promote cooperation between different disciplines, the treatment bias was toward radiotherapy. As H. H. Schlink and colleagues at Royal Prince Alfred Hospital stated in 1947, surgeons, physicians, and pathologists generally did not attend the prewar Canberra conferences but left the field to the radiotherapists (Schlink, Chapman, and Chenhall, 1947, 397).

As mentioned earlier, Ralston Paterson and Edith Paterson, both doctors at the Christie Hospital and Holt Radium Institute in Manchester, accepted the invitation of the New South Wales government to visit Sydney in 1944 to advise it on the establishment of a specialist cancer center. The Labor premier, William (later Sir William) McKell, had appointed an advisory committee on the future of services. While there, they also visited Melbourne and Brisbane to discuss cancer treatment developments. Ralston Paterson pointed out that the principal advantage of such centers was the greater opportunity for learning about treatment because of the large numbers of patients they attracted. Soon afterward, McKell became governor general, and, since the new premier, J. J. McGirr, did not favor a specialist center, no such facility was established in New South Wales.

With the creation of the Queensland Radium Institute (QRI), the Queensland Cancer Trust was dissolved, and the QRI took over the facilities at the Royal Brisbane and the Mater Misericordiae hospitals. In accordance with Paterson's advice, peripheral clinics were set up in provincial centers. In Victoria, following Paterson's recommendation for a centralized unit, the Cancer Institute was opened in 1949, and the treatment section was named the Peter MacCallum Clinic in honor of a man who had long campaigned for better facilities. Peripheral clinics were created in all of Melbourne's teaching hospitals and in provincial centers such as Bendigo that were large enough to have a base hospital.

The Australian and New Zealand Association of Radiologists was formed in 1935. In 1949 this became the College of Radiologists (Australia and New Zealand); in 1952, the College of Radiologists of Australasia; and in 1972, the Royal Australasian College of Radiologists. In 1978, to promote radiation oncology, the Radiotherapy Standing Committee was set up within the college, and in 1994 the Faculty of Radiation Oncology was created.

The arrival of the first linear accelerator at the QRI in 1956 marked the beginning of the megavoltage era in Australia, and over the next decade and a half, units were installed in all of the capital cities. However, opposition to the development of radiotherapy remained significant, partly because, in the past, deep therapy equipment could not achieve adequate dosage without damage to normal cells and in part because better surgery, hormone therapy, and then chemotherapy seemed likely to render radiotherapy obsolete.

By the mid-1990s there were only 5.4 radiation oncologists per million in Australia when the rate should have been 7. Between 1986 and 1994, fewer than 40 percent of newly diagnosed cancer patients were treated with radiotherapy despite increases in the number of megavoltage machines, and the situation was much worse outside the capital cities. As in Britain and Canada but unlike in the United States, in Australia radiation oncology is practiced mainly in public hospitals, although funding through Medicare, the national health insurance program, has allowed some growth in the private practice sector. A basic obstacle to the expansion of radiation oncology has been doctors' ignorance of its role in the management of cancer patients (Morgan, 1996, 224–31).

I have already referred to the passing of Victoria's 1948 Cancer Institute Act and New South Wales's 1955 State Cancer Council Act, both of which led to major developments in cancer therapy facilities. However, the immediate postwar years saw other new developments. Sydney's Rachel Forster Hospital for Women and Children provided Australia's first cancer detection clinic for women. Following standard practice in the United States, women who were 25 years of age and older were encouraged to visit their doctor every six months for vaginal, rectal, and breast examinations. The need for early detection was clear when evidence demonstrated that 10–12 months might elapse between the appearance of symptoms and the commencement of treatment. The blame for such a dangerous delay had to be shared by both patient and doctor (*Medical Journal of Australia,* 1944, 31–32; 1948, 192).

Tables 3.3–3.5 illustrate the "cure" rates for cervical cancer patients treated at the Royal Prince Alfred Hospital in Sydney between 1930 and 1940.

H. H. Schlink and colleagues at the Royal Prince Alfred Hospital proposed combined treatment for cervical cancer whenever surgery was possible, believing the better outcomes over those of radium treatment alone were largely due to extirpation of the lymphatic glands. In 1955 H. J. Ham of Sydney noted that only surgery plus radiotherapy (X-rays, radium, and radioactive isotopes) still offered the possibility of cure, as chemotherapy and hormone therapy were essentially palliative. He complained that, at two of Sydney's teaching hospitals, about 40 percent of patients treated with deep X-ray therapy suffered from inadequate bed accommodation. B. T. Edye of Sydney claimed that hormone therapy and radiotherapy had in recent times pushed surgery more and more into the background, while Sir Albert Coates of Melbourne noted that the current level of collaboration between radiotherapists and surgeons in treatment had not existed 20 years earlier (Schlink et al., 1947, 399; *Medical Journal of Australia,* 1955a, 527; 1955b, 913–14).

Table 3.3. Five-Year Cure Rate, Cervical Cancer, 1930–1940

Condition of Patients	Royal Prince Alfred Hospital		Aggregate of 16 World Centers		Holt Institute, Manchester, 1934–1938	
	Number	%	Number	%	Number	%
Patients examined	371	–	9,051	–	899	–
Patients treated	357	96.2	7,958	87.8	826	91.6
Without recurrence after 5 years	111	31.0	2,194	27.6	214	25.9
With recurrence after 5 years	2	0.5	128	1.6	8	0.96
Died of cancer	214	59.9	5,368	67.5	572	69.2
Died of intercurrent disease	11	2.9	163	2.0	21	2.5
Lost	19	5.1	105	1.3	11	1.3

Source: Schlink, Chapman, and Chenhall, 1947, 398.

Table 3.4. Ten-Year Cure Rate, Cervical Cancer, Royal
Prince Alfred Hospital, 1930–1940

Condition of Patients	Number	%
Patients examined	197	–
Patients treated	188	95.4
Without recurrence after 10 years	41	21.8
With recurrence after 10 years	1	0.5
Died of cancer	125	66.5
Died of operation	2	2.4
Died of radium treatment	3	2.9
Died of intercurrent disease	8	4.3
Lost	8	4.3

Source: Schlink, Chapman, and Chenhall, 1947, 398.

In 1956 B. A. Stoll of Melbourne's Peter MacCallum Clinic reported on the use
of the chemotherapeutic agent Nitromin (nitrogen mustard N-oxide) in the treatment of 19 patients (male and female) with advanced cancers in various sites and
malignant lymphomas. Immediate regression of the cancers took place in six cases.
After two months 10 people were still alive. Three years later Stoll reviewed the
state of chemotherapy and found that, whereas in the past, it had been mainly palliative, in recent years it had been tried as a prophylactic during or just after radical
extirpation of cancer tissue. In 1965 D. P. Ewing and colleagues of the radiotherapy
department at Saint Vincent's Hospital in Sydney reported the results of a prospective randomized trial comparing radiotherapy alone with radiotherapy plus the use
of Nitromin with 44 patients with lung cancer in each group. Although there was
an apparent increase in the survival rates of those receiving the combined treatment, it was not statistically significant (Stoll, 1956, 884–87; Stoll, 1959, 242;
Ewing, McEwen, and Atkinson, 1965, 400).

In 1962 a survey of 1,106 women who had been referred to the radiotherapy
department at Royal Adelaide Hospital found that androgens were more useful
than estrogens in treatment; about 50 percent of adrenalectomies were beneficial;
and peripheral radiation was no more helpful than other radiological techniques
after radical surgery. Brisbane surgeon I. Burt pointed out in 1966 that, in breast

Table 3.5. Treatment of Cervical Cancer at Royal Prince
Alfred Hospital, by Duration and Treatment Type

	Type of Treatment	
Duration of Cure	Radium and Surgery	Radium Alone
Five years	54%	14%
Ten years	44%	8%

Source: Schlink, Chapman, and Chenhall, 1947, 398.

cancer, chemotherapy was still only palliative treatment; the order of treatments remained first, surgery; second, radiation; third, hormones, where appropriate; and finally, chemotherapy for palliation. In 1975 R. G. Bourne and K. S. Mowatt of the Queensland Radium Institute in Brisbane warned that recent favorable results from the use of chemotherapy as adjuvant to radical mastectomy involved only short-term follow-ups and that the usefulness of 1-phenylaline mustard was not yet conclusively proven (*Medical Journal of Australia,* 1962, 204; 1966, 1127–28; 1975b, 282).

The *Medical Journal of Australia* pointed out in 1972 that the team approach to the treatment of cancer was now accepted by most patients and many doctors. The approach had various advantages—availability of a spectrum of expertise; ease of meaningful assessment of results; higher motivation for long-term follow-up because the patient is committed to the group; and, with conflicting opinions over the most effective primary treatment mode, great opportunities for prospective trials. Few tumors had greater than a 50 percent, five-year survival rate; thus such advantages were most welcome. The journal expressed regret that the growth of teams had been slow in Australia but stated that this was understandable given that, until recently, most tumors had been treated either by surgery or radiotherapy but not by both. L. Atkinson and N. C. Newton, doctors at the Prince of Wales Hospital in Sydney, rejected the claim of Australian tardiness in developing a team approach, pointing out that multidisciplinary management was so widely accepted that the Clinical Oncological Society of Australia had been set up five years previously to ensure regular meetings at which members could share their experiences. A. Freedman of Kings Cross in Sydney pointed out that combined clinics had been operating at the Special Unit for Investigation and Treatment of Cancer in Randwick since 1960 and that, within the University of New South Wales, consultative clinics had been performing cancer therapy since 1967 (*Medical Journal of Australia,* 1972a, 558; 1972b, 828).

Treatment in New Zealand

In New Zealand, too, the therapeutic application of X-rays was begun at an early date. Thus, in 1909 they were being used at Christchurch Hospital. However, except for P. D. Cameron's work in Dunedin in 1911, radium was not used until after World War I. Christchurch Hospital took the initiative with regard to radium, proposing to hospitals in Wellington and Dunedin the idea of a radon emanation plant to make the glass capsules filled with radium gas that were then being used to treat cancer. A public fund was established in Wellington and endorsed by the Wellington health authorities. A similar public appeal for funds was started in Auckland, and money was also raised in Dunedin.

Christchurch authorities were advised to spend a conservative amount on radium and also to install a deep therapy plant. In 1924 the Christchurch hospital offered both radium treatment and deep therapy. In 1934 the old conflicts between surgeons and radiotherapists were minimized by the introduction of a consultation clinic where surgeons, radiotherapists, dermatologists, and, on occasion, pathologists could jointly discuss cases. In 1947 nitrogen mustard and later other chemotherapeutic agents were used, as were hormonal treatments. In 1948 radioactive iodine, the first of the isotopes, was employed. In the 1950s a high-voltage unit was donated by Sir Arthur Sims (who had earlier funded the purchase of radium) and, soon afterward, such units were also installed in Auckland, Dunedin, Wellington, and Palmerston North (Bennett, 1962, 199–208).

THE EMERGENCE OF MEDICAL ONCOLOGY IN THE UNITED STATES, THE UNITED KINGDOM, CANADA, AND AUSTRALIA

In the United States, the 1960s and 1970s saw an increasing use of chemotherapy in the treatment of a wide variety of cancers, and, as physicians focused on the drug treatment of cancer, medical oncology emerged as a subspecialty. The American Board of Internal Medicine decided in 1971 to provide certification, and the first examinations were held in 1973; just over a decade later there were 3,000 certified oncologists who acted not as consultants but actually managed therapy, sometimes in cooperation with other specialists. From the outset, oncology was linked with laboratory work and research in specialties such as pharmacology, cell biology, biochemistry, and endocrinology. The cultural tradition of settlers battling opponents on the frontier easily translated into doctors aggressively fighting cancer.

The war on cancer, initiated by the Cancer Act of 1971, was generously funded; over the next three years $1.6 billion was to be spent on experimentation with new drugs. Medical oncology thus became a specialty that relied heavily on clinical trials. Indeed, in 1990 the leading centers boasted that there were so many trials that virtually every patient with advanced cancer could participate in one, and enrollment became a routine aspect of treatment.

Although the preeminence of the United States in basic and clinical research meant that the U.S. model greatly influenced management in Europe, local medical and cultural traditions, as well as local policy, health services organizations, and funding affected national responses. In Britain, comparatively few medical oncologists were trained; indeed, in 1981 there were only 40–50 consultants. While complaints surfaced about the lack of oncologists, the U.S. approach, believed to show the dangers of excessive medicalization, was not popular. In 1981, for example, the *Lancet* said that development of a specialty based on the use of a few drugs was hardly justified. In the end the solution was seen to involve dual training in medical oncology and radiation therapy, although those who were trained remained relatively few, and they continued to act as consultants to those who had primary responsibility for the care—general practitioners and specialists in internal medicine, hematology, and gastroenterology.

Differences in resources and health services organizations played their part. British spending per capita on chemotherapy in the early 1980s was only one-fifth of the amount spent in the United States, and patients with solid tumors in the United States were five to six times more likely to be treated with drugs than British patients. The fee-for-service system in the United States put its own pressure on doctors to be active—actually to be doing something for patients. In Britain the publicly funded care system put pressure on doctors to be cost effective in therapy, and chemotherapy was not widely considered as contributing significantly to increasing the period of good-quality life. Moreover, where affluent Americans might shop around for new experimental treatments, the regional organization of health services (and perhaps a greater inclination to trust the doctor's judgment) did not encourage the same quests in Britain. Even so, institutional differences within countries may also be important. Leading teaching and research hospitals in the West, irrespective of country, tend to pursue an experimentalist approach, which is furthered by the competitiveness of the international scientific culture (Lees, 1974, 7; Del Vecchio Good, 1991, 121–22; Löwy, 1996, 63–72).

In theory, then, whether a patient with advanced incurable cancer went into experimental drug therapy or palliative care depended on the values and beliefs of the patient and the attending physicians. In reality, it was also very much affected by medicine's professional and institutional structures, which were themselves influenced by national cultures. The U.S. approach to therapy probably reflects a can-do heritage left over from pioneering days, whereas the British doctors' paternalism and less interventionist approach probably reflect the values of a traditional, class-conscious society. America's industrial organization of research and treatment and the competition of doctors and institutions for patients again point toward larger cultural and social influences. In Britain the weaker hold of individualism and the acceptance of central control, as expressed in the National Health Service, is perhaps reflected in the comparatively small growth of medical oncology.

In the late 1990s a Canadian expert could still lament the inadequate degree of collaboration between oncologists and palliative care physicians in that country. Where interdisciplinarity was integral to palliative care, the concept of the patient care team had yet to become universal in oncology, despite the fact that interdisciplinarity had become more common as treatments increased in complexity. Some palliative care doctors still underestimated the value of chemotherapy and radiotherapy in symptom relief, while many oncologists failed to point out how often their activities were palliative. However, there had recently been progress partly because of the recommendations of the Expert Panel on Palliative Care to the Cancer 2000 Task Force. Symptom control clinics now often worked with cancer centers.

The departments of oncology at McGill University and the University of Alberta included divisions of palliative medicine. Calgary's Tom Baker Cancer Center had a pain management program and a community palliative care service, and similar cooperative arrangements were being developed at cancer centers in British Columbia, Winnipeg, Ottawa, and Halifax (Löwy, 1995, 209, 224–25).

By the mid-1970s medical oncology was flourishing in North America as a subspecialty of internal medicine, having shown the effectiveness of multidrug, cytotoxic therapy against leukemia, lymphomas, and Hodgkin's disease, either alone or in combination with surgery and radiotherapy. In Australia, however, while many physicians and hematologists employed chemotherapy, full-time medical oncologists were few. There was a movement toward regional or statewide centers because of the high capital cost of radiation equipment and the continuing dearth of trained radiotherapists. Social workers were now seen as essential staff at such centers to give emotional support to patients and facilitate patient-doctor communication. The only comprehensive cancer center in the country was Melbourne's Cancer Institute, which ran the Peter MacCallum Hospital and Clinics. The clinics were located in provincial cities throughout Victoria and in Launceston and Hobart in Tasmania. The hospital was a teaching institution for Melbourne and Monash universities and an Australia-wide trainer of radiotherapists. It was accredited for postgraduate training in pathology, diagnostic radiology, hematology, gynecology, and reparative surgery. Moreover, it instructed postgraduate students in science, medical technologists, diagnostic radiographers, nucleographers, and oncology nurses (*Medical Journal of Australia,* 1974, 513–14; Ilbery, 1978, 574–75).

Reviewing cancer management in the 1980s, Martin Tattersall, professor of cancer medicine at the University of Sydney, pointed out that many Australian hospitals had multidisciplinary cancer clinics. New diagnostic and therapeutic developments were changing the management of cancer. Noninvasive staging techniques such as ultrasound and CT scanning allowed greater accuracy in diagnosing tumor spread and size. These techniques had decreased the need to resort to radical surgery because, if the cancer had progressed beyond local therapy, such surgery was not justifiable, although surgery generally remained the keystone of cancer treatment.

While about 70 percent of patients were treated when the cancer appeared to be local, about half were still not cured by local therapy, mostly because microscopic metastases had not been identified. Adjuvant chemotherapy immediately after local treatment had extended disease-free survival time in children with various solid tumors. Clinical studies were in progress on various cancers in adults. The best timing and best duration of adjuvant chemotherapy were still undetermined. However, adjuvant hormonal treatment of localized tumors was justifiable only with hormonally sensitive primary tumors such as breast, prostate, and endometrial cancers. Most hormonal treatments, of course, had the advantage of being less toxic for normal tissue than cytotoxic therapy. With advanced cancer, chemotherapy remained palliative, and a balance had to be struck between toxicity on the one hand and greater survival and symptom relief on the other. The multidisciplinary cancer clinics were ideal for doing clinical trials, which had not been well organized in the past. A new national clinical trials data center would greatly assist in the future conduct of clinical experiments.

The growth of health care costs in recent times had evoked greater emphasis on prevention. Oncology centers could play an important role in community preventive education, as well as the ongoing professional education of physicians and surgeons doing oncology in other hospitals. Although general practitioners now treated few cancer patients, their role as advisors to patients and family concerning therapy options, their involvement in the process of chemotherapy, and their knowledge of the patient's domestic situation when terminal care had to be arranged were a vital part of modern cancer management.

At the end of the 1990s, Tattersall and colleagues investigated the extent to which Australian patients with incurable cancer were informed of their treatment options and prognosis by their oncologists, using a sample of patients from two Sydney teaching hospitals. They noted that Australia, like the United States, Canada, and the United Kingdom, had developed guidelines for disclosure of information, and patients in Australia shared similar information and involvement preferences. They found that Australian patients were well informed except about alternatives to treatment and prognosis: 85 percent, about the treatment objective; 75 percent, about the fact that their disease was incurable; and 58 percent, about life expectancy. However, only 44 percent were told of an alternative such as supportive or palliative care; 36 percent, how treatment would impact their quality of life; and 30 percent, of a choice in management (Tattersall, 1981a, 10–15, 41; Tattersall, Gattellari, Voigt, and Butow, 2002, 314–21). Cooperation between practitioners of oncology and palliative care was improving. Thus, the Ashford Cancer Center in Adelaide had set up a joint service with the hospice at the Repatriation Hospital to enable the palliative care team to work with treatment professionals well before the patient reached the terminal stage. The clinical manager at Ashford observed that, historically, oncology and palliative care had been seen as being at opposing ends of the health care continuum. In the past, only when there were no more therapy options were patients referred to palliative care (*Australian Nursing Journal*, 1997, 26).

MEDICAL EDUCATION ABOUT CANCER

In the 1970s and 1980s, surveys in North America, Europe, and Australia revealed the need to improve cancer education in medical schools. The American Association for Cancer Education had surveyed programs between 1975 and 1980, and, as a result, cancer educators had developed a list of educational objectives in basic science and pathology. A second survey was carried out in 1992 and showed among other things that more curriculum time was needed for oncology.

In 1988 the European Economic Community (EEC) and the European Organization for Research in Treatment of Cancer (EORTC) conducted a workshop that had been approved by the deans of medical schools in 17 European countries. The participants made 10 proposals, one of which was that pain control and care of the terminally ill should be part of every oncology course. In the late 1970s London's Middlesex Hospital Medical School was already including seminar topics such as care of the dying for second-year oncology students. In 1976 the school's long-established chair of radiotherapy had been changed into an academic department of oncology.

In 1986 an Australian survey of various medical schools found considerable differences in the courses they offered and between what staff members thought should be taught and what students actually experienced. In 1989 the Australian Cancer Society (ACS) produced guidelines for a model cancer curriculum that was similar in content to the program proposed by the workshop organized jointly by the EEC and the EORTC. Few schools had cancer medicine or oncology departments, and none fully followed the ACS guidelines for a program of study in oncology, whereas most EEC countries required a full-time course of 10–14 days. Moreover, a survey of graduates who were beginning their internships at 13 hospitals revealed that they lacked important knowledge: slightly more than 29 percent rated their instruction in palliative care of cancer patients as poor or very poor; just over 8 percent rated their instruction in cancer prevention as poor or very poor; and 14.5 percent rated their instruction in the treatment of cancer as poor or very poor. Included among the objectives of the ACS model compulsory course in oncology was possession of skills and knowledge sufficient to enable students to participate in palliative care and the management of dying patients (Berry and Johnson, 1979, 398–400; Tattersall and Langlands, 1993, 224–25; Wright and Tattersall, 1994, 104–5; Robinson, 1994, 2–5).

MODERN TREATMENTS

Most advances in chemotherapy were based on the information provided by studies of acute leukemia, mainly in childhood. Table 3.6 shows the great improvement by the mid-1970s in the prognosis for acute lymphocytic leukemia in children.

By 2000, cure was possible for many children with acute lymphoblastic leukemia. Contemporary treatment offers a 75 percent, event-free survival for these children

Table 3.6. Improvement in the Prognosis for Acute Lymphocytic Leukemia in Children

Period	Drugs Available	Complete Remission Rate (%)	Median Survival Time (Months)	5-Year Survival Rate (%)	10-Year Survival Rate (%)
To 1948	0	5*	1–2	0	0
To 1959	1	25*	5	0	0
To 1960	3	45*	12	0	0
To 1965	5	80	19	3**	0
To 1970	9	90	28	15**	1**
To 1975	11+	95	36	30+**	2**

* Estimated because bone marrow assessment was not routinely done.

** Calculated from patients starting 5 or 10 years before the year named (e.g., the 10-year rate to 1975 was 2% of patients starting treatment in or before 1965).

Source: Colebatch, 1978, 268.

(Smith, 2000, 568–69). In 1985 a study of pediatric patients treated at the Department of Hematology and Oncology at the Prince of Wales Children's Hospital in Randwick between 1964 and 1987 for a range of cancers—363 with acute lymphoblastic leukemia, 126 with tumors of the central nervous system, 86 with acute nonlymphoblastic leukemia, 81 with lymphoma, 79 with neural crest tumors, 69 with renal tumors, 66 with bone sarcomas, 53 with soft tissue sarcomas, and 77 with other diagnoses—revealed an actual survival rate of 79 percent at five years. Survival from Hodgkin's disease and Wilms' tumor was high during that period, while significant improvement in survival occurred for acute lymphoblastic leukemia, nonHodgkin's lymphoma, and osteogenic sarcoma. However, chances for survival in patients with neuroblastoma and acute nonlymphoblastic leukemia continued to be poor.

Since conventional chemotherapy was often almost as toxic to normal tissue as to cancer, natural anticancer substances were of great interest. Two that turned out to be disappointing were the bacillus Calmette-Guérin (BCG) vaccine against tuberculosis and interferons (antivirus substances naturally produced in the body). Another substance naturally produced in the human body was tumor necrosis factor. Discovered in 1975 at Memorial Sloan-Kettering Cancer Center in the United States, it was then produced by gene-splicing techniques in quantities sufficient for treatment purposes. Although used since the late 1940s, the mode of action of corticosteroid agents began to be understood in detail only in the 1970s. By the late 1980s, these agents were recognized as having a major part to play in treatment, although long-term use was contraindicated because of serious side effects. Corticosteroid agents were seen as specifics for malignant lymphoproliferative conditions and breast cancer. They were considered to be very useful in controlling the effects of common complications—hypercalcemia, increased intracranial pressure, and pulmonary lymphangitic carcinomatosis (Schmeck, 1985, 450–51; Lowenthal and Jestrimski, 1986, 81–84; McCowage, Vowels, Brown, O'Gorman-Hughes, White, and Marshall, 1993, 453–56).

Responsible for almost 18 percent of cancer mortality worldwide, lung cancer has until recently evoked an attitude of therapeutic nihilism. With small-cell and advanced non-small-cell cancer, chemotherapy is viewed as helpful, although most patients succumb to the disease. There is now much interest in agents that are capable of suppressing tumor angiogenesis (thus reducing the blood supply to tumors) and drugs influencing the cancer cell's microenvironment. Improved surgical and radiographical techniques, as well as improved selection of patients for resection or radiotherapy, promise better treatment outcomes, while improved screening means that more cases will be identified early (Hoffmann, Mauer, and Vokes, 2000, 479–84).

NATIONAL CANCER CONTROL POLICY AND PALLIATIVE CARE

In the 1990s the evolution of a national cancer control policy in each of our Anglo-Saxon countries was based on the recognition that the growth of epidemiological and medical knowledge in the previous two decades or so offered great possibilities for controlling cancer, even in the absence of a capacity to cure all cases. Above all, epidemiology's demonstration since the 1950s that the smoking of tobacco correlates with increased incidence of lung cancer and that large-scale cessation of smoking reduces the incidence convinced health authorities that preventive interventions could be combined with treatment and other remedies in coherent control programs. This represented a significant departure from the obsession with the total defeat of cancer, which the research and treatment "war" on cancer that was conducted for much of the twentieth century implied. Integral to the more measured approach of containment was the provision of palliative care for those dying of cancer.

In 1995 a publication of the World Health Organization (WHO) on national cancer control pointed out that control did not mean eradication in the way that immunization, properly done, can "eradicate" an infectious disease. Instead, effective control meant that at least one-third of cancers were preventable; a further third, diagnosed early enough, were potentially curable; and the remaining one-third of patients, through appropriate palliative care and pain control, could enjoy a substantially improved quality of life even in the face of imminent death (WHO, 1995, xiii–xviii, 1–4; Pinell, 2000, 685).

Australia

In 1987 Robert MacLennan of the Queensland Institute of Medical Research prepared a major report for the Australian Cancer Society (ACS) on a national prevention and research policy. He pointed out that in the previous two decades the government had barely considered such a policy. The impetus for a national policy was now coming from the states, especially Victoria and Queensland, and in light of the federal government's commitment to health improvement following the Better Health Commission's report, cancer control had to be integrated with other areas of disease prevention and health promotion.

In 1991 the Commonwealth Department of Health, Housing, and Community Services decided to revise the national health goals. From a range of objectives, the state and federal health ministers collectively chose four priority areas—cancer, cardiovascular disease, mental health, and injury. Implementation groups were created for each area, and they were to develop targets and strategies covering the continuum of care. The Australian Cancer Society's Public Affairs and Behavioral Interventions Committee (PABIC) was charged with preparing a background brief for the cancer implementation group. It was to provide information on, first, health promotion strategies; screening activities; clinical diagnosis and treatment; best practice; rehabilitation; and palliative care; and second, key stakeholders and leading agencies; epidemiology and demography; and available data, including incidence and prevalence data for cancer and associated risk factors (Australian Cancer Society and Hall, 1995, 1). The PABIC developed the National Cancer Prevention Policy (NCPP) that the federal health minister, Brian Howe, inaugurated in December 1992. Some experts hailed the measure as the dawn of a new approach to cancer prevention because it called for the explicit setting of goals, appreciation of the social determinants of health, and integration of prevention into the delivery of health care (Ward and Henry, 1993, 502).

The ACS, established in 1961 to foster national and international coordination of all activities concerning cancer in Australia, redefined its aim three decades later to be leadership in the development and promotion of national cancer control policy. In 1995 the ACS and the Clinical Oncological Society of Australia brought into being the Australian Cancer Network. This was to encourage collaboration among professional organizations ranging from basic research to clinical care to public health, and it included representatives of governments and consumers. To complete the circle of collaboration among all of the stakeholders, the ACS in early 1997 negotiated an agreement with the Commonwealth Department of Health and Human Services to establish the National Cancer Control Initiative (NCCI) to help create a nationally coordinated cancer control plan. The ACS also worked with the NHMRC to identify strategic directions in the funding of cancer research.

The NCCI was commissioned to identify priorities in improving cancer control, and the years from 1997 to 2002 were designated as the period of concern. After extensive consultation with stakeholders across the country, the NCCI management committee identified priority actions in light of demonstrated and perceived benefits, time frame, immediate cost, and potential to allow the formation of strategic partnerships for their implementation. The whole priority-setting process resulted in the identification of 21 actions, from which those deemed to have top priority were chosen (Table 3.7) (Coates, 1998, 8–9; Sanson-Fisher, Campbell, Ireland, and Lovell, 1999, 7–9).

The NCCI proposed that future development of cancer control should arise from an examination of existing activities, especially from identifying gaps in provision such as those in palliative care. Clinical outcomes in Australia in terms of five-year survival rates compare favorably with those of other economically advanced countries—female survival is the best in the world, and male is second only to that in the United States. However, healthcare professionals and consumer groups believe that both survival and patients' quality of life can nevertheless be improved.

New Zealand

In New Zealand, similar developments were taking place in the late 1990s. These were spurred on by the awareness that, since 1960, the New Zealand cancer mortality rate had been growing faster than that in Australia, Canada, the United States, or the United Kingdom. In 1999 a widely representative Workshop on Cancer Control unanimously proposed the development of a national cancer control strategy.

With funds provided by the Cancer Society of New Zealand and the Child Cancer Foundation, the New Zealand Cancer Control Trust came into being in 2000 in order to speak for the nongovernment sector in the process of devising the control strategy. A discussion document, *Toward a Cancer Control Strategy for New Zealand Marihi Tauporo,* was made publicly available in 2002. Its publication fol-

Table 3.7. Actions Proposed by the Priority-Setting Process

Primary Prevention	
1. ★Tobacco	Preventing tobacco-related cancers
2. Skin cancer	Reducing risk
Population-Based Screening and Early Detection	
3. Breast cancer	Improving BreastScreen Australia
4. Breast cancer	Promoting prompt diagnosis
5. Cervical cancer	Improving Pap smear programs
6. Cervical cancer	Handling Pap smear results
7. ★Colorectal cancer	Developing fecal occult blood testing
8. ★Prostate cancer	Rationalizing prostate-specific antigen testing
9. Skin cancer	Improving diagnostic skills
Treatment	
10. ★Guidelines	National approach
11. ★Multidisciplinary care	Evaluation and facilitation
12. ★Palliative care	Filling gaps
13. ★Prostate cancer	Dealing with treatment uncertainties
14. ★Psychosocial care	Defining, implementing, and monitoring
General	
15. ★General practice	Promoting participation in cancer control
16. Equity	Implementing culturally relevant cancer control measures
17. Consumers	Facilitating involvement
18. ★Research	Continuing the national commitment
19. ★Familial cancers	Organizing education and resources
20. ★Data collection	Meeting urgent national needs
Clinical trials	Encouraging participation of doctors and patients

★ Recommended for priority implementation.

Source: Sanson-Fisher, Campbell, Ireland, and Lovell, 1999, 9.

lowed a lengthy process of consultation with people involved in developing control strategies in Australia, England, Canada, and Norway, as well as New Zealand stakeholders (New Zealand Ministry of Health, 2002, v, 3; Elwood, McAvoy, and Gavin, 2003, 1–3).

The New Zealand Cancer Control Strategy was made public in August 2003. Listed as one of its goals was the improvement of the quality of life of cancer sufferers and their families through support, respite, and palliative care. Additional goals were to reduce cancer incidence through primary prevention; to ensure effective screening and early detection to reduce incidence and mortality; to ensure effective diagnosis and treatment to reduce morbidity and mortality; to improve service delivery across the continuum of cancer control; and to advance the effectiveness of control through research and surveillance.

Among the first priorities of the New Zealand Palliative Care Strategy of 2001 was ensuring the availability of palliative care to all dying people; and the operation of at least one palliative care service in each district health board area. The Expert Working Group on Palliative Care of 2003 identified the following as barriers to appropriate care for everyone: the lack of a palliative care approach by some cancer service providers; uneven distribution of palliative care services throughout New Zealand; difficulties of access, especially for Maori and Pacific Island peoples; and a lack of services designed for children and adolescents (Frizelle, 2003, 1–2; New Zealand Cancer Control Strategy, 2003, 16, 31–32).

Canada

In 1999 a consortium composed of the Canadian Cancer Society, the National Cancer Institute of Canada, the Canadian Association of Provincial Cancer Agencies, and Health Canada (the federal health department) launched the Canadian Strategy for Cancer Control. The objectives of the strategy were to lower the risk of developing cancer and of dying of cancer and to improve cancer care (including screening, treatment, and the patient's quality of life and access to services).

The strategy employed six working groups staffed by experts to draw up priorities. One such group was the Palliative Care Working Group, which presented its final report at the beginning of 2002. The report observed that the focus in cancer care had moved from tertiary care centers back into the community, so that the patient's family now carried more of the burden of care. Indeed, a study of trends in the care of cancer patients dying in Nova Scotia between 1992 and 1997 found that the proportion of those dying outside the hospital had increased from 19.8 percent in 1992 to 30.2 percent in 1997, although a large majority continued to die in hospitals. The working group maintained that palliative care should be part of anticancer treatment throughout the course of the illness and not be seen as simply end-of-life care. It proposed seeking to achieve the following outcomes: better integration of palliative care delivery within cancer and other health care delivery systems; affirmation of palliative care as a basic part of cancer control; improved control of pain and other symptoms though better education of health professionals; and greater capacity to carry out palliative care research (Canadian Strategy for Cancer Control Palliative Care Working Group, 2002, 3–4; Burge, Lawson, and Johnston, 2003, 2; Comeau, 2004, 2–3).

Indeed, in mid-2000 a Canadian senate subcommittee reported on end-of-life care and made 14 recommendations to improve such care. In a November 2001 submission to the Commission on the Future of Health Care in Canada, the Canadian Hospice Palliative Care Association strongly endorsed the following of those recommendations: assessment by the federal government of home care and pharmacare for the dying; provision of funding by the federal and provincial governments; implementation of income security and job protection for family members caring for the dying; investigation into ways to improve the training of health professionals involved in end-of-life care; joint discussion of funding of end-of-life initiatives by federal and provincial health officials; establishment of an institute for end-of-life issues by the Canadian Institutes of Health Research; and the development of indicators of high-quality end-of-life care by the Canadian Institute for Health Information. The association also pointed out that as few as 5 percent of Canadians had access to hospice palliative care, and most of this care was directed toward people with cancer (Canadian Hospice Palliative Care Association, 2001, 4–5).

By 2004, Canadian experts were complaining about a lack of government leadership concerning cancer control strategy. The chief executive officer of the Cancer Society, Barbara Wylie, said that support was needed across government agencies and not just from Health Canada. The need for a coordinated approach was urgent since it was expected that, by 2010, cancer would replace heart disease as the leading cause of death in Canada. The financial cost could be expected to be huge; even in 1998 the direct cost of treatment, care, and rehabilitation was $2.5 billion, while the indirect costs (mainly lost productivity) amounted to $11.8 billion. Noting that Sen. Sharon Carstairs, a liberal, was the only federal figure to strongly support the cancer control strategy, Dr. Andrew Padmos, the commissioner of Cancer Care Nova Scotia, stated that all those involved in advancing the plan were disappointed with the federal government's poor level of engagement (Comeau, 2004, 2–3).

The United States

In the mid-1990s, much public attention in the United States was given to developing palliative care. In 1997 the prestigious Institute of Medicine of the National Academies of Science issued a report, *Approaching Death,* that identified four broad deficiencies in the care of people with incurable conditions: too many suffered from the failure of caregivers to offer effective palliative and supportive care; from caregivers who pursued aggressive treatments known to be ineffectual and even harmful to the dying patient; from regulations and other issues that frustrated the administration of adequate pain control; from fragmented organizations that complicated the coordination of care; from Medicare hospice benefits requirements that could not be reconciled with the progression of many terminal illnesses that lack the steady progression of incurable cancer; from fee structures that induced overuse of procedural services but underuse of patient management and supportive services; from deficiencies in the education of health professionals that meant they did not know how to adequately care for dying patients; and, finally, from insufficient research (biomedical, clinical, epidemiological, and health services) into end-of-life care. The committee agreed that it would not comment on the morality or legality of physician-assisted suicide, but it did believe that concern with this matter should not prevent health care reforms aimed at improving end-of-life care (Field and Cassel, 1997, 5–6, 13).

In 2001 the Institute of Medicine produced a second report, *Improving Palliative Care for Cancer.* This report was concerned with the management of cancer symptoms and appropriate referral of the patient to palliative and hospice care. The document was sponsored by the National Cancer Institute, the Centers for Disease Control and Prevention, and the American Cancer Society.

Kathleen Foley (of the Death in America Project of the Open Society Institute and the Memorial Sloan-Kettering Cancer Center in New York City), coauthor of the report, pointed out that 3 percent of the population had been living with cancer but that the pursuit of cure had taken attention away from the need for palliative care The report pointed out that the National Cancer Institute, the federal funder of cancer research and training, spent only $26 million of an annual budget of $2.9 billion on research and training for palliative and end-of-life care in 1999. It proposed that any facility seeking to be recognized by the NCI as a comprehensive cancer center should be required to do research on palliative care and symptom control.

Further, the report stated that the NCI should identify appropriate facilities as centers of excellence in palliative care. One basic problem was that active treatment and palliative or hospice care remained unintegrated. Another obstacle was the Medicare hospice benefit, which, in its failure to cover life-extending treatment and its requirement that patients be at a stage where they could expect to live for no longer than six months, deterred many patients from seeking hospice care. Endorsing the report, Joanne Lynn, president of Americans for Better Care of the Dying, stated that, until recently, in the national war on cancer, all efforts had been devoted to treatment, prevention, and survivorship. However, the new recommendations offered hope that all of those who were suffering from a fatal disease would benefit from better pain and symptom management (*Improving Symptom Control and End-of-Life Care for Cancer Patients Requires Stronger Federal Leadership*, 2001, 1–2).

There was some response to the report's calls for better professional education. The American Medical Association, assisted by the Robert Wood Johnson Foundation, developed a curriculum called Education for Physicians in End-of-Life Care. A similar program became available to nurses, and nurse educators have begun training a corps of specialist nurses. The Joint Commission on the Accreditation of Healthcare Organizations, in cooperation with 17 medical subspecialty societies, has worked to include palliative care courses and guidelines within the range of expertise of the various subspecialties. The Veterans Administration, which provides care for the military (and under the auspices of which 14 percent of deaths occur), has a curriculum for physicians in residency and offers a fellowship program as part of its training program. Medical schools have been introducing pain management courses and palliative care rotations. The Project on Death in America has provided funds for just under 90 faculty scholars who act as leaders in their home centers in the development of palliative care in medicine and nursing. Similarly, it has funded more than 42 social workers to do the same thing in their discipline. Indeed, the American Board of Hospice and Palliative Medicine has certified more than 900 physicians, while the Hospice and Palliative Care Nurses Association has certified more than 10,000 nurses.

The Robert Wood Johnson Foundation has funded community-state partnerships. As a result, more than 30 states have created programs for community discussions of end-of-life care. Both the Johnson Foundation and the Project on Death in America have assisted in the development of national guidelines for the care of dying prisoners in jails and of initiatives to rectify inequities concerning care for African Americans (*Improving Symptom Control and End-of-Life Care for Cancer Patients Requires Stronger Federal Leadership*, 2001, 1–2; Foley, 2003, 89–91).

The United Kingdom

The 1990s were a period of strong policy development on cancer control in Britain. A white paper titled *The Health of the Nation,* published in 1992, identified five key areas of action for health improvement. Through prevention and screening, the potential for reducing cancer mortality was considerable, the white paper stated. However, for almost two decades, professional groups and health authorities had been calling for improvement in cancer services: *Cancer Care and Treatment Services* (Royal College of Radiologists and Royal College of Physicians); *Review of the Pattern of Cancer Services in England and Wales* (Association of Cancer Physicians); *Protocol for Investment in Health Gain* (Welsh Office); *Management of Nonsurgical Cancer Services in Scotland* (Scottish Office); and *Report of an Independent Review of Specialist Services (Cancer) in London*.

Concerns about how outcomes of treatment for cancer varied geographically prompted the chief medical officer of England, Kenneth Calman, and the chief medical officer of the Welsh Office, Deirdre Hine, to establish an Expert Advisory Group on Cancer (EAGC). The EAGC produced a report on cancer services in 1995 that recommended significant changes in organization and provision of services: a new structure based on a network of expertise extending from primary care teams through cancer units in district general hospitals to cancer centers providing specialist diagnostic and therapeutic techniques including radiotherapy; and justification on scientific or logistical grounds of any units or centers employing different treatment methods. Among other recommendations were several that addressed palliative care: in order that patients (and their families) may have the best possible quality of life, palliative care should be integrated with cancer treatment at an early stage and no longer be seen simply as terminal care; the palliative care team should include specialist medical and nursing staff, social workers, physiotherapists, and occupational therapists, and it should work closely with other specialists such as dieticians; spiritual care should be available when wanted; historically, the evaluation of services had been couched in terms of survival, but another important outcome was the patient's quality of life (Expert Advisory Group on Cancer, 1995, 2–7, 18–30; Mathew, Cowley, Bliss, and Thistlewood, 2003, 273; Lewis, 2003b, 199).

The Calman-Hine report and the subsequent NHS executive clinical outcomes guidelines, while primarily concerned with cancer, also reviewed palliative care research. Developed in consultation with clinicians, NHS managers, patients' groups, cancer charities, and researchers, the NHS cancer plan was launched in September 2000 with four stated aims: to save more lives; improve quality of life by ensuring professional support and care, as well as therapy; reduce inequalities; and improve education, training, and research to accommodate an expanding workforce. It was the first comprehensive national program in England and Wales and covered prevention, screening, diagnosis, treatment, research, and palliative and supportive care. The plan identified district nurses as the key to provision of palliative care in the home, and £2 million was to be allocated for educational initiatives for these professionals. While palliative care thus continued to be connected with cancer services, it was clear that education of community nurses would also help improve the quality of care for those with incurable conditions other than cancer (Richards, 2000, 1; Mathew et al., 2003, 273, 279).

The increase in funding for cancer services that resulted from the plan was the largest ever. In the first year, an additional £280 million was spent, while between 2003 and 2004, £570 million more a year was to be spent than in 2000–2001 (when the plan was released). By mid-2001, the waiting times for treatment were being cut. Consequently, 92 percent of those with suspected cancer were seeing a specialist within two weeks of referral by their general practitioners. Clinicians and managers were being furnished with evidence-based guidance on good practice and treatment benefits, including the need for teams of multidisciplinary specialists. The plan called for almost 1,000 more cancer consultants by 2006 and for staff members who were trained in skills usually applied by other specialists in fields such as endoscopy, therapeutic radiography, breast screening, and histopathology.

Cancer patients themselves were being invited to contribute to the cancer networks through patient partnership groups (involving patients and caregivers in decisions about treatment services). In response to the overwhelming desire of people with advanced cancer to remain at home, various initiatives were introduced: one in four district nurses was being trained to support people who wished to stay at home as long as possible; £45 million was made available to improve access to adult palliative care, especially for disadvantaged groups; eight palliative care beacon partnership projects were set up to spread good practice throughout the NHS and voluntary sectors; funds were provided for the National Council for Hospices and Specialist Palliative Care to assist cancer networks in working with voluntary hospices to assess local needs for palliative care and to develop plans to meet such needs; and an evidence-based review of supportive and palliative care services was commissioned. Initiatives were also started in research: a new National Cancer Research Network was established that would greatly increase the number of patients in research trials for new treatments; and a National Cancer Research Institute was set up to bring together funders of research from the government, private sectors, and industry to develop a strategic approach to supporting new cancer research (Department of Health, 2001, 1–10).

OBSERVATIONS

In Britain in the 1890s, the cancer hospitals, recognizing the special needs of dying patients, had planned to set up hospices for the dying. However, the plans for these Friedenheims were not implemented, and the funds were put instead into research in the hope that a cure (which was expected soon) would make such institutions redundant. For many more decades, the overwhelming priorities were research and new modes of treatment. Specialist care of the dying disappeared from cancer control objectives. Then, in the 1960s, the hospice movement independently resurrected care of the dying as a primary clinical responsibility in the face of a medical establishment so intent on curing that it had seemingly lost the capacity to deal humanely with death and dying (Murphy, 1989, 221–22).

By the 1990s, so successful had the palliative care movement become that national cancer control policy in each of these Anglo-Saxon countries included proper care of the dying as an integral part of treatment for cancer.

4 Development of Palliative Care Services

The Development of Modern Palliative Care

Those who ran institutions established specifically for the care of the dying in the late nineteenth century focused their efforts on the salvation of souls. Indeed, the early hospices had three primary types of concerns—religious, philanthropic, and moral. Unlike the modern hospice, they were not centers of sophisticated medical care.

Between the 1970s and the 1990s, palliative care services grew considerably in Britain, North America, and Australasia. In Britain, the number of hospices increased to about 700, and in the United States to 1,500. In contrast with Britain, hospice in the United States became a concept (rather than a place) of care, with care being provided in the patient's home wherever possible. The term "palliative care" became in many ways a synonym for hospice. In the same period, national and international bodies (such as the European Association for Palliative Care [EAPC]) were established, and several journals came into being, textbooks on palliative medicine were published, and chairs in palliative medicine were set up in universities.

"Palliative" is derived from the Latin for cloak or mantle, "pallium." Metaphorically, palliative care may be seen as a cloak of warmth and protection for the terminally ill. Robert Twycross, a British pioneer of hospice, has used the term in another way: the symptoms are "cloaked" with treatments whose only aim is to make the patient comfortable. Indeed, as early as the sixteenth century doctors used the term "palliation" to describe alleviation or mitigation of suffering. The first modern, "official" definition of palliative medicine was offered in 1987, when the practice was recognized in Britain as a specialty; palliative medicine is the study and management of patients with far-advanced disease for whom quality of life is the focus of care. Later, the definition was widened to include the notion of life-threatening disease. In 1989 the EAPC said that palliative care is active total care when disease is not responsive to curative treatment; it neither hastens nor postpones death; it provides relief from pain and other distressing symptoms; it integrates the psychological and spiritual aspects of care and helps the family cope during the patient's illness and in bereavement.

In 1990 the World Health Organization (WHO) stated that palliative care includes the active total care of patients whose disease is not responsive to curative treatment; that control of pain and other symptoms and of psychological, social, and spiritual problems is paramount; that the goal is promotion of the best possible quality of life for patients and families, and that aspects of palliative care are applicable earlier in the illness in conjunction with anticancer treatment. In 1997 Twycross proposed that palliative care be seen as active total care by a multiprofessional team at the point when the patient's disease is not responsive to curative treatment and life expectancy is short; it provides for physical, psychological, social, and spiritual needs and, if necessary, for support in bereavement. The WHO definition (more than EAPC's) emphasizes the matter of the patient's quality of life, and in 1997 Twycross expanded on his 1987 definition by introducing the idea of the multiprofessional team, life expectancy, and bereavement support.

Historically, palliative care evolved from hospice care, but it may differ in the following ways: provision of care concerning the comfort of patients and families at all stages of the illness; strong and continuing involvement of physicians; willingness to use tertiary interventions such as primary anticancer treatments and invasive therapies for symptom control where appropriate; and acceptance of research on the improvement of quality of care. It may be used for any life-threatening condition during and after the period of aggressive primary therapy; when applied at a nonterminal stage, it may be any mixture of symptom control, function-oriented therapies, and psychosocial support; in the terminal stage, it will usually follow hospice principles.

Palliative care may be provided in homes or inpatient and outpatient settings and by day care and consultation services. In Britain and the United States, home services are primarily the responsibility of general practitioners, family physicians, and community nurses who coordinate the care, which may also be provided by social workers, physiotherapists, psychologists, chaplains, and volunteers. In Britain, Marie Curie Cancer nurses and Macmillan nurses provide palliative care as well. If a medical problem cannot be solved by the primary care team, the patient is referred to hospital specialists. Home teams advise the primary care teams.

In the United States most palliative care programs provide home care. These community-based programs are composed of independent units or office-based services that do the coordinating; "back-up" beds are negotiated with hospitals or nursing homes. The heart of the team is the family physician and community nurse. Nurses may coordinate services with a hospice doctor and provide advice on pain and other symptom management.

Inpatient services are offered in hospices, which may be independent within a hospital or nursing home, or be an independent unit. In Britain about 20 percent of hospices are conducted by the National Health Service; the rest are funded in part or completely by charitable funds. In the United States hospice is provided mainly in the home, although some teaching and other hospitals have set up hospices. Because independent hospices proliferated so early in Britain, only a limited number of hospital-based palliative care units have developed; in 1998, there were 240 in university and district hospitals, with Saint Thomas's Hospital in London being the first to establish one (1976). The first hospital-based team in the United States was set up at Saint Luke's Hospital in New York in 1975. There a nursing home may contract with a hospice program for the latter to provide services; some nursing homes have special units for care of the dying, but most permit dying people to remain in their own room (Abu-Saad, Huijer, and Courtens, 1999, 9–17).

In the first five to six decades of the twentieth century, the capacity of medicine to cure some types of chronic disease or prolong survival in others advanced considerably. Not only did the capacity to treat disease increase markedly, but more areas of everyday life also became the province of medicine, from pregnancy and childbirth, through aging, to dying. The people of modern urban-industrial societies learned to look to an ever-more confident and technological medicine to solve their life problems. If medicalization of life increased, then so did medicalization and institutionalization of death. Thus, by 1990, 24 percent of all deaths in Britain still took place at home, but 72 percent now occurred in hospitals, hospices, or other institutions.

This marked institutionalization and medicalization of death in the later twentieth century is related to important social, epidemiological, and demographic changes. In the United Kingdom (as in the other Anglo-Saxon countries), life expectancy at birth had greatly increased, climbing in 1991 to just over 73 years for men and just over 78 years for women. The principal causes of mortality were now chronic diseases of the circulatory and respiratory systems and cancers. A very large percentage of the terminally ill were people aged 75 years and over. Similarly, there were changes in family and household organization. With families now much smaller, many women in the paid workforce (and the fragmentation of families resulting from high divorce rates), there were simply fewer unpaid caregivers to look after the chronically and terminally ill (Field, 1994, 58–59).

Britain

The principles of hospice care developed by Cicely Saunders at Saint Christopher's Hospice in London in 1967 were quickly taken up by pioneers in other countries, and it was realized that they could be applied not only in freestanding hospices but also in home care, day care settings, and indeed in hospital units. Suggested in 1974 by Canadian oncologist Balfour Mount, "palliative care" became the term that identified the set of principles and practices used in relation to this new style of caring for the dying (Clark, 2002, 905–6).

When, in 1948, the National Health Service (NHS) was set up in Britain, it provided free health care for all as a matter of citizenship; it was intended to replace the dependence of the poor on charity. However, in a long-term perspective, for the public hospitals it represented their final era of growth, which had begun in the mid-eighteenth century. By the end of the 1930s, these accounted for more than 50 percent of acute services. The hospitals dominated the first decades of the existence of the NHS, and clinical goals remained cure and rehabilitation. Aneurin Bevan himself said, when piloting the NHS legislation through the House of

Commons, that he would rather be kept alive in the efficient if cold environment of a large hospital than die in the warm and caring embrace of a small one. Terminal care was of little interest, although the situation began to change in the 1950s, when two major surveys of services for the dying were made.

In 1951 a national survey of cancer patients living at home (7,050 cases in England, Wales, Scotland, and Northern Ireland) was carried out by a joint committee of the Marie Curie Memorial and the Queen's Institute of District Nursing. The committee was chaired by surgeon Ronald Raven. The survey revealed that failure to seek treatment was common, as was psychological suffering. Poor living conditions and ignorance of aid available through the NHS and the National Assistance Board were not uncommon. The committee proposed the provision of more residential homes, night nurses, and domestic aides. Soon afterward, Marie Curie homes for dying cancer sufferers began to be created, and in 1958 Marie Curie night nurses became available.

The second survey, carried out by former army doctor H. L. Glyn Hughes for the Calouste Gulbenkian Foundation in 1957 and 1958, focused on the terminally ill. The report was more concerned with policy and services than the earlier inquiry had been. Hughes pointed out that, since the advent of the NHS, aged care had received more attention. However, the 1954 Phillips Committee report and the 1957 Boucher report had not dealt with terminal care.

In 1957 the Ministry of Health identified the division of responsibility between local authorities and hospitals: the first were to care for the aged in welfare homes; the second, for the chronic needing prolonged nursing. Since hospitals were not required to admit all terminal cases, a serious gap in provision existed. Where would these people go?

Hughes obtained information from medical officers of health, senior administrative medical officers responsible to regional hospital boards, many voluntary bodies, religious orders, philanthropic organizations, 150 local councils of the National Council of Social Services, and more than 600 family doctors. In 1956, 40 percent of deaths took place in NHS hospitals, and of the rest, more than 82 percent took place at home; 46,000 cancer deaths and 120,000 deaths from circulatory disease occurred at home, and many of these people needed ongoing medical and nursing care. Hughes was critical of the quality of the care in the small number of homes for the dying (run by religious orders or charities) and the larger number of for-profit nursing homes. The former provided loving attention but lacked trained nurses. In many nursing homes, skilled nursing of the terminally ill was lacking, and in some, outright neglect was found. Hughes saw value in beds for the dying in acute care hospitals and closer relations between homes for the dying and hospitals.

The period also saw the stirring of clinical interest. The *Practitioner*, in late summer of 1948, published a series of papers on the care of the dying, the most important of which was that of W. N. Leak. Leak stated that, just when death was becoming commonly located in old age and resulted from a chronic condition, families were neither able or nor willing to provide care. Yet, with so many deaths happening in large hospitals and with medicine's drive to prolong life waxing strong, the clinical skills for dealing with the dying were disappearing. A plenary session of the British Medical Association's 1957 conference was devoted to the care of the dying. The *British Medical Journal* reported that one general practitioner with 30 years of experience had said that the doctor's role is to make the patient as comfortable as possible; morphine was still the answer to pain, but its use should not be such as to induce addiction; and more hospital accommodations for the dying should be a high priority.

In 1961 evidence-based discussion of the care of the dying was beginning to appear. In that year, A. N. Exton Smith, a physician at Whittington Hospital in London reported his study of 220 older people who died in the hospital. In 1959 he had visited Cicely Saunders at Saint Joseph's Hospice in Hackney, and they had remained in contact.

By the early 1960s Saunders was promoting the modern hospice as the institutional solution to the deficiencies identified by Hughes and others. In proposing a multidisciplinary approach, she drew on her own experience as, successively, nurse, social service worker, and physician. In building the new discourse on hospice, she drew on evidence from various sources—a survey of people suffering from lung cancer at the Brompton and Royal Marsden hospitals; a survey of public opinion on cancer; and a study of cancer patients' reluctance to seek treatment. She also drew on work on psychosocial issues, especially that done in the United States and by British psychiatrist Colin Murray Parkes.

In the mid-1960s Eric Wilkes, a general practitioner who later founded Saint Luke's Hospice in Sheffield, began publishing in the *Lancet* his research on home care for people with terminal cancer; he called for "terminal care units" for those unable to stay at home. Another British doctor who helped shift the basis of the field from anecdote to systematic observation was psychiatrist John Hinton. In 1963 he published works on the physical and mental distress of the dying, using interviews with 102 hospitalized patients (and controls), which showed the dying were more often depressed and anxious. He noted that Exton Smith notwithstanding, one had to go back to William Osler in 1906 for material on the incidence, severity, and relief of distress among those dying in hospitals. Welcoming his work, the *British Medical Journal* observed that there was a lack of such systematic studies. In response, Saunders sent a letter saying there was a need for more research and teaching in this neglected field.

However, at this stage, specialist institutional care of the dying remained in the hands of a small number of homes and hospices inspired by older traditions of Christian charity. They mostly functioned outside the NHS and with very limited medical input. In London, there was Saint Columba's Hospital, which had begun as Princess Alexandra's Friedenheim in 1889; the Hostel of God (conducted by Anglican orders), which had begun as the Free Home for the Dying in 1891; Saint Luke's Home for the Dying Poor, established by the Methodist West London Mission in 1893 and absorbed by the Saint Mary's Teaching Group of Hospitals when the NHS was inaugurated (Saunders worked there as a volunteer in the late 1940s and used the writings of Howard Barrett, who had run the hospice until 1921, to begin to develop her own ideas); and Saint Joseph's Hospice, established by the

Irish Sisters of Charity in 1905 (Saunders worked there from 1958 to 1965). Outside London, there were just a few homes: under the NHS, the Taylor Memorial Home of Rest, Birmingham, established in 1910 for women with incurable cancer, became part of the Dudley Road Group of Hospitals; the Tarner Home in Brighton was established in 1936; in 1950 the Sisters of Charity opened Saint Margaret's Hospice in Clydebank; and in 1952 the first of eight Marie Curie cancer center homes was opened at Hill of Tarvit in Fife, although these homes were not completely devoted to end-of-life care.

While outside the mainstream, some of these homes and hospices had developed practices that, channeled through Saunders's work, came to have an important effect: for example, Saint Luke's regularly administered small injections of morphine to relieve intractable pain rather than pursue the then common practice of withholding relief until very large doses were needed; and the quality of the highly personalized care at Saint Joseph's was widely appreciated.

The pursuit of self-help, often in a religious context, set these facilities apart from the socialized, secular medicine of the NHS. However, their values and practices integrated into Saunders's new synthesis—"total care" (physical, social, psychological, and spiritual)—quickly spread first throughout the Anglo-Saxon world and then globally. John Hinton recalled that the spiritual aspect of Saunders's total care, expressed in her Christian commitment, was seen as something of a barrier to wide acceptance of her approach. It was believed that evidence coming from people with a religious vocation would be biased.

Attendance as a speaker at a Royal Society of Health conference in 1961 marked a transition point for Saunders. There she talked with the deputy secretary of the health ministry, Dame Enid Russell-Smith, about the location of her planned terminal care home. Dame Albertine Winner, the deputy chief medical officer, came away from a visit to Saint Joseph's impressed by Saunders's work. Even before Saint Christopher's opened, Saunders was advising the medical advisory committee of the Regional Hospital Board about how to extend terminal care.

David Clark, a medical sociologist, has identified four important innovations in the two decades before the opening of Saint Christopher's that helped prepare the way for the modern hospice concept. The first is the shift in medical studies about care of the dying from anecdote to systematic inquiry, making the quality of the evidence more compelling. Both the *Lancet* and the *British Medical Journal* used the new evidence to argue that good terminal care was an alternative to euthanasia. The second is the attempt to promote dignity and meaning in the dying process and death as an integral part of life. The third is the tendency for medicine, with its emphasis on cure, to be passive in the face of the need for a good death and a new call for commitment. The fourth is identification of the interaction of physical and psychological (and spiritual) suffering; her concept of total pain was a great challenge to the dualism of body and mind underlying contemporary medicine.

Clark also sees two significant continuities between the earlier traditions and the new discourse on terminal care. The first is how the presence and personality of the physician were viewed as therapeutic. Saunders wrote of a patient's gratitude for her caring, as well as her technical assistance. Second is the debt that terminal care owed to traditions of religious and charitable care, the provision of which the NHS and the rest of the welfare state were intended to replace.

In a context of postwar financial constraint, the priorities of the NHS were acute care and rehabilitation, and hospital specialist medicine was highly valued. However, those who developed early terminal care came from general medicine and psychiatry—Saunders, Hinton, Wilkes, and Murray Parkes. Until 1960, terminal care medicine did not exist as a branch of medicine. The lack of truth telling about imminent death and inadequate pain control were obstacles. Only 29 percent of patients in 1969 were told about their diagnosis of cancer, but by 1987 the percentage had risen to 73. Two historians of general practice have noted that few doctors talked about death and dying or were taught anything about it; the district nurse in some cases played a larger part than the general practitioner; often the only training that general practitioners received was what they picked up from senior partners or other colleagues. However, the coming of the hospice movement changed all of this.

In 1980 a working group (of the cancer subcommittee of the Standing Medical Advisory Committee), chaired by Eric Wilkes, produced a report on terminal care. The report advised against allowing the expansion of inpatient hospices to take precedence over that of hospital- and community-based accommodation and urged the coordination of general practice, hospital, and hospice services. In 1969 Saint Christopher's introduced a home nursing service, and in 1975 the Macmillan nurses began to work with primary care teams. By the mid-1990s there were 1,200 Macmillan nurses, 384 home care teams, and 5,000 Marie Curie nurses providing 24-hour home care. In 1987 the National Association of Health Authorities issued guidelines for health authorities on standards and services for dying people. The Department of Health requested that they work with the public to plan palliative care services, and £11.25 million in public funds were provided in 1988 and 1989 for public services (Glyn Hughes, 1960, 9–63; *Principles and Provisions of Palliative Care,* 1992, 3; Clark, Malson, Small, Mallett, Neale, and Heather, 1997, 62; Jackson and Eve, 1997, 146; Loudon and Drury, 1998, 121–22; Clark, 1999a, 225–43).

The establishment of palliative care in an acute hospital setting was initiated in 1976 at Saint Thomas's Hospital in London, and soon afterward a team was introduced at Saint Luke's Hospital in New York. Some hospital teams grew out of pain relief or symptom control units. Others developed from independent hospices or community services. Hospitals in Britain that had a full team or a single palliative care nurse specialist increased from 5 in 1982 to 40 in 1990. By 1996 the number was 275. The core of the team is the nurse specialist and the palliative medicine physician, while the other members are the chaplain, social worker, pharmacist, and psychologist, and there is also access to physiotherapy, occupational therapy, dietetics, and complementary therapies. The team provides specialist advice and support for other clinical staff, patients, and families, offers formal and informal education, and liaises with other services both within and without the hospital. It was clear by the end of the 1990s that nursing homes were becoming a more common site of deaths and yet had inadequate resources. By 1997 there were 5,559 registered homes with more than 153,000 beds in England. Where in 1990, 13 percent of deaths were in nursing or residential homes, in 1995, it was 18 percent. Two approaches had been tried; one was for palliative care practitioners to advise home staff; the other was the provision of education through courses for home staff or training of link nurses (those nurses with palliative care skills who can act as links between patients in homes and external palliative care services), who applied their new expertise in the home (Glicksman, 1996, 3–4, 7; Jackson and Eve, 1997, 146; Froggatt, 2001, 43–46).

In this era considerable development of professional structures took place. In 1987 Britain became the first country to recognize palliative medicine as a specialty, when the Joint Committee on Higher Medical Training approved a four-year course for senior residents. Two years earlier the Association for Palliative Medicine of Great Britain and Ireland was formed as an organization for doctors working in hospices and hospital units. A decade and a half later the group had 800 members. The first peer-reviewed journal, *Palliative Medicine,* appeared in 1987. The National Council for Hospice and Specialist Palliative Care Services began work in 1991 as an umbrella organization for the various professional associations, the NHS and public sectors, the national charities, and, via regional representatives, all palliative care providers.

The first edition of *The Oxford Textbook of Palliative Medicine* came out in 1993, and the next year the first issue of the *European Journal of Palliative Care* was published. At the beginning of 1995, the *European Journal of Palliative Nursing* first appeared. By the end of the 1990s *Palliative Medicine* had an impact factor large enough to appear in the Journal Citation Reports league tables (rankings of journals according to how frequently their articles are cited in other publications). The factor is calculated by dividing the total number of citations of a journal in one year by the number of items published in that journal in the previous two years. With an impact factor of 1.86, it ranked 19/100 in the general medicine category and 14/100 in the public health category. These figures suggest it was being used by health professionals outside as well as inside the specialty. The impact factors of the palliative medicine journal compared well with those of other specialist journals such as the *British Journal of General Practice* (2.01) or *Medical Care* (2.17), but they fall far below those of the leading medical journals—the *Lancet* (16.14) and the *New England Journal of Medicine* (27.77) (Doyle, 1997, 7; Higginson and McGregor, 1999, 273).

In Britain, academic palliative medicine developed within internal medicine, but elsewhere departments of family or community medicine, oncology, pediatrics, geriatrics, and anesthesia have also been sites of growth. In 1992 the Association for Palliative Medicine (APM) published the *Palliative Medicine Curriculum for Medical Students, General Professional Training, and Higher Specialist Training.* This was the basis for the development of a palliative care curriculum for Europe produced by the European Association for Palliative Care. In 1991 a chair in palliative medicine was established in London. By 1996 more chairs had been established—in Bristol, Sheffield, London, Wales, Sunderland, and Glasgow universities, while in 1988 a clinical readership had been established at Oxford. Senior lectureships were instituted at five London medical schools and in universities in six cities. In

1991 the APM nominated an educational representative in each health region of Britain.

By 1992, 22 of 28 medical schools taught palliative medicine; at 22 schools students might visit a hospice or palliative care unit; 16 schools stated that a question on palliative medicine was a regular or an occasional item on the final examination. Postgraduate courses also developed: in 1991 the University of Wales offered a degree in palliative medicine that soon attracted hospital and hospice doctors, general practitioners, and trainees from overseas; in 1994 Glasgow and Trent universities and in 1995 Dundee University offered a multidisciplinary degree, while master's courses could be taken in four nursing schools in 1995; and in 1992 a degree in psychosocial palliative care was available at Southampton University. In 1987 specialist training for senior residents was available, involving placements in oncology, radiotherapy, neurology, anesthetics, ear, nose and throat (ENT) medicine, and pain medicine. This instruction led to the accreditation needed for appointment as a medical director or consultant. In continuing education many seminars and courses became available: for example, vocational trainees for general practice might do a one-day intensive rotation every six months at Saint Christopher's, where clinical aspects, communication, and bereavement were addressed, while the Royal College of General Practitioners appointed palliative care facilitators to develop continuing education in other districts of the country (Scott, MacDonald, and Mount, 1997, 1176, 1184; Smith, 1999, 1188–89).

Historically, palliative care has focused mainly on people dying of cancer. A 1990 survey of services in the United Kingdom and Ireland found that, of 95 units with at least five beds, 67 percent cared for people with motor neurone disease (MND); 40 percent, those with multiple sclerosis (MS); 40 percent, those with AIDS; 21 percent, those with Parkinson's disease; 23 percent, those with heart or chest disease; 14 percent, those who had had a stroke; and 8 percent, those with Alzheimer's disease (patients with multiple conditions are counted separately for each condition). Only five units provided for all of these conditions but AIDS, and one accepted people with any of the conditions.

A second survey in 1991 found that, of 139 inpatient units (88 percent of those listed in the 1991 Directory of Hospice Services), more than 50 percent looked after people with MND and almost the same number would care for people with AIDS. However, as few as 6 units said they would care for persons with any condition. Of the 129 day care units in the survey, 82 took patients with MND, while 56 took AIDS patients. Hospital support teams were asked whether they took people with noncancer conditions. Virtually all who responded took people with MND and AIDS. About 66 percent took those with multiple sclerosis (MS) or heart disease. Just under 50 percent were willing to care for anyone with a terminal condition.

The 1992 report on palliative care of the Standing Medical Advisory Committee and the Standing Nursing and Midwifery Committee recommended that palliative care services for noncancer patients be developed. A random sample of 639 adults dying in 1987 revealed that only 44 were provided with hospice services, and only 2 of these had conditions other than cancer. General practitioners in the Thames Valley who were surveyed in the early 1990s said that the largest demand from noncancer patients came from people with strokes, cardiovascular disease,

MS, and rheumatoid arthritis; every year 11 noncancer patients per practice needed respite or continuing care, and this level of unmet demand required more bed days per year than were available for the mostly cancer patients (George and Sykes, 1997, 241–42).

The 1995 Calman-Hine report on cancer services required NHS commissioners and providers to ensure that people with cancer could access palliative care services if needed. In early 2000, the NHS brought out the National Service Framework for coronary heart disease. This proposed that the local palliative care team provide support for patients with chronic heart failure (CHF), representing a basic change in the focus of services from the preoccupation with cancer; in 1994 and 1995 cancer was the condition of 96.3 percent of those receiving community palliative care. Whereas disease progress in cancer is more or less predictable, in CHF reliable prognosis is difficult because some people die suddenly, but others appear to be no sicker at the terminal phase than during earlier stages of the illness (Addington-Hall, Simon, and Gibbs, 2000, 361–62).

Traditionally, palliative care was reserved for those in the dying stage after cure was no longer possible. As it became clear that, in terms of quality of life, its cost-effectiveness was greater than efforts to cure, palliative care was introduced at an earlier stage of the disease. Moreover, palliative medicine specialists may find they have patients referred to them with "incurable" metastatic cancer who would benefit from curative or other interventions because the referring doctor simply failed to appreciate curative opportunities. Misdiagnosis may occur since, for example, infections such as tuberculosis can resemble cancer, and chronic conditions such as Addison's disease or advanced pulmonary disease can give rise to cachexia or, like verterbral collapse due to osteoporosis, cause pain similar to that associated with a recurrence of cancer (Finlay, 2001, 437–38).

In World War II, the scale of the killing, the horrors of the Nazi concentration camps, and the shocking destructiveness of the atomic bombs over Japan disturbed social scientists and health professionals in the United States and Britain both personally and professionally. Just as deep concern about preserving human dignity at the species level led to the Universal Declaration of Human Rights in 1948, it also prompted some people in health care to think about the often alienating conditions under which people died in hospitals and other health care locations. As noted earlier, in the 1950s, some social workers, psychologists, psychiatrists, and physicians became interested in investigating terminal care, and thanatology later emerged as the name for the study of grief, dying, and death.

Herman Feifel organized a session on death and dying at the annual conference of the American Psychological Association in 1956. Gardner Murphy called it a bold move. Feifel's book *The Meaning of Death* (1959) greatly influenced social scientists, health professionals, and laypeople alike. In England, psychiatrists John Bowlby and Colin Murray Parkes investigated bereavement processes, while John Hinton pursued empirical work involving dying patients. In the United States, nurse educator Esther L. Brown in 1952 asked a group of health care workers whether they saw a role for themselves in comforting the dying or whether this should be left to the clergy. When she found that they, as well as other nurses, saw no role, she began to include in her workshops discussions of the needs of the dying and their families.

In New York two medical social workers obtained funds from the National Cancer Foundation to establish Cancer Care, which provided psychological support for cancer patients and their families. The American Cancer Society, which had until then focused on medical research, now also funded psychological support. In 1956 the National Cancer Foundation sponsored a symposium on terminal illness and, two years later, on a constructive approach to terminal illness. The 1959 National Conference on Social Welfare saw the first discussion of social work intervention involving dying patients and their families.

In 1948 Cicely Saunders began working at Saint Luke's Hospital (mentioned earlier as one of the late nineteenth-century hospices in London) as a volunteer nurse. When she qualified as a doctor in 1958, she began full-time work at Saint Joseph's Hospice in Hackney. For pain control she introduced the practice of regular administration of oral opioids, a practice that she had observed at Saint Luke's and that had existed there since about 1935. This new practice aimed to prevent pain and replaced the less satisfactory giving of drugs by injection as required. Wanting to combine scientific medicine with the traditional compassionate nursing style of the Sisters of Charity, she sought to establish a third way between treating the disease as if cure were realistic and legalized euthanasia. The aim was to attain a level of opioid dosage that kept the patient between the pain relief and sedation thresholds. Long-established medical concerns about drug dependence, rising tolerance to drugs, and respiratory depression were discovered to be unfounded.

Saunders developed the concept of total pain in response to patients' own descriptions of the nature of their pain. She understood both the significance of helping patients to face the truth of their situation as a means of regaining a sense of control and the significance of providing support for the whole family. Responding to the latter, she developed plans for home care, involving good liaison with the family doctor. The contemporary appearance of psychotropic drugs, nonsteroidal anti-inflammatories, and synthetic steroids meant that there were now available many adjuvants to the traditional analgesics. Moreover, palliative radiotherapy and oncology were also developing.

The issue of establishing a new hospice where all of these elements of the plan to provide an environment in which symptom-free patients could pursue the meaning of their terminal situation was resolved with the setting up of Saint Christopher's in 1967. Two decades later there were 2,300 hospice beds in the United Kingdom, as well as home care services. At the heart of Saunders's approach was symptom control in order to offer dying patients freedom from the physical discomfort and fear that prevented them from coming to terms with their situation and from resolving long-standing interpersonal relations issues, where these existed.

Cicely Saunders had a direct influence on the development of hospices in North America. She visited there three times—in 1963, 1965, and 1966. However, the connection began earlier. In 1959 she began to correspond with Dr. Robert Loberfield of the New York City Cancer Committee and then with Prof. W. Bean of the University of Iowa. American clergyman Rev. Benjamin Holmes, who had read her *Care of the Dying* (1959), visited Saint Joseph's Hospice when she was a research fellow there and urged her to go to the United States. She wrote to the American Cancer Society that she and some others had plans for an interdenominational hospice in London and that, while in the United States, she wished to investigate the following issues—pain control, patients' psychological problems, training of hospital chaplains, bereavement, and any hospice that might offer ideas for the planned London establishment. She made clear that her field was not the treatment of cancer but the care of the dying.

During her 1963 visit to the West Coast, she met Herman Feifel and social anthropologist Esther Lucille Brown; on the East Coast she met with Florence Wald, dean of nursing at Yale University; Gordon Allport, professor of social psychology at Harvard University; and Carleton Sweetser, chaplain at Saint Luke's Hospital in New York.

Allport introduced her to the ideas of Viktor Frankl (*Man's Search for Meaning,* 1962; originally published in German in 1946 after his release from a concentration camp), which had a profound effect on her thinking. During her 1966 visit, she went to Yale to lecture to nurses, to Cleveland, and also to Vancouver to visit a pain clinic. While at Yale she met Elisabeth Kübler-Ross and English psychiatrist Colin Murray Parkes (who was at Harvard for a year). Yale was a continuing source of contacts and the sharing of ideas. Her friendship with Dean Wald was to deepen as plans developed for the Connecticut hospice, the first U.S. hospice of the modern era.

During this period Cecily Saunders published a number of pieces in the United States directed variously toward church, nursing, medical, and psychiatric audiences. By late 1965 she was prominent enough for an article on her to appear in *Time*. At the same time thanatology itself and public concern with death and dying were emerging in the United States. In mid-1966 at Western Reserve University in Cleveland, she gave one of five lectures on death and dying. The other lecturers were Lawrence Leshan (psychotherapy with the dying patient), Anselm Strauss (awareness of dying), Robert Kastenbaum (psychological death), and Richard Kalish (the dying person's impact on family dynamics).

In the 1950s Saunders had read U.S. physician Alfred Worcester's classic, *The Care of the Aged, the Dying, and the Dead* (1935), as well as reports of terminal cancer care in Boston in the 1940s. In the United States she encountered the traditional Catholic hospice (familiar to her from her stint at Saint Joseph's) in New York at the House of Calvary (descended from Jeanne Garnier's nineteenth-century Dames de Calvaire), Rosary Hill Home, Saint Rose's Home, and Saint Vincent's Hospital. She also encountered U.S. mainstream medicine with its aggressive approach to treatment, as well as doctors, nurses, and others who were searching for an alternative, such as chaplain Carleton Sweetser, who was trying to humanize the care of the dying in an urban acute care hospital; pain specialist S. L. Wallenstein at Memorial Hospital in New York; and Harold Beecher at Massachusetts General Hospital.

Before the Vietnam War protest era, the United States encouraged Saunders to be optimistic and adventurous, and she appealed to liberal reformist Americans seeking better conditions for the dying. As David Clark has observed, out of this interaction in the 1960s came a new social movement and a new medical specialty in Britain, the United States, Canada, Australia, New Zealand, and many other countries (Wald, 1997, 65; Clark, 2001, 16–27).

Canadian Balfour Mount spent a sabbatical at Saint Christopher's and returned to Montreal to establish a palliative care unit in a teaching hospital in 1975. This new model of hospice care involved a visiting team that consulted in the hospital and the home alike. At virtually the same time, the first continuing care unit, established by the National Society for Cancer Relief in England, began its work. Yet another model was perfected at a New York hospital, where a consulting hospital team without its own beds began work in 1975 (Saunders, 1988, 167–76). The hospice ethos in the United States was to evolve differently from that in Britain.

The United States

If Saunders was a charismatic leader in both Britain and the United States, Elisabeth Kübler-Ross was a charismatic leader of the U.S. movement but in a different way. Kübler-Ross turned hospice into a nationally known concept but was not active in the planning of programs. Saunders gave advice in the United States on the development of hospice care programs, conferring on them the face of acceptable medical care. Saunders's approach impressed health professionals. Kübler-Ross impressed the public at large with her interest in making Americans confront their denial of death, dying, and grief. To her, hospices were important because they would provide environments where the dying and their families could better communicate about the fact of impending death. If Saunders spoke of the spiritual and physical aspects of dying, Kübler-Ross talked of the psychological processes involved.

Kübler-Ross's early work led to a stage theory (the stages of denial, anger, bargaining, depression, and acceptance) of the psychological process of dying, implying the need for a supportive environment for the dying person to use to move toward a healthy acceptance of death. In 1965 theological students at Billings Memorial Hospital requested that she give a seminar on psychological processes in death and dying. Physician colleagues at Chicago Medical School were hostile to her ideas, but other health care professionals were receptive, and she was soon conducting lectures throughout the United States. Her book *On Death and Dying* (1969) and an interview published in *Life* in 1970 raised her public profile even higher.

Florence Wald did much to bring structure to the loose international social movement concerned with death and dying. She brought together Cicely Saunders, Elisabeth Kübler-Ross, and Colin Murray Parkes to talk about the care of the dying in the United States. She developed the Yale Study Group and then approached individuals around the United States to form a group to develop hospice programs on a national scale. The group assumed a formal guise in 1974 with the first official meeting of the International Working Group on Death, Dying, and Bereavement (IWG) in Baltimore. The people who set up the first three hospice programs in the United States were all members of this group. The IWG was basically a think tank to discuss issues related to thanatology and to make recommendations to governments and other influential organizations. It still meets every couple of years in different parts of the world. North Americans and Britons form a large part of its membership, while the majority of the remaining members come from Western European and other first-world countries such as Australia.

Each of the first three hospice programs in the United States followed a different model of care. Founded by the Yale Study Group in Branford, Connecticut, Hospice Inc. followed the Saunders model. The founders decided early on that they did not want to affiliate with the Yale University Hospital, and it became the only hospice to be unconnected with the acute health care system; the founders were anxious to avoid conflicts over values with acute health care people and to steer clear of financial entanglements that might rebound on them in times of constraint.

Awarded a 1969 grant, Wald conducted a study that showed that those who were dying wanted to do so at home and also to be as free of discomfort as possible, and by 1973 funds were sufficient to initiate a home care service. The National Cancer Institute provided $800,000 in a grant that year. In the second round of grants in 1977, Hospice Inc. secured more funds and, with these and state and local endowments, built a 44-person facility. The personal interest of Connecticut governor Eleanor Grasso, a cancer sufferer herself, had brought not only state funding but also public legitimation as a health care service. The first modern hospice in the United States, Hospice Inc. was also a leader in promoting training. In 1975 the first National Hospice Symposium was held at the Connecticut facility.

Rev. Carleton Sweetser was the driving force in the formation of the second hospice, Saint Luke's at Saint Luke's Hospital in New York. It was the first of many hospital-centered programs. As a chaplain at Sloan-Kettering, a well-known cancer treatment center, Sweetser had heard Cicely Saunders speak during her 1963 lecture tour. He subsequently joined the death and dying movement and became involved with IWG. When he became head chaplain at Saint Luke's Hospital, Sweetser eventually won the support of the hospital board for the establishment of a hospice. Saunders herself assisted in the task of raising funds. When physical space for a hospice was not forthcoming at the hospital, it was decided that the multidisciplinary hospice team would care for designated hospice patients within normal wards under what was later termed the "scatter bed" model.

Working within an existing acute care hospital environment, the team at Saint Luke's won recognition for its expertise in pain management and symptom control. As the hospice team expanded, home care services were offered. Cicely Saunders introduced the scatter bed model to those English facilities that offered an environment similar to that of Saint Luke's Hospital. While this model offered an opportunity to humanize acute care practices, it also encountered entrenched values unsympathetic to hospice objectives. The price might entail less discussion about dying and less willingness to offer postmortem bereavement support to the family.

The Hospice of Marin in California, founded by psychiatrist William Lamers, represented another type of program: the volunteer community support team. Lamers originally had in mind a clinic where grieving people might be helped to work through their loss. However, Kübler-Ross persuaded Lamers that a hospice would better fulfill his goals. In 1975, with a volunteer staff, the hospice began to offer home support services. Seeing how difficult it was to obtain funds for an independent facility, the hospice board incorporated the hospice as a home health agency. Other groups also saw the wisdom of containing costs by using volunteer professionals and laypeople in a home care service. Thus, the Hospice of North Carolina in the late 1970s established home care services throughout the state.

The different models that evolved in the first phase of hospice development had characteristic strengths and weaknesses; for example, home care services were limited in their capacity to provide advanced methods of pain control and to offer continuity of care after hospitalization; conversely, hospital-based services usually presented less opportunity for honest communication about dying and for grief counseling (Siebold, 1992, 61–74, 87–88, 97–107).

Saint Christopher's in London became a center of learning, as well as inspiration, for international visitors, who came in a steady stream from throughout Europe and North America. By the mid-1980s about 100 hospices had been set up in Britain, plus home support services and the earliest hospital-based, palliative care units. In the United States, 516 hospices had been established. While organizational form differed, the international hospice movement shared certain basic values and practices—respect for personhood, advanced pain and symptom control, and multidisciplinary staffs.

Early hospices in the United States embodied many values similar to those of the alternative institutions of the counterculture of the 1960s and 1970s. Thus, supporters of the free school movement said that traditional public schools did not properly educate children, and hospice advocates said that general hospitals failed to care properly for the dying. The hospices wanted to curtail the physician's traditional authority over other health care professionals; further, they saw the quality of interpersonal relations as critical, so the empathic nonexpert—the volunteer—was as valued as an expert. Consumer rights were sovereign, so dying patients were entitled to honest communication and a say in their care. Valuing the natural, they rejected the heroic interventions of scientific medicine and approached death as a normal part of life. They also rejected the bureaucratic organization of modern health care. The needs of the individual patient were paramount, so round-the-clock home care was fundamental. Support for the family was also integral. They were proud of their historical forerunners: just as food cooperatives pointed to the nineteenth-century cooperative movement and free schools linked themselves to the earlier schools of the Progressive educational reformers, so the hospice pioneers saw their origins in the tradition of the religious hospices of medieval Christendom, where travelers were housed and also nursed if sick.

Like the counterculture generally, they were wary of the cash economy and sought to avoid dependence on third-party payers, whether private health funds or government agencies. Instead, they sought private and public grants and donations and used the labor of volunteers extensively. Also like the counterculture, they were the products of middle-class white idealism and effort. Located mainly in suburban areas, they were staffed by middle-class volunteers and professionals. Thus, while the first hospices were part of the international movement to humanize dying, they were also part of the world of the counterculture; in particular, they shared with holistic health care advocates the objective of a holistic approach to the patient; with the women's health movement, criticism of the excessive authority of the doctor and medicine's heavy reliance on technology; with the home birth movement, rejection of the medicalization of major life events; and with the self-help movement, demystification of expert knowledge and egalitarianism in relations between laypeople and professionals (Abel, 1986, 72–82).

It was in the United States that the advantages and disadvantages of absorption into the mainstream of health care were first experienced and discussed. In the 1980s two important shaping forces were the National Hospice Study and the Medicare hospice benefit; the first revealed how hospice could contain costs by keeping people in their homes; the second provided major public funding. By the 1980s in the United States and Britain, fears were being expressed that the power of hospices was being sapped by the medicalization resulting from integration into the health care system. However, elsewhere in Western Europe, palliative care, whether hospital based or home care, was made part of the mainstream of health care from the outset.

One indicator of this integration or mainstreaming was the appearance of national and international organizations. These served both to educate the general community and to lobby governments. In 1991 the National Council for Hospice and Specialist Palliative Care Services served as the British national body, while the European Association for Palliative Care (established with 42 members in 1988, a decade or so later it had 9,000 members from more than 50 countries) played the same type of role at the European level. Some key figures such as Jan Stjernsward, head of the WHO Cancer and Palliative Care Program, consistently argued that only through integration might equity of access and cost containment be achieved, especially for those suffering from chronic diseases less notorious than cancer. Others were worried that while pain and other symptom control might flourish in integrated services, spiritual and psychosocial support would fall by the wayside (Clark, 2000a, 53–54).

By the end of the 1970s, hospice was popular with the national media in the United States. Articles appeared in national newspapers and journals such as the *New York Times* and *Newsweek,* and there were frequent advertisements, as well as in-depth opinion pieces on television. In 1979 *Index Medicus* listed hospice as a separate category. Republicans and Democrats publicly endorsed it. In 1982 Pres. Ronald Reagan proclaimed a week in November National Hospice Week, while Sen. Edward Kennedy accepted an invitation to speak at the first National Hospice Meeting in Washington, D.C., that same year.

The demand for training was national in scope and growing quickly: where in 1975, 70 people attended a training seminar at Hospice Inc., in 1978 more than 1,000 attended the National Hospice Organization's annual conference. It was becoming evident that health care insurance funding was necessary if facilities were to be provided on a nationwide scale. Foundation grants and private funding alone could no longer sustain an expanding program. While some members of the movement were uneasy about integration, most were eager to see hospice care become an alternative benefit under Medicare. A national organization was needed to pursue the key tasks of obtaining ongoing funding, integrating hospice into the acute care system, and educating the public. When the National Hospice Organization (NHO) was incorporated, it established an office in Washington, D.C. The search for funding soon dominated its efforts. However, the quest for insurance reimbursement and the necessary standardization of care alienated some hospice groups, and by 1982 about 50 percent of hospice programs had not joined the NHO.

Although there was concern about the price of integrating with hospitals, by 1980, 46 percent were so affiliated. Funds for independent facilities were just too hard to access. In 1978 Joseph Califano of the U.S. Department of Health, Education, and Welfare stated that Medicare and Medicaid would fund a two-year hospice demonstration project. At the same time, Blue Cross/Blue Shield insurers said they would support demonstration projects in the belief that hospice could reduce health care costs. The hospice movement, on very little hard evidence, commonly asserted that hospice care was cheaper than hospital care because it was low tech.

Using assumptions concerning hospice developed by IWG in 1979, NHO published the first official hospice-care standards. However, a majority of hospice providers rejected these guidelines, preferring to provide care in their own way. Some saw hospital practice as incompatible with hospice care, and they wished to gradually increase the growth of hospice facilities. Others accepted the need to integrate with acute health care to obtain funds but wished to do so slowly and carefully. Others again, the optimists, said that integration must go ahead, and they saw the speedy public acceptance of hospice as evidence that a more compassionate attitude to the dying was emerging in the United States.

In 1982 Medicare, Blue Cross/Blue Shield, and other insurers introduced a hospice benefit. The Medicare hospice benefit was made permanent after a favorable evaluation was presented in 1986. The benefit undoubtedly represented an improvement in terminal-care services. Hospice providers, nevertheless, had four criticisms:

1. The total reimbursement was capped at $6,500 for the six-month period of the benefit; clearly, volunteers and family members were expected to provide most of the physical care.
2. The patient was expected to die at home as acute and respite care were restricted.
3. Patients had to acknowledge that they were terminal; they had to be willing to forgo curative therapies to receive the hospice benefit.
4. The benefit did not include bereavement and pastoral care services, yet clergy and the religious had been central to the growth of early services.

In the end, access to funding through the health care system overshadowed care ideals such as normalizing grief and death; the potential conflict between this ideal and the desire to control pain and other discomforts of dying was never properly addressed.

In 1990, hospice programs numbered 1,450, according to the NHO. At least 16 insurers provided a hospice benefit, and 39 states had instituted licensing for hospice programs. There was a breakaway national organization started by those who believed NHO did not properly represent hospice ideals: the American Society of Hospice Care and the Hospice Association of America (HAA). The HAA claimed that the increased hospice benefits in 1989 resulted from its lobbying of members of Congress.

By the 1980s it was clear that financial problems were making initiation or indeed continuation of hospice programs very difficult. Providers tried to respond to what they identified as community needs, but insurers wanted home care services. Medicare rates were such that they compelled providers to offer only supportive care; they could not admit patients needing palliative radiation or surgery. A new type of business-oriented provider offered programs in which spiritual or psychosocial matters were subordinated to treatment protocols.

Under Medicare, home care programs did best, but for cost reasons they used nursing homes for inpatient purposes. These homes, however, lacked proper pain control services. Independent hospices had to find funding to supplement the Medicare benefit in order to continue. Hospital programs had problems with servicing distant patients and usually needed extra funding from the hospital to continue to function. The use of volunteers declined. They were used more by independent than institution-based programs. The medicalization associated with health care institutions meant there was less room for volunteers, who were often disillusioned by the medical approach. The early innovators such as Cicely Saunders, Elisabeth Kübler-Ross, Florence Wald, and William Lamers were now less prominent.

Physicians tended to resist involvement in hospice programs, often referring only for the home support services they offered. There were, however, some efforts to introduce hospice care into medical education. Medicare regulations sharpened physician opposition by requiring that patients be classified as terminal before admission to hospice and that the recommendations of the hospice team take precedence over the physician's.

Hospices were often in competition for referrals with area hospitals, nursing homes, and home health agencies in a period when health care as a whole was facing financial cutbacks resulting from the federal government's wish to contain expenditures. In 1989 Medicare reimbursed hospice day care services, and these were a way to increase referrals to the main hospice program. Some hospices marketed a consulting service to train personnel from nursing homes in their vicinity in terminal care.

Educated, middle-class people disproportionately used the hospice programs. Neither ethnic minorities nor rural patients had adequate access to them. The National Hospice Study carried out at Brown University revealed a number of strengths and weaknesses. The study involved 25 demonstration hospice programs, 14 nondemonstration hospice programs, and 14 conventional care programs. The major findings were that hospice did not greatly improve quality of life or reduce pain; that, for patients who spent only a short time in a hospice, hospice care was less costly than conventional health care; and that families in receipt of inpatient hospice services were less stressed than those involved in nonhospice care.

Two decades after the first hospices came into being in the United States, conventional health care structures were apparently more able to co-opt hospice than hospice was able to change traditional medical care. The leaders of the hospice movement assumed that their aims were widely understood by the public, but most citizens remained ignorant of what hospice was. Moreover, the government, restrictive in its funding, was primarily interested in what hospice could do to contain health care costs. After the advent of the Medicare benefit, hospice services took different paths—some conformed to the restricted view of hospice entailed by Medicare, others went their own way, and a minority adhered to their fundamental values (Siebold, 1992, 109–13, 132–36, 145–63).

At the end of the 1990s, Andrew Billings, director of the palliative care service at Massachusetts General Hospital in Boston, stated that "palliative care" and "palliative medicine" had become commonly used terms in the United States and elsewhere in the world for programs based on the hospice philosophy. Indeed, in 1997 the prestigious Institute of Medicine (IOM) in the United States had recommended that palliative care should become at least a defined area of expertise, education, and research.

For Billings, palliative care in the United States aimed to apply the hospice philosophy to a larger population than that served by the hospices as such. As we have seen, federal regulations had restricted both the services that hospices could provide and the actions of health maintenance organizations and insurers, which financed their work. Hospice patients had to be satisfied with comfort care rather than life-prolonging measures, prefer home care, and possess health insurance that included hospice. These constraints meant that hospices cared for those who were very close to death and, in all, only about 20 percent of dying people. Billings, however, stated that palliative care should become involved at the time of diagnosis. The strength of hospice lay in quality home care and provision for progressive terminal illness. Palliative care had other strengths.

Based on acute care hospitals, hospices could contribute to the work of the emergency wards and intensive care units, as well as in the case of deaths from acute conditions. Moreover, since services were often located in teaching hospitals, they could train physicians, other health care professionals, and students in providing quality terminal care. Being neither organ-based specialists such as nephrologists nor disease-based specialists such as oncologists nor age-based specialists such as pediatricians, palliative care physicians were generalists who were able to offer comprehensive care to a particular population group. Palliative care units offered a range of consultative and primary-care services on an interdisciplinary basis; indeed, a consultative service dealing only with physical symptoms and not psychosocial and spiritual matters was not a proper palliative care service (Billings, 1998, 73–79).

In the late 1960s medical schools in the United States began to provide education in end-of-life care. In the early 1990s, 89 percent of schools provided some teaching, although as few as 11 percent had a full-time course; 52 percent provided modules in required courses, while 30 percent offered one or two classes. In 83 percent of these, teaching was primarily through lectures, and fewer than 33 percent involved patients in teaching. Education of residents was similarly restricted. Only 26 percent of programs routinely included a course on end-of-life care. Physicians who were training in family medicine, internal medicine, pediatrics, and geriatrics on average cared for 28 terminally ill patients a year. When the American Board of Internal Medicine surveyed more than 1,400 residents, 72 percent said they were adequately trained in the management of pain and other symptoms; 62 percent reported adequate training in communicating bad news to patients; 38 percent in educating patients and families about the process of dying; and 32 percent in dealing with patients wanting help to die.

Calling for a better educational response in the late 1990s, Andrew Billings and Susan Block (Brigham and Women's Hospital, Boston) put forward a comprehensive, evidence-based approach to improving education in end-of-life care: (1) care of the dying is a core obligation; (2) areas to be dealt with include effective communication, skillful management of pain and other distress, accessible and quality home and hospice care as alternatives to acute hospital care, appreciation of the limits of treatment in advanced conditions, respect for patients' values and cultural and spiritual concerns, capacity to work in an interdisciplinary team, response to stress in fellow professionals, and development of an awareness of one's own attitudes and feelings concerning death and loss; (3) students should be encouraged to develop positive feelings toward the dying; (4) teaching about death and dying should be tailored to students' developmental stage and included in various courses; (5) dealing with patients and families must be at the core; (6) teaching should emphasize humanistic attitudes; (7) teaching must include communication skills; (8) students should be exposed to excellent physician role models; (9) respect for patient values and cultural and spiritual diversity must be demonstrated; (10) values such as compassion inherent in quality care must be shown in teaching; (11) ways in which to work well in a multidisciplinary setting must be demonstrated; (12) teachers must model ideal behaviors and skills; (13) student competence in management and the teaching itself must be evaluated; and (14) costs can be reduced by using programs evaluated elsewhere. Unhappily, at the beginning of the new millennium, Andrew Billings reported that no meaningful standards of certification existed and that anyone who was licensed to practice medicine could become medical director of a hospice (although Billings also pointed out that the American Board of Hospice and Palliative Medicine had committed itself to raising the standards of educational testing) (Billings and Block, 1997, 734–37; Billings, 2002, 644).

Australia

The original British model of hospice influenced the beginnings of palliative care in Australia, just as it had the early developments in the United States. However, as in the United States, with the passing of time, a local mix of services developed, so there too a new Australian amalgam was created, although not all of the early commentators saw the need for specialists in care of the dying. Thus, G. W. Milton of the Department of Surgery at the University of Sydney addressed his 1972 discussion of the "problem of the dying patient" to doctors and nurses in general and said that special wards, or even special hospitals, for the dying were not desirable because their occupants felt cut off from the world of the living. Similarly, Paul

Valent, a consultant liaison psychiatrist at Prince Henry's Hospital in Melbourne, decried the specialist approach, aiming his 1978 discussion of issues concerning dying patients toward all doctors, but particularly hospital doctors (Milton, 1972, 177–82;Valent, 1978, 433–37).

Attending the Second World Congress of Palliative Care organized by Balfour Mount at the Royal Victoria Hospital in Montreal in October 1980 were about 30 nurses and doctors from throughout Australia. Although most of them did not know each other, they decided to form an Australian society to share their ideas and establish training. They met in Adelaide in February 1981, deciding first to set up state branches.

However, even in the 1970s individual Australian health care professionals, particularly nurses, were bringing back new ideas about hospices and humane care of the terminally ill from the United Kingdom and Canada. Thus, senior nurses in the Anglican hospices in Sydney—Marion Peters, Blanche Lindsay, and Barbara Fox—tried to introduce the new approach to their institutions. Teresa Plane, a nurse proprietor of Mount Carmel, a private hospital in Sydney, funded her own small palliative care unit with medical aid from specialist physician Murray Lloyd and, later, her husband, general practitioner Carl Spencer. General practitioner Gordon Coates, brother of Alan Coates, professor of oncology at Royal Prince Alfred Hospital in Sydney, pursued palliative care in his private practice, but despite his enthusiasm, it failed to support him, and he moved away. Specialist physician Paul Laird and nurse Bethne Hart initiated a part-time, consultative service at Royal Prince Alfred, but when Laird moved to Lismore after a few years to practice, the service closed. Brian Pollard, director of anesthetics at the Repatriation Hospital in Concord, who set up one of the first palliative care consultative facilities in the country, visited Saint Christopher's Hospice in London in September 1980. Throughout 1981 he discussed plans with the medical superintendent of his hospital and taught himself more about palliative care. In May 1982 the service was becoming sufficiently large for an oncology nurse, Eileen James, to join him.

In March 1982, on the initiative of Brian Dwyer, director of anesthetics, a palliative care service was established at Saint Vincent's Hospital in Darlinghurst. Dwyer had already been working with John Woodforde for some years in the hospital's pain clinic. The Palliative Care Service was to offer consultation in symptom control for terminal cancer patients and, although having no hospital beds of its own, worked closely with the long-established Sacred Heart Hospice, which was located nearby. Jocelyn Kramer, who had worked at Saint Christopher's Hospice in London and the Palliative Care Service of the Royal Victoria Hospital in Montreal in 1982 and 1983, became a full-time resident in 1984. By 1985 the Palliative Care Service doctors were involved in combined hospital rounds with the director of radiation oncology and the medical oncologist (the first full-time medical oncologist was appointed in late 1983) and attended the head and neck cancer clinic, the oncology team meeting, and the surgical oncology conference every week.

Visits to Australia by Cicely Saunders and Elisabeth Kübler-Ross increased local enthusiasm and the inflow of ideas. In September 1977 Dr. Saunders presented a week of seminars and public lectures in Perth. People with backgrounds in areas of academic medicine as diverse as internal medicine, anatomy, clinical pharmacology, anesthesia, and medical oncology became committed to changing the way terminal care was provided. In 1974 Albert Baikie, founding professor of medicine at the University of Tasmania, initiated multidisciplinary instruction in the care of the dying. In the late 1970s F. W. Gunz, hematologist and director of medical research at the Kanematsu Institute of Sydney Hospital, became interested in palliative care and set out to bring together like-minded people from around the country to advance the cause. He initiated the organizational process in September 1981 by holding a meeting to establish the Palliative Care Association of New South Wales. David Allbrook, professor of anatomy at the University of Western Australia, had been in contact with Saint Christopher's Hospice in London in the 1970s. He later played a significant role in New South Wales (NSW) as director of palliative services in the Hunter Valley region.

In 1982 Allbrook, Gunz, and Gordon Coates (vice president of the Palliative Care Association of New South Wales) each wrote a leading article on hospice and palliative care in the November issue of the *Medical Journal of Australia:* Allbrook on the doctor's role in the Australian hospice movement; Gunz on hospices in Australia; and Coates on the concept of palliative care (Pollard, n.d., 3–4; Coates, 1982, 503; Gunz, 1982, 501; Allbrook, 1982, 502; Cavenagh and Gunz, 1988, 51–52; Oliver, 1992, 9–13; Lickiss, 1993, 388; Dalley and Hickie, 2000, 437–40).

It was no accident that it was Sydney anesthetists Brian Pollard and Brian Dwyer who established palliative care consultative services in major teaching hospitals in the early 1980s. Pollard has stated that he faced much skepticism from heads of other departments at his hospital and that they were highly dubious that an anesthetist had anything of value to teach real doctors about patient care. As discussed in the chapter on pain control, cancer pain management had for a long time been of concern to anesthetists. The Australian Pain Society came to be usefully complementary in this area of palliative medicine.

Cancer medicine specialists were also calling for better palliative care in teaching hospitals. Trevor Malden and others from Royal Prince Alfred Hospital concluded a 1984 report on factors influencing where cancer patients died by pointing out that a substantial number still died in major hospitals and that therefore improvement of palliative care services in these institutions was as important as progress in services elsewhere. In 1985 the service at Royal Prince Alfred was reorganized with the creation of an inpatient hospice unit and, later, a community consultative service serving central Sydney. This was the first of a new model of palliative care that developed throughout the country.

F. W. Gunz was a particularly important medical pioneer. As mentioned earlier, the New South Wales Palliative Care Association had been inaugurated with him as president. He recognized from the outset that a balance had to be struck between the ideal of hospice and political and economic realities. By the third meeting, in early February 1982, the association had drawn up a constitution. Inspired by Gunz, the group immediately began raising funds for research. Among others, he invited the director of the State Cancer Registry, Joyce Ford, to the first meeting of the association's research committee. He pointed out the need for more information on where people died and for research on the quality of life of the dying (before 1982 very little research had been done on this issue).

The association's education committee held its first seminar in June 1982 at Concord Repatriation Hospital. The following year the committee prepared papers on palliative care in medical and nursing education. At the second annual general meeting, Eric Wilkes, professor of palliative care at Sheffield and medical director of Saint Luke's Hospice, was guest speaker. The educational mission of the association progressed further in April 1984, when it sponsored a conference on education concerning the care of the dying. Opened by the NSW minister of health, this meeting was attended by doctors, administrators, and academics from all of the states.

Gunz also pursued the cause of palliative care at the Commonwealth level. When the federal health department said in 1983 that it would not recognize palliative care as a separate area of medicine, he assembled working parties to look at the key issues of personnel, teaching, and funding. In November, a paper drawing on their work and titled "The Role of the Doctor in the Provision of Palliative Care" was completed and distributed to all relevant government departments.

Having consulted with doctors from throughout Australia at the association's 1984 conference on education regarding the care of the dying, Gunz pressed for the creation of a national body. All of the states agreed to establish the Affiliation of Australian Palliative Care/Hospice Programmes. This was a loose federation that Gunz saw as a means of developing a national policy. The administrative office was at first in New South Wales but moved to Victoria in 1986. One of the first achievements of the organization was the adoption by the Australian Council of Hospital Standards of provision for special facilities for the dying as a condition of the accreditation of large hospitals. In 1990 the Australian Association for Hospice and Palliative Care, a multidisciplinary body, was formed. Three years later the Australian and New Zealand Society of Palliative Medicine (ANZSPM) was established. It occupies the ground between the multidisciplinary bodies and medicine's Royal Australasian College of Physicians.

When, at the end of 1985, Gunz discovered that the New South Wales Cancer Council was to be reconstituted, he persuaded its director, Elaine Henry, to establish a committee on patient care as one of its new groups. This set up its own subcommittee on palliative care, and Gunz served as the chair of both committees. From this development came grants for nurses and doctors to assist them in obtaining advanced education in palliative care. Ever busy in the cause of the care of the dying, at his death in 1990 Gunz was concerned with two issues—ways to achieve accountability for the use of Medicare incentive funds and ways to overcome the lack of interest in palliative care in the New South Wales Department of Health, a position that contrasted markedly with that found in other states (Pollard, n.d, 1–4; Gunz, 1982, 501; Cavenagh and Gunz, 1988, 52–53; Lickiss, 1993, 389; Maddocks, 1994, 670; Pollard, interview by Lewis, 1998).

In November 1985 the caucus of Labor members of the federal parliament established a working group, chaired by Wendy Fatin, on hospice and palliative care. Dr. Neal Blewett, federal health minister, and Dr. Ric Charlesworth, a physician, were members. The group explored the questions of whether hospice should be based in the community, hospitals, or nursing homes and the respective roles of the Commonwealth and the states. Although in 1985 Blewett had not been eager to fund anything having to do with palliative care, by mid-1987 he was ready to have Commonwealth-state Medicare agreements amended to include home and coordination services in hospice and palliative care. This change appears to have been produced by pressure to fund the care of AIDS patients because, as Blewett himself recognized, if this were to be done, the community would demand the funding of the care of non-AIDS patients as well.

In 1988 the Commonwealth Labor government provided funds—$37.8 million over five years—to the states under the Medicare agreements for projects aimed at improving palliative care, particularly that available in the home. While this might have been intended in part to contain rising hospital costs, it had the effect of widening access to palliative care. Unlike in the United States under the Medicare benefit, there was no criterion concerning an expected prognosis of fewer than six months for participation. Every patient could access community nursing (supported by public funds) for a small fee or without payment. The palliative care services were mostly without cost.

The 1987 Victorian parliamentary inquiry into dying with dignity recomended, among other things, that education in palliative care be included in professional development programs provided for all health care professionals. The 1988 Commonwealth inquiry into medical education also recognized that universities should educate medical interns in the care of patients suffering from advanced diseases.

By the late 1970s and early 1980s, a number of the larger faculties of medicine were already aware of this responsibility. Flinders, Sydney, and Newcastle appointed staff members at the level of professor or associate professor, and in the early 1990s the University of New South Wales followed suit. The College of General Practitioners took on the responsibility of educating general practitioners who needed new skills to care for their own terminal patients or to act as consultants to home hospice programs. The Royal Australasian College of Physicians (RACP) established training in palliative medicine, and in 1989 the Medical Oncology Group of Australia sponsored a national conference with the theme of palliative care in the 1990s. In large city hospitals, it was not uncommon in the early 1990s for consultant physicians to head palliative care services or to act as palliative care consultants. Besides the developments in undergraduate medical education in the 1980s and the early 1990s, an interdisciplinary master's program was established at Flinders University in Adelaide, and a training program was introduced by the Institute of Palliative Medicine in Sydney (Lickiss, 1989, 28; Oliver, 1992, 45–46; Lickiss, 1993, 389; Kasap and Associates, 1996, ix).

By the 1990s various inquiries into medical education had revealed a need for more attention to palliative care in the curriculum. The ANZSPM began developing an Australasian Undergraduate Medical Palliative Care Curriculum. With Prof. Michael Ashby (Monash University, Melbourne) as convener and Dr. Mary Brooksbank (Adelaide), Dr. Paul Dunne (Tasmania), and Dr. Rod MacLeod (Wellington) as members, the ANZSPM committee produced a core curriculum in late 1996 that would ensure that graduating students were aware of the basic principles of caring for the dying: pain control, common symptom management, communication, family support, ethics, decision making, grief and bereavement, multidisciplinary teamwork, and emotional care of the self.

The committee also identified a number of core values to be discussed with students: the best possible pain and symptom relief as a patient's right and a doctor's duty; dying as a natural part of life; loss and bereavement as integral to one's life; the concept that the time of dying is as valuable as the rest of one's life; the patient's needs as the basis of care (rather than a collection of medically defined body systems); the concept that negotiated symptom relief does not constitute causing death; and the understanding that care is focused on the individual, but bereavement support should be offered to family and friends (Ashby, Brooksbank, Dunne, and MacLeod, 1996, 1–6). In 1997 Prof. Peter Ravenscroft, president of the ANZSPM, attended meetings of the education committee of the National Cancer Advisory Committee, which was assessing undergraduate teaching on cancer care in medical schools. He saw to it that the survey of teaching included questions on palliative care and presented a copy of the ANZSPM Palliative Care Curriculum to the committee for use in devising a national cancer curriculum (*ANZSPM Newsletter,* 1998, 2).

Representatives of the ANZSPM, the Royal Australian College of General Practitioners (RACGP), and the Australian Council of Rural and Remote Medicine (ACRRM) came together in 2000 to discuss ways to assist general practitioners (who care for most dying patients) to provide better palliative care. They developed the Joint Position Statement on Palliative Medicine in General Practice, which was then approved by the RACGP, the Royal New Zealand College of General Practitioners, and the ACRRM. Included was a proposal for a clinical degree in palliative medicine similar to the degree in obstetrics developed by the Colleges of General Practitioners and the Royal Australian and New Zealand College of Gynecologists (*ANZSPM Newsletter,* 2000b, 1; 2000–2001, 2).

The New Zealand branch of the ANZSPM did much to promote palliative care education in New Zealand through its annual conferences and workshops. By 2000 it had 58 members, and in 2001 the total membership was 272. In September 2001 the Chapter of Palliative Medicine of the RACP was accepted in New Zealand law as a specialty group, and fellows of the chapter could then apply for specialty status (*ANZSPM Newsletter,* 2000a, 1; 2001a, 3).

Some pioneers of palliative care education in Australasia have already been identified. Others included Douglas MacAdam, who came from England in 1980 to accept a lectureship with the University of Western Australia Faculty of Medicine. There MacAdam established a unit on palliative medicine in the Department of Community Practice; last-year students learned about symptom control, visited a dying patient, and drew up a care plan. In 1985 the Cancer Foundation created the country's first senior lectureship in palliative care, and the director of the palliative care unit at the Hollywood Repatriation General Hospital in Perth, Rosalie Shaw (just as Cicely Saunders, a nurse before she became a doctor), occupied the position part-time from 1986 to 1988. Unhappily, her hospital would not give her specialist status, and faculty support was not strong.

MacAdam followed her in the lectureship, and the Department of Community Practice sponsored workshops for health professionals in 1985 and 1986. Derek Doyle, medical director of Saint Columba's Hospice in Edinburgh, was the keynote speaker in 1986. The Hospice Support Organization (later the Western Australian Association for Palliative Care/Hospice Programmes) sponsored the workshops in 1987. In the 1990s the Edith Cowan University in Perth appointed a nurse researcher as professor of palliative care, and this fostered the growth of Perth as a significant center for research and for efforts to advance the standard of practice, such as the development of the recent guidelines for palliative care in residential, aged-care facilities.

The efforts of pioneers of postgraduate education are more recent. In 1988 Flinders University in Adelaide established the first chair of palliative care in Australia, which was occupied by Ian Maddocks. A multidisciplinary course leading to a diploma, or master's degree, was established, and in 1992, 45 students were enrolled. Distance learning enabled doctors and nurses in remote areas to participate in the challenging course.

Similar developments were occurring in other cities. The University of Melbourne established a postgraduate degree in 1996 and a chair in palliative medicine. Chairs were also created in the 1990s at Monash and La Trobe universities. In 2003 the University of Queensland appointed a professor of palliative care. A chair in palliative medicine was then established at the University of Newcastle.

In the late 1980s the Sydney Institute of Palliative Medicine, established by Norelle Lickiss, head of palliative care services at Royal Prince Alfred Hospital, a teaching hospital of the University of Sydney, provided clinical training for doctors. It was then incorporated into the curriculum at the Prince of Wales Hospital, a teaching hospital of the University of New South Wales. There it met the training needs of various groups—those preparing for certification by the Royal Australasian College of Physicians; those preparing for the institute's own certificate; those training in family medicine; and international fellows. Three training contexts were available—inpatient units, hospital consultancy, and community consultancy (Oliver, 1992, 64–65; Maddocks and Donnell, 1992, 317–19; Lickiss, 2005, 5–10).

Growth of Services in Australia

In Victoria, the Sisters of Charity had opened a mainly inpatient hospice service, Caritas Christi Hospice, in the 1930s. The Little Company of Mary Hospital (formerly Bethlehem Hospital) offered some terminal care in 1964, and in 1982 it became an inpatient 46-bed hospice.

In the late 1970s interest in home-based services developed. In 1981, with grants from the W. K. Kellogg Foundation in the United States and the Commonwealth government, the Melbourne City Mission Hospice program was launched. The dual program involved home care hospice and a 10-bed inpatient facility at the Harold McCracken Nursing Home in Fitzroy. At the same time, the first extrametropolitan home care program, located in the provincial city of Geelong, opened its doors.

A 1985 ministerial committee on cancer services, chaired by Prof. R. Lovell, accepted a proposal by the oncology subcommittee of the Victorian Anti-Cancer Council that regionalized palliative care units be established in all large metropolitan and provincial hospitals. Between 1983 and 1985 five home care programs had already been established in Melbourne, and two small inpatient programs in extrametropolitan areas.

By 1989, there were 16 hospice programs in the state, of which only 4 were run by organizations specifically designed to provide hospice care. Besides these 16, home care services in Melbourne were offered by the Royal District Nursing Service (RDNS) and the Visiting Nursing Service (VNS) of the Peter MacCallum Cancer Institute. In 1950 the latter had begun assisting outpatients and potential patients. The RDNS had been a provider of home terminal care (along with other care) in Melbourne since 1885.

The Victorian Health Minister endorsed the following propositions in a policy statement of 1987: that all terminally ill Victorians with six months or less to live should have access to palliative care; no more independent hospices would be established, and palliative care should be developed in hospitals; regional, home-based systems should be developed; an identified doctor should coordinate any multidisciplinary care team; and all health care professionals should receive postgraduate education and training in palliative care.

As a result of the statement, the Palliative Care Council was set up by the minister, David White, in May 1988 to monitor the development of services, advise the minister of health, and act as a forum for the discussion of issues. The speedy growth of facilities in Victoria was supported by Commonwealth funding from 1988 to 1989. Under the Medicare Incentive Package, $6.6 million was approved from 1988 to 1989 for palliative care facilities and other postacute community services (mainly home nursing). Funding was guaranteed under the Medicare agreements in the early 1990s. In mid-1995 a Palliative Care Task Force appointed by the Victorian government reviewed the state's palliative care provision. Four subcommittees were created to implement the task force's recommendations concerning the integration of services, quality assurance and accreditation, cultural issues in Australia's multicultural society, and the promotion of community and professional education (Cavenagh and Gunz, 1988, 53–54; Bird, Humphries, and Howe, 1990, 2–6, 121; Kasap and Associates, 1996, 9).

In the late 1970s various groups were discussing the establishment of a hospice in Perth. Anglican Archbishop Geoffrey Sambell supported the idea of a church-run hospice, while the Anglican Homes Incorporated explored the need for such a service. The Christian Medical Fellowship sponsored the 1978 visit of Reg Luxton, a retired consultant who was involved in the British hospice movement. Prof. David Allbrook played a key role in the fellowship and the Perth hospice group that was formed in 1980 to promote the establishment of a hospice. He won the support of the Western Australian Cancer Council for the idea after the Anglican Homes withdrew from the project.

In 1980 the Cancer Council commissioned Dr. David Frey to carry out a feasibility study on hospice. He recommended a three-year pilot home hospice program, and this was begun in Perth in mid-1982. The part-time medical director, Douglas MacAdam, a medical academic and ordained minister of the Uniting Church of Australia, who had worked in hospices in England, recommended that the Silver Chain Nursing Association (the only comprehensive home nursing body in Perth) be involved. While only 28 percent of cancer deaths in Western Australia in 1981 took place outside hospitals, the decision was made to establish a home care service. The Hospice Palliative Care Service (HPCS) was the offspring of the Cancer Council and the Silver Chain Nursing Association, and it received funding from the state health department. To allay any concerns of general practitioners about encroachment, the HPCS took patients only on referral from a general practitioner or hospital doctor. The patient's spiritual needs were met, if expressed, by Father John Ryan, Roman Catholic chaplain at Royal Perth Hospital, who acted simply as a minister of the Christian Church unless the patient was a Catholic.

By the mid-1980s the service covered the whole metropolitan area. It had promoted considerable change in patients' place of death, with more than 60 percent of those admitted to the service now dying at home. As a backup, inpatient beds were made available, at first in a private hospital. A larger palliative care unit was established at an acute care hospital. In 1987 a cottage hospice was opened so that patients thereafter had a complete range of services available. In December 1993 the State Planning Committee on Palliative Care presented its report to Western Australia's commissioner of health. In addition, a working party of the Western Australia Hospice Palliative Care Association, in collaboration with the state health department, produced a report on palliative care that would extend to 2001. The reports provided a basis for the organization of services to the beginning of the new millennium (*Care of the Terminally Ill,* 1986, 33–35; Cavenagh and Gunz, 1988, 53; Oliver, 1992, 13–21; Kasap and Associates, 1996, 10).

In 1964 the Mary Potter Home for the Dying, Calvary Hospital, Adelaide, was at the forefront of hospice development in south Australia. The Royal District Nursing Service of South Australia and the State Cancer Foundation were also pioneers in the provision of terminal care. Indeed, since the 1890s, in south Australia, as in other states from around the same time, district nursing had provided home care for the aged and chronically ill (and thus terminal) patients. However, in the late 1970s, district nurses became more conscious of their role as hospice care professionals. In 1985 the South Australian Health Commission published a "Hospice Care Policy," pledging its support for improvement in services. The Flinders Medical Center, a major Adelaide teaching hospital, had a palliative care team, and its members had access to inpatient beds at Kalyra Hospital. It also ran an outreach program.

In the early 1990s, as a result of the inquiry of the South Australian parliament into laws and practices concerning death and dying, the minister of health was to prepare an annual report on the care of the dying in that state. Areas of ongoing concern identified in the later 1990s were the following: rural areas lacking designated palliative care professionals; nursing homes with insufficient resources to provide adequate palliative care; and private hospitals requiring better links with community and specialist palliative care services.

By the 1990s New South Wales offered palliative care services in every region, rural and urban. A health department discussion paper of the period made a commitment to equity and universal access, as well as continuity of care. Emphasis would be placed on better cooperation between hospital and community services, on enhanced community services, and on promotion of the cause of palliative care in mainstream health care. Deficiencies included too few medical and nursing consultants to advise general practitioners and community nurses who were caring for home care patients. Considerable difference existed between palliative care services—some were narrow in focus, whereas others, like that at Royal Prince Alfred Hospital, provided inpatient beds in the acute hospital and the hospice unit, as well as consultation services in various settings (e.g., wards, emergency departments, nursing homes, clinics, family homes).

In Brisbane, Mount Olivet Hospital, which was run by the Sisters of Charity, pioneered palliative care in the 1950s. More recently, it had established connections with Brisbane teaching hospitals. In the 1990s the Queensland Cancer Fund assisted with the introduction of services at the Mater Hospital in Brisbane and also in the northern provincial city of Townsville. Hospital outreach programs were the means by which community services developed in this state, but privately insured patients did not have access to home care funded by public hospitals. The pain management expertise of pain clinics at the Royal Brisbane Hospital, Princess Alexandra Hospital, and Greenslopes Repatriation Hospital was particularly valuable in the absence of proper palliative care services in hospitals until the 1990s.

As in the other states in the same decade, the health authorities and palliative care experts in Queensland worked together to produce a statewide plan for adequately resourced provision of palliative care. In Tasmania, in addition to designated palliative care services, community and clinical services were available through oncology units. The Repatriation Hospital in Hobart offered an inpatient unit, while two private hospitals provided inpatient care when called upon to do so. Also in the 1990s Tasmanian health authorities were busy planning the delivery of palliative care services on a regional basis (Cavenagh and Gunz, 1988, 54–55; Lickiss, 1993, 390–92; Kasap and Associates, 1996, 9–10).

By the early 1990s, as one well-informed observer has noted, palliative care was becoming part of mainstream health care. Although a Christian orientation marked some of the well-established facilities, there had also been a strong growth in "secular" services funded by public monies. Thus inpatient facilities ranged from those in which, at a minimum, patients needed to be comfortable with a religious ambience, where procedures such as blood transfusions and the intravenous administration of antibiotics were not commonly carried out, and where people normally came to die; to busy urban hospital-based units from which religion (but not necessarily spirituality) was absent, patients were not well known, the attitude toward interventions was flexible, and a large percentage were discharged in order to return home (Lickiss, 1993, 393).

During the five years of Commonwealth funding beginning in 1988, more than $37.8 million went to support 86 projects chosen through priorities set by the states and territories. In the financial year 1993–1994, Commonwealth funding for the Palliative Care Program (PCP) was renewed, and $55 million was made available for a period of four years. The continued funding enabled the following to be achieved: extension of services to communities not previously able to access them; daily provision of services 24 hours per day in some areas; both community and hospital-based medical and nursing consultancies; inpatient beds in hospitals previously lacking designated beds; statewide programs for education, evaluation, and provision of information (for clinicians and the public); and national projects on a range of service infrastructure and delivery issues.

In mid-1998 the federal coalition minister for health and family services, Dr. Michael Wooldridge, launched the National Strategy for Palliative Care in Australia 1998–2003. He promised the Commonwealth would commit $10 million during this period to fund national activities such as the development of performance indicators, as well as education and research on palliative care services, and to support the work of the national organization, Palliative Care Australia, formerly the Australian Association for Hospice and Palliative Care (Kasap and Associates, 1996, ix–xv; Media Release, 1998, 1).

In the United States, the Institute of Medicine published a report in 1997 on improving care at the end of life. The report proposed a "mixed management" model of care that involved the continuation of efforts to extend life while at the same time preparing for death and comforting both the patient and family. The model has considerable implications for palliative care practice in Australia, which has historically been provided in hospices or at home for people with advanced cancer who were no longer receiving curative treatment. The IOM report recognizes the need to institute palliative care at an earlier stage; thus the specialist in palliative medicine will have to possess greater knowledge of the natural history and the choice of treatments for a range of ultimately fatal diseases such as end-organ failure, Alzheimer's disease, HIV/AIDS, and other diseases in addition to cancer (Glare and Lickiss, 2000, 453).

Paul Glare and Stephen Clarke, palliative care physician and medical oncologist, respectively, at the Royal Prince Alfred Hospital (RPAH) in Sydney, have identified three historical models of palliative care: (1) in the 1960s and 1970s, the sequential model, in which oncology and palliative care are clearly separated and palliative care enters only when treatment options have been exhausted; its disadvantages were median survival of only a few weeks, with no time for the patient and family to prepare for death, limited access to palliative care (in Britain in the 1980s only 20 percent of those dying from cancer received palliative care), and insufficient access to other specialties; (2) from the 1980s to the early 2000s, the concurrent model, which flourishes where specialist palliative care services exist and in which palliative care personnel have some training in oncology and can communicate with oncologists from the time of diagnosis. This is the case at the RPAH palliative care service, where about 30 percent of patients are still receiving disease-controlling treatment and the median survival is two months. The disadvantages of this model are that oncology still dominates the earlier stages and palliative care the later ones, and the latter is not involved in cancer treatment planning.

The mixed-management model was proposed by the Institute of Medicine to rectify problems in the United States, where specialist palliative care services have not flourished but community-based hospice teams, usually a nurse and a social worker with almost no medical input, have, and these follow the old, sequential model, with the result that median survival is three weeks. The latest model assumes that (a) patients want disease control and concurrent palliative care irrespective of prognosis; (b) treatments are often arbitrarily distinguished as preventive, curative, rehabilitative, and palliative (for example, bisphosphonates to prevent fractures, treat hypercalcemia, and relieve pain); (c) end-of-life care should not be provided only by palliative care specialists and palliative medicine should not be recognized as a specialty; rather, all clinicians should be trained in the specifics of symptom control, psychosocial support, and disease-controlling treatments so that the two-phase structure of the first two models disappears.

While a small number of Australian practitioners become qualified in medical oncology and palliative care, Glare and Clarke do not see this as heralding the beginning of the mixed-management model in Australia. In the foreseeable future, oncology and palliative care there will remain distinct, which is all the more reason for the interface to be maintained by good communication and an exchange of ideas (Glare and Clarke, 2002, 6–8).

Implicit in the proposed model is the idea of palliative care as an adjunct rather than an alternative to other specialties. The approach of palliative care may then creatively permeate other areas of medicine, and especially geriatrics, because it submits that each patient is unique, everyone dies, comfort and happiness are very important, there are many unmeasurable adverse consequences of medical treatments, and caregivers have an ability to treat without excessively diagnosing (Maddocks, 1999, 64; Goodwin, 1999, 1283).

New Zealand

Hospice principles and practices were introduced to New Zealand in Wellington through the work of the Community Health Nursing Service (CHNS), the Mary Potter Hospice, the Te Omanga Hospice, and the Wellington Division of the Cancer Society of New Zealand. In 1968 the Community Domiciliary Nursing Trust provided home nursing for terminally ill cancer patients. Seven years later the Calvary Hospital dedicated five beds for such patients in the Mary Potter ward, from which the Mary Potter Hospice developed in 1979. In 1976 the first oncology nurse was appointed by the Wellington Hospital board, and by 1981 the CHNS had three such nurses. Two years later the CHNS introduced a "cancer phone service," which became a source of referrals, and it worked closely with local district nurses, general practitioners, hospitals, and hospices. One year later the community-based Te Omanga Hospice opened in the Hutt Valley.

With hospice services proliferating, Wellington Hospital's Department of Radiotherapy and Oncology, supported by the Cancer Society, proposed the development of a regional policy on the care of the dying. A working group, created in 1981, made recommendations for services: both citizens and health professionals needed to be better informed about services; hospital staff needed education in the hospice approach; more public funds should be advanced for both community and institutional services; and palliative care was integral to the health services as prevention and cure (*Care of the Terminally Ill,* 1981, 1–31).

Local pressure coming from the community and various professionals shaped the development of services, so that by 2000, provision varied widely among areas—from 0.64 inpatient beds per 100,000 population in the Waikato to 7.73 in Wellington, with the national average at 4.03 (compared with 5.1 in Britain). Of

37 services in New Zealand, only 19 had inpatient beds, and there were only four hospital units in the country. Most of the work was done in the community by general practitioners and community nurses who could consult with hospital services. Maori and Pacific Islanders and all those who were suffering from nonmalignant conditions (90 percent of recipients were cancer patients) suffered from a lack of access to services.

In 1992 the New Zealand government began a process of central planning, having received a report from the core health and disability support services committee of the Ministry of Health, which recommended that regional health authorities give priority to hospice service development. In 1993 the ministry received the report of a consensus forum on hospice and palliative care services. Composed of people experienced in palliative care, the forum made recommendations similar to those in many other countries: services must be available to everyone in need; people should be referred early; services ought to be free; and the family, as well as the patient, should be the focus of care.

In 1998 the National Advisory Committee on Health and Disability, in the face of failure to advance the provision of, and access to, services, formed a working group on the care of the dying. The next year the Health Ministry and Health Funding Authority, assisted by an expert group, began to work on a five-to-ten-year strategy for the development of palliative care services. In 2000 a discussion document was distributed to stakeholders, and a consultative process, involving written submissions and public meetings, was completed.

In 2001 the government released the national palliative care strategy, which aimed to build on existing services and to establish two interlinked levels of care throughout the country; it also aspired to set up specialist services with links to both regional cancer centers and local centers provided by each of 21 district health boards. The main political parties endorsed this more equitable system.

The first initiatives were to be the development of units for assessment and care coordination and specifications for existing services; a review of support services by the Department of Social Services; development by each district health board of a plan to coordinate services; encouragement of specialist services in teaching hospitals able to advise on care, education of local providers, cooperation with cancer centers and other specialist services, the advancement of research in the region; development of hospital units; and education of the community about palliative care. The government would fund essential clinical services, but hospices would still use the labor of volunteers and work with donated funds (The New Zealand Palliative Care Strategy, 2001, 1, 34–37; MacLeod, 2001, 71–73).

Opportunities for professional education and career advancement increased in this period. Hospice New Zealand, the national organization promoting hospice and palliative care, published *Standards for the Provision of Hospice and Palliative Care* and *Guidelines for Nurses in Palliative Care*. It also worked with the New Zealand Nurses Organization to develop a career path for hospice nurses. More than 25 fellows of the Chapter of Palliative Medicine of the Royal Australasian College of Physicians work in New Zealand, and about half of them are full time in palliative care.

The Australia and New Zealand Society for Palliative Medicine introduced a curriculum for medical students, but the development of academic positions in the country's two clinical schools has been slow. In late 2002 the University of Otago announced that it would be establishing the South Link Health Chair in Palliative Medicine, the first chair in New Zealand. Another area just beginning to receive attention is services for dying children. With 29 percent of child deaths occurring in hospitals, many children spend a long time in the care of a hospital team. New Zealand's small population—3.8 million—means the provision of quality care throughout the country may always be difficult as teams outside large urban centers struggle to build up the requisite expertise (MacLeod, 2001, 73; MacLeod, 2002, 1–2; Otago Unveils Innovative Campaign to Advance as a World-Class University, 2002).

Canada

A study of palliative care in Canada has found that, in various ways, it is similar to care in Britain, Australia, and Ireland (Gaudette, Lipskie, Allard, and Fainsinger, 2002). In Canada 92 percent of patients had cancer; in Britain and Ireland, more than 90 percent, and in Australia, 70–90 percent. The median length of stay (LOS) for each care episode was 13 days in Canada, although it varied from 7 in a dedicated unit to 54 in chronic care settings. Care was available in acute wards, dedicated units, tertiary care and chronic care settings, and at home. In the United Kingdom and Australia, the LOS averaged 13–15 days for each inpatient episode but 10–26 in Canadian inpatient settings. Where 46 percent in Canada were discharged at death and 26 percent to home, in Australia 46 percent of hospital patients were discharged at death and 43 percent to home.

The Canadian senate's 2000 report on quality end-of-life care stated that palliative care was the right of every citizen, but fewer than 5 percent of dying people received such treatment. Access for urban cancer patients had improved: in Edmonton in 1992 and 1993, 22 percent saw a team, in 1996 and 1997, 82 percent did so; in Halifax, 36 percent of terminal cancer patients were in a palliative care program, but only 14 percent elsewhere in Nova Scotia were seen (ibid., 1–10).

Palliative care began in Canada in the mid-1970s, as noted earlier. In late 1974 the first palliative care unit, under the direction of Paul Henteleff, opened at Saint Boniface Hospital in Winnipeg. The Sisters of Charity of Montreal, the Grey Nuns, had established the hospital in 1871 in what was then a frontier district of Manitoba. The hospital, with more than 500 beds, is affiliated with the University of Manitoba and is the second largest in the province, serving the people of Manitoba, northwestern Ontario, and parts of Saskatchewan. Reviewing the development of this unit a decade or so after its inauguration, Henteleff noted that palliative care in Canada was inspired by the hospice movement in England and identified Elisabeth Kübler-Ross and Cicely Saunders as the two great advocates of modern care of the dying. He also stated that the unit could not provide for everyone with cancer and only rarely took noncancer patients.

In January 1975 the second palliative care unit, under the direction of Balfour Mount, was opened at Royal Victoria Hospital in Montreal. With 800 beds, this hospital is a teaching hospital of McGill University. In Canada, "palliative" is the descriptor of hospice care and was first employed at the Royal Victoria Hospital so that Francophones, who differ from Anglophones in their notion of "hospice," would not misunderstand the modern concept. Further, the palliative care unit in Canada evolved within an acute care hospital context, enjoying the same autonomy as an intensive care or coronary care unit. This model has involved physician leadership and close relations with oncology from the outset; thus "care" and "cure" have closely interacted.

Establishment of the 13-bed unit at Royal Victoria and the 22-bed unit at Saint Boniface Hospital was followed by the January 1979 opening of a 15-bed unit in the Salvation Army Grace Hospital, a chronic care institution in central Toronto; in May, a 12-bed unité de soins palliatifs at the Hôpital Notre-Dame, an 800-bed teaching hospital of the Université de Montreal; and in November, a 10-bed unit at Saint Clare Mercy Hospital, Saint John's, Newfoundland, a 325-bed teaching hospital of Memorial University. Only in April 1980 was the first independent hospice opened. La Maison de Sillery in Quebec was funded by the provincial branch of the Canadian Cancer Society. It was directed by oncologist Louis Dionne and affiliated with the Hôtel-Dieu de Québec, a Laval University teaching hospital (Scott, 1981, 176–78; Henteleff, 1986, 81–82; MacDonald, 1998b, 1710).

The origins of the Royal Victoria unit may be traced to an invitation in 1973 to some members of the hospital staff to talk on death and dying at a local church. Those invited decided to go beyond anecdotes, and they set up an ad hoc committee on thanatology to study the needs of dying patients, identify deficiencies in care, and look for ways to remedy these. Health care professionals, clergy, and some terminally ill people were surveyed. The committee found that there were serious inadequacies in care and that staff members were ignorant of the suffering of both patients and families.

Balfour Mount has recorded how he saw the similarities between the findings and Elisabeth Kübler-Ross's list of deficiencies in hospital care discussed in her classic, On Death and Dying (1969), and those he had encountered when a cancer patient himself. Having noted her references to the work of Cicely Saunders, he arranged to spend a week at Saint Christopher's in London. This visit had a life-transforming impact on him. He was deeply impressed by the following aspects of care at Saint Christopher's—pain relief in individually optimized doses of opioids; management of bowel obstruction; the atmosphere of peace and security; the skilled and caring staff; attention to the needs of families; concern with psychosocial and spiritual matters; competence in home care; respect for what the patients and families themselves taught; and the integral role of teaching and research. He believed that in Canada the provision of hospice for all those who were then dying in institutions would be prohibitively expensive.

Saunders was doubtful, but Mount felt confident the quality care at Saint Christopher's could be provided in a large, acute care hospital. He later identified the advantages of his marriage of hospice and hospital: the proximity of palliative care and acute care units may mutually encourage improvements in care; the need to build costly independent facilities would be obviated; it would be possible to use existing resources such as radiation therapy for palliation; and the hospital would be able to show it could care for those in the terminal stage of life, as well as every other stage.

The board of the Royal Victoria agreed to a two-year trial of the proposed unit. The gamble was considerable since the hospital had built its international reputation on the quality of scientific medicine practiced there. In addition to inpatient facilities, the unit had a home care program, a consultation team, and a bereavement follow-up group. As at the Saint Boniface Hospital unit, the initial focus was on cancer patients. Research and teaching (in McGill's medical, nursing, and social work schools) were integral to the work of the unit, as were the services of volunteers. When a centralized oncology department was developed in 1991 to serve all of the institutions affiliated with McGill, Palliative Care McGill was designated one of its divisions so that the quality of care could be standardized throughout the hospitals. It came to embrace programs in 10 hospitals and in the community (Mount, 1997, 73–84; Wilson, Ajemian, and Mount, 1978, 3–19).

The multidisciplinary Canadian Palliative Care Association began to promote the cause of service development, research, and education in the early 1980s, organizing two national congresses and launching a journal. However, financial problems forced it into inactivity. In 1987, when only three provincial associations existed, an attempt was made to revive the national organization. In 1990 the first Canadian Palliative Care Directory was produced on the initiative of the Royal Victoria Hospital Palliative Care Services. The following year the Canadian Palliative Care Association (CPCA) was formally inaugurated, and in 1993 it was incorporated. By the mid-1990s it had a membership of 250 individuals, provincial associations, and affiliate members such as the Canadian Society of Palliative Care Physicians.

In 1998, with the assistance of the GlaxoWellcome Foundation, the CPCA mounted an educational campaign, producing pamphlets, a guide for family physicians, and one for caregivers. In that year, the first National Hospice Palliative Care Week was launched by the honorary patron of the CPCA, Her Excellency Mme. Diana Fowler-Le Blanc. In 2003 another awareness-raising event, the National Hike for Hospice Palliative Care, was initiated by the CPCA, which in 2001 was known as the Canadian Hospice Palliative Care Association (CHPCA) in recognition of the fact that hospice and palliative care had ceased to be seen as separate matters.

After a decade of work, in 2002 the CHPCA produced *A Model to Guide Hospice Palliative Care: Based on the National Principles and Norms of Practice,* which spelled out nationally accepted practice norms. In 1989 Ottawa University and the University of Alberta offered one-year palliative medicine fellowships. However, at the end of the 1990s, medical education in palliative care remained underdeveloped. The Canadian Committee on Palliative Care education produced a common curriculum in 1991, and an accompanying textbook, edited by Neil Macdonald, was published in 1998. However, none of the 16 medical schools had fully introduced the curriculum. Dr. Macdonald told the Special Senate Committee on Euthanasia and Assisted Suicide inquiry of the mid-1990s that part of the problem was that medical academics tended to regard palliative care research and education as lacking in academic rigor. Another problem was the continuing isolation of many programs from mainstream medical care and their focus on a particular group of patients—cancer sufferers. He wanted to see palliative care more integrated into disease control programs. Thus, cancer control should have four phases—prevention of occurrence (for example, quit smoking campaigns); prevention of invasive cancer (for example, PAP tests); prevention of death or severe morbidity (surgery, radiotherapy, and chemotherapy); and prevention of suffering (palliative care).

The Canadian Senate Committee's inquiry into euthanasia and assisted suicide discussed palliative care and in its report said that palliative care reflected a return to person-centered medical care from scientific medicine's excessive concern with the disease. The committee stated that demand for services still exceeded supply and that universal access was desirable; thus, the committee concluded, palliative care should be integrated with other health services. Indeed, it should be a first priority in restructuring the health care system. National standards should be maintained, training of health professionals expanded, coordination of delivery (whether in the home, hospice, or institution) established, and research, especially into pain control and symptom relief, encouraged (*Of Life and Death,* 1995, 17–18, 23–24; Bruera, 1998, 134–35; Canadian Hospice Palliative Care Association, 2004, 1–3).

While euthanasia and physician-assisted suicide were prominent as public issues, development of comprehensive palliative care services was not. A national survey carried out in 1997 revealed that only about 50 percent of respondents knew of the existence of hospice or palliative care, and only 33 percent could accurately describe them. In 2000 the senate revisited palliative care. In mid-2000 a report titled "Quality End-of-Life Care: The Right of Every Canadian" stated that little progress had been achieved with the recommendations contained in *Of Life and Death.* The 2000 report contained a number of recommendations aimed at improving end-of-life care, including the development of a national strategy jointly by the federal and provincial governments; better access to home care; income security and job protection for caregivers; and greater support of research into palliative care issues.

In March 2001 Sen. Sharon Carstairs, leader of the government in the senate, became minister with special responsibility for palliative care and adviser to the federal minister of health. Work on a national strategy began. In June the administrative office on end-of-life and palliative care was set up within Health Canada. The previous December 24 national stakeholders had met to plan a strategy, and from this meeting emerged the Quality End-of-Life Care Coalition and a report titled "Blueprint for Action."

In March 2003 the administrative office of Health Canada convened a national action-planning workshop attended by more than 150 people, representing stakeholders such as health care professionals, federal, provincial, and territorial governments, consumers, native peoples, researchers, health charities, professional associations, advocacy groups, and nongovernmental organizations. At the workshop the following issues were explored—availability of and access to services; education of health care professionals; ethical, cultural, and spiritual matters; education of the community; research; support of families, caregivers, and significant others; and supervision.

The creation of new research capacity was begun with the appointment of Harvey Chochinov of the University of Manitoba as the first research chair in palliative medicine. He received $1.5 million in federal funds for his work at Cancer-Care Manitoba. Greater support for caregivers was provided with the introduction of a compassionate family care benefit under which, as part of the employment insurance program, a person could take a six-week leave of absence to care for a dying child, parent, or spouse. To further assist caregivers (and patients), the Canadian Virtual Hospice was made available online, providing educational resources, bulletin boards, and chat rooms (Fainsinger, 2000, S24; National Action Planning Workshop on End-of-Life Care Report, 2002, 2–3, 21; Palliative Care Week, 2003, 1–2; *Quality End-of-Life Coalition,* 2003, 1–2).

While much has been achieved in policy formation, at the grass–roots level progress has been much slower, as a study, based on mortality records for 1997 and published in 2000, has shown. It found that most Canadians, like most Americans, Britons, and Australians, died in hospitals (or in long–term care facilities): 73 percent in 1997. The study authors stated that, despite the rhetoric about moving care out of hospitals, their findings suggest, at least with respect to end-of-life care, that success has been limited. Deaths in hospitals varied from 87 percent in Quebec to 52 percent in the Northwest Territories. A substantial proportion of hospital deaths took place in special care units, where the proportion varied from 25 percent in Manitoba to 7 percent in the Northwest Territories (Heyland, Lavery, Tranmer, Shortt, and Taylor, 2000, 1–10).

OBSERVATIONS

The hospice and palliative care movement began in the United Kingdom and quickly spread to the other Anglo-Saxon countries. The original model was modified to meet local conditions and constraints. Thus, from the outset in the United States, hospice was a home- and community-based service with a comparatively small input from physicians, whereas in Britain it was a service provided in an independent institution with not only a large role for doctors but also fairly prompt recognition of palliative medicine as a medical specialty. Australia and New Zealand also accepted palliative medicine early on as an accredited area of specialist practice. In Canada the first services were hospital-based units that only later provided community services. However, in the longer run each country tended to develop a mix of independent, hospital-based, and community-based services. Moreover, by the close of the twentieth century all of these countries were developing national policies on palliative care and recognized the problem of socially and geographically uneven access to services (even if they did not always do enough about it).

At the heart of modern palliative care is effective pain management. Indeed, as I relate in the following chapter, Robert Twycross and other leading figures in palliative care have made basic contributions to clinical knowledge and practice concerning pain control. However, modern pain medicine itself has origins different from those of the palliative care movement and has to a large extent developed independently, although they share a deep concern with the patient as person and with reduction of suffering as primary goals of medicine.

5   DEVELOPMENT OF PAIN CONTROL

Effective pain control is vital in modern palliative care, even if a small number of patients, perhaps 5 percent, do not find relief. Some critics of modern medicine—Ivan Illich is a good example—have focused on its preoccupation with technology and have called for a return to greater patient responsibility, including the bearing of pain in the face of death. Yet, as the hospice movement in Britain showed from the outset, effective pain management is the key to a quality of life that allows a dignified, or even a tolerable, death. As Roy Porter has observed, effective control of pain may well be one of the more substantial, if less glamorous, triumphs of modern medicine (Porter, 1993, 1599).

LAY AND MEDICAL EXPLANATIONS OF PAIN

Pain is one aspect of the larger phenomenon of suffering. Anthropologists have spent considerable time on the cross-cultural study of explanations of suffering. At the global level, the three most important forms of explanation for, and responses to, suffering are the interpersonal, the moral, and the biomedical. Other causal ontologies are the sociopolitical (suffering results from adverse economic, social, or political conditions as, for example, in colonialism); the psychological (frustrated desires or fears cause suffering); the astrological (inauspicious alignments of planets, moon, and stars or inauspicious periods of time are responsible for suffering); and the stressor (environmental stress causes suffering).

Of the "big three," the interpersonal causal ontology in traditional societies posits spirit attack or sorcery and, in contemporary societies, abusive (or "toxic") relationships as the explanatory factor. Protective devices, counteraggression, and restitution of interpersonal relationships are the common therapeutic mechanisms.

The moral causal ontology involves ethical failure, whether by omission or commission, and transgressions of obligations. Therapy involves confession, reparation, purification, and the pursuit of behavior deemed correct by the prevailing authority. The biomedical causal ontology, as expressed in modern scientific medicine, looks to genetic defects, hormonal imbalances, diseased organs, and physiological problems as explanatory factors; in Ayurvedic or traditional Chinese medicine and complementary (or alternative) Western medicine, causes are expressed as dangerous or imbalanced bodily fluids or life forces. Cure results from the intake of recommended agents, whether modern pharmaceuticals or traditional vegetable or mineral substances. It also results from the rehabilitation of organs or damaged fibers, whether by surgery, joint manipulation and massage, or purgatives, emetics, and bloodletting.

A key question in Judeo-Christian metaphysics is, if God is both omnipotent and good, why does evil (including suffering) exist in the world? One answer is that ultimately suffering is not evil because people can learn from the experience to be morally stronger. Another answer is that given by modern science (of which biomedicine is a part). In this view suffering is divorced from the patient's personal narrative. It is essentially an accident, a random event, and thus devoid of existential meaning. It is to be dealt with pragmatically, and the aim is to relieve and cure, not to establish ultimate responsibility or to discover why a particular person is suffering. This, however, may not be satisfactory for the individual patient who wants to make sense of a very intense, personal experience, even more so if that person has a terminal illness.

In Western culture, we have historically tended to move between polar extremes in our explanation of suffering. At one extreme, the sufferer is blamed for character defects or misbehavior that brings on the suffering. At the other, the sufferer is free of all fault and simply a victim. Currently, the dominant view tends to be that sufferers are passive victims. While this has the merit of removing blame from the victim, it has also removed recognition of the sufferer's capacity for remedial action. That person must rely wholly on the power and knowledge of experts (Shweder, Much, Mohapatra, and Park, 1997, 121–64).

THE EVOLUTION OF THE UNDERSTANDING OF PAIN IN WESTERN MEDICINE

The Greeks were the first to offer naturalistic explanations of pain. A follower of Pythagoras, Alcmaeon of Croton said the five senses resulted from the passage of external elements through sensory ducts to the "sensorium" located in the brain. Anaxagoras (500–428 B.C.) proposed that pain was an element in all sensation. Democritus (460–362 B.C.) held that emanations from external objects acted through the body's ducts to activate the different senses. The Hippocratic view was that pain resulted when one of the four bodily humors was out of balance.

Plato saw pain and pleasure as opposed to each other; an unnatural or violent affection was painful, while reversion to a natural condition produced pleasure. Aristotle saw pain as greater sensitivity of the touch sense. The heart is the site of the "sensorium commune," and pain, felt in the heart, is the opposite of pleasure.

Galen distinguished "soft" nerves having sensory functions from "hard" nerves, which had motor functions; the smallest nerves, a third type, dealt with pain sensations. The brain was the recipient of all sensations. However, Galen did not try to locate the soul as Aristotle did, and so the Christian Church preferred the latter's sensory physiology. During the Renaissance, the ideas of Plato and Aristotle gained renewed impetus from their being available in Greek. Leonardo da Vinci (1452–1519) believed that pain sensations travel through the spinal cord to the "sensorium commune" in the third cerebral ventricle, which, he maintained, is the location of the soul.

In the view of René Descartes, the nerves were tubes containing fine threads beginning in the brain and reaching to the skin or endpoints in other tissues. Sensations moved along the threads to the brain's ventricular walls, then via the ventricular fluid to the pineal gland. Pain resulted when central threads were pulled to the point of rupture. In the pineal gland, where the *res cogitans* and the *res extensa* were connected, consciousness of sensations occurred (Procacci and Maresca, 1984, 2–6; Procacci and Maresca, 1998, 213–19).

Other eminent thinkers concerned themselves with sensation and pain, including Thomas Hobbes (1588–1679), Baruch Spinoza (1632–1677), and Isaac Newton (1642–1727). However, within medicine, it was the Italian iatromechanical school that advanced a materialist conception. Members of the school saw all sensory phenomena as vibrations along nerve fibers, and they tended toward a conception of nerve impulses as a chemical flow through their concern with "nerve juices." Giovanni Borelli (1608–1679) said the sensation of pain was produced in the brain by agitation of the nerve juice.

Albrecht von Haller (1708–1777) replaced mechanical and chemical speculations with physiological experiment. He distinguished nerve impulses from muscle contractions and said that anything that irritated the nerve produced a sense of pain. His claim that the nervous juice producing the impulses was like electricity marks the first time electricity was identified as the means of conveying impulses (Ackerknecht, 1982, 115–118, 133–35; Procacci and Maresca, 1998, 222–24).

During the first half of the nineteenth century, recognizably modern scientific knowledge about pain developed. François Magendie (1783–1855) demonstrated the sensory function of the dorsal spinal roots and the motor function of the ventral roots. The German physiologists could draw on the expertise of physicists in experiments. E. H. Weber (1795–1878) differentiated touch from pain by describing the former as a sense of the skin and pain as *gemeingefühl* (literally, common sensation or feeling); sensitivity was common to the skin and internal organs. Johannes Mueller (1801–1858) proposed the law of specific nerve energy, in which information was carried to the brain by the sensory nerves; for each of the five senses it was carried through a particular form of energy; thus stimulation of the optic, acoustic, sensory, or motor nerves could elicit only optic, acoustic, sensory, or motor responses.

In 1858 Moritz Schiff advanced a specific theory of pain; pain was a specific sensation independent of touch and the other senses. In 1874 W. H. Erb proposed the intensive theory of pain (which Charles Darwin had suggested): if intense enough, every sensory stimulus could produce pain. In the mid-1890s A. Goldscheider argued that intensity of stimulus and central summation determined pain. At the close of the nineteenth century, the specificity and the intensive theories remained in opposition to each other.

The conflict persisted into the 1920s. In the 1950s G. Weddell and colleagues proposed the pattern theory, in which different sensory modalities did not have specific skin receptors. Rather, different kinds of stimuli excited nonspecific receptors via different spatiotemporal patterns of activation, and these patterns elicited different sensations in the central nervous system.

The pattern theory was supported by neurologists and neurosurgeons who could not easily explain the pain in conditions such as postherpetic neuralgia and causalgia in terms of specific receptors and pathways. This model was not popular with neurophysiologists, who knew that some receptors and nerve fibers had high specificity for some kinds of stimuli. In 1959 W. Noordenbos suggested the sensory interaction theory. The central nervous system has different ascending pathways, and Noordenbos himself identified the significance of a multisynaptic afferent system. D. Albe-Fessard differentiated within the ascending system both nonspecific and specific pathways. Descending systems (coming from different brain structures) played an inhibitory role. The discovery of endogenous opioids led to the realization that the release of these substances controls afferent impulses.

Receptivity to pain results from a feedback system. In 1965 Ronald Melzack and Patrick Wall described the working of the feedback system in their gate control theory. This showed how large-diameter, afferent fibers have an inhibitory effect on small-diameter, nociceptive fibers and on the way the descending control systems function. The dynamic nature of the theory has rendered the long-standing debate about the specificity of afferent fibers less significant. Melzack and Wall pointed out that the main site for modifying pain impulses is the dorsal horn of the spinal cord. This offers a means of explaining why pain may be modulated by cortical, subcortical, and other spinal activity such as psychological factors, pain located elsewhere, and simultaneous stimulation of sensory fibers in the same peripheral nerve (Ackerknecht, 1982, 158, 161–65, 173; Procacci and Maresca, 1984, 6–8; Woodruff, 1996, 44–45; Procacci and Maresca, 1998, 224–26).

CULTURAL ATTITUDES TOWARD PAIN

Enlightenment thinkers, shifting the center of the world from God to people, wanted to minimize pain. Above all, the utilitarians suggested that humans were essentially motivated by the stimulus of pleasure or the fear of pain; thus, through an applied science based on such a "felicific calculus," their behavior might be most effectively managed. Indeed, for Jeremy Bentham (1748–1832), the utilitarian philosopher, the only evil was pain. At the turn of the century, William James, the American philosopher, noted the long-term cultural influence of the humanistic attitudes born in the age of the Enlightenment, pointing out that people at the end of the nineteenth century no longer had to accept physical pain as an immutable fact of existence (Caton, 1999, 9; Porter, 1999, 369–74).

That playing out of the ideas of the Enlightenment—the French Revolution—promised, through the pursuit of human rights, to advance the material welfare and the happiness of all humankind. The British Romantic poets and writers, like all progressive democrats, at first welcomed the revolution, but as the Reign of Terror and the autocracy of Napoleon dashed their hopes, they turned to the free self and an individuality that was open to the adventure of life as the way forward for humanity.

The Romantics saw pain and suffering as a means by which to reconstruct the self, providing a new human being for a new era. Shelley (who suffered from melancholia and suicidal feelings) expresses through his poetic hero, Prometheus, the wish that no living being suffer pain. He envisages a future free of suffering and where love overcomes pain. That such attitudes to pain had wider resonance is seen in the fact that in 1807 Britain ended the slave trade and in 1833 abolished slavery itself. In 1835 Queen Victoria became a patron of the new Society for the Prevention of Cruelty to Animals.

The personal suffering of poet Samuel Taylor Coleridge was both physical—he was prone to injury and experienced withdrawal symptoms because of opium addiction—and psychological and emotional. His emotional pain was related to an unsatisfactory marriage and his attraction to Wordsworth's sister-in-law, Sara Hutchinson. He also feared in an ongoing way the disappearance of his creative ability. He believed that reconnecting with the beauties of nature would lead to self-healing.

Byron's existential pain had no basis in physical lesions. It is not explicable in terms of the materialism of the emerging medical approach to pain. As David Morris has noted, Byron's experience throws light on a historical drama in which medicine and the Romantic reconstruction of selfhood moved toward collision. The conflict is still with us. Patients who today accept a biomedical account of their pain also want to describe it in personal accounts that use mental and emotional language. Pain then is located at the interface of biology and culture. It arises from the interaction of body, mind, and feelings. This significant epistemological legacy may be said to contribute to the contemporary problem of undertreatment of pain. If fear of encouraging drug addiction and the alleged inhumanity of doctors are inadequate explanations of the longevity of this problem, we might then look to the persistence of conflicting conceptualizations of pain and the privileging in medicine of biology and objective evidence over the culture and subjective experience (Papper, 1990, 176–81; Porter, 1993, 1584; Morris, 1999, 4–6).

ANESTHESIA

According to Roy Porter, neither Classical nor Renaissance doctors saw pain control as a primary responsibility. However, the situation began to change in the seventeenth century at a time when opium became more easily available.

In the 1790s physician Thomas Beddoes and his assistant, Humphrey (later Sir Humphrey) Davy, seeking a remedy for consumption, experimented with nitrous oxide and discovered its anesthetic capacity. Nothing immediately came of Davy's idea of using it in surgery. In 1818 physicist William Faraday demonstrated the anesthetic property of ether. In 1842 Crawford Long, a doctor from rural Georgia, used ether to anaesthetize a boy while he excised a cyst. In 1844 Connecticut dentist Horace Wells was anaesthetized with nitrous oxide while a tooth was extracted. A Bostonian, William Morton, experimented on his dog, on himself, and on a patient and in 1846 used ether during an operation to remove a tumor from a patient's neck.

Within a couple of months, the use of ether in surgery had been adopted in Europe. James Young Simpson, Edinburgh professor of surgery, used ether extensively in midwifery practice beginning in 1847. The disadvantage of ether was that it caused vomiting and lung irritation, and in Britain it was quickly replaced by chloroform, although it remained popular in the United States.

Chloroform anesthesia won the endorsement of Queen Victoria in 1853 after John Snow anaesthetized her during the birth of Prince Leopold. A few years later Snow published *On Chloroform and Other Anesthetics* in an effort to give a scientific basis to anesthesia, but medical critics remained concerned about the safety of the procedure. The *Lancet* strongly advised against its use in childbirth (Porter, 1993, 1588–89; Porter, 1997, 269, 365–68).

THE USE OF OPIATES AND OTHER ANALGESICS

In the nineteenth century the new pharmaceutical industry made available a range of analgesics, sedatives, and narcotics. Opiates remained the treatment of choice for both recurrent and acute pain. In 1804 F. W. Serturner isolated the active principle in opium and called it morphine in honor of the classical god of dreams, Morpheus. Soon afterward, codeine was produced. In the 1820s the industrial production of morphine was under way in Germany and, 10 years later, in the United States. In the 1850s Alexander Wood invented the hypodermic syringe, which enabled heavy concentrations of opiates to be injected into the body. Morphine was then used for minor surgery, postoperative pain, and chronic pain. Florence Nightingale, pioneer of modern nursing, observed with regard to one of her many episodes of illness that she had obtained relief from the new procedure of putting opium under the skin.

By the 1870s doctors in Britain and elsewhere were condemning narcomania. Ten years later the Bayer Company synthesized heroin (diacetylmorphine), contending that it was more powerful than morphine and less susceptible to abuse. Within a few years, young working-class people in the United States were inhaling the powder obtained from crushing heroin pills. In 1903 Bayer marketed barbitone as Veronal and phenobarbitone as Luminal in 1912. A Canadian general practitioner said that in the interwar period he had purchased Luminal tablets in batches of 5,000 every few months. Salicylic acid was used in headache powders in the later nineteenth century. Felix Hoffman acetylated salicylic acid, and the new product, aspirin, first marketed in 1899, was safer. Aspirin became the most-used drug of all time, replacing the opiates for mild to moderate pain (Poynter, 1974, 6; Brownstein, 1993, 5391; Porter, 1997, 448, 663, 675; Meldrum, 2003, 2470–75).

Arab traders took opium to India and China as early as the eighth century, and it was transported from Asia Minor to various parts of Europe between the tenth and thirteenth centuries. Around 1680 it was consumed as laudanum (opium in sherry or port to disguise the bitter taste). In the eighteenth and into the following century, laudanum was purchasable over the counter. With the supply from the East expanding massively between the seventeenth and the nineteenth century, opium consumption grew significantly (Porter and Porter, 1989, 279).

For various reasons, it is impossible to give totally reliable figures for opium consumption in Britain and the United States in the nineteenth century. However, there are figures for the period before higher tariff levels encouraged smuggling: opium imports into Britain averaged a little more than 36,000 pounds a year between 1831 and 1842 and into the United States, somewhat more than 27,000 pounds a year between 1827 and 1842. On a per capita basis, British imports increased from about 2 pounds per 1,000 population in the early 1840s to about 2.8 pounds in the mid-1850s. U.S. imports rose more steeply, from 1 pound to 4–5 pounds per 1,000 population in the same period. If allowance is made for opium imported for smoking by Chinese immigrants, large numbers of whom began to arrive in the United States in the 1850s, the U.S. increase in per capita consumption is not a great deal more than that of Britain. Within the United States, the South had the greatest incidence of opiate addiction because the swamplands and alluvial plains gave rise to malaria, fevers, and rheumatism, and opium was effective for the pain these maladies caused.

During the last three decades of the nineteenth century, in Britain, North America, and Australasia the sales of patent medicines increased markedly. The ingredients of many such medicines included opiates. From 1880 to 1910, the U.S. population grew by about 83 percent, but the sale of patent medicines increased by 700 percent.

As in North America and Britain, in Australasia the habit of self-treatment was widespread. The earliest official efforts to control the use of drugs aimed at preventing poisoning, suicide, and murder, and they did not restrict mass access: for example, the popular cough mixture Bonnington's Irish Moss contained opium and morphine, and Atkinson's Royal Infant Preservative was full of opium. The Commonwealth Royal Commission on Secret Drugs, Cures, and Foods, established in 1907, found a dangerous lack of control of the ingredients used in proprietary medicines. In 1900 Octavius Beale, the royal commissioner, claimed that Australia consumed more proprietary medicines per capita than any other Western country. However, it was the small Chinese community and its opium smoking that were targeted. From the 1890s colonial and state laws against smoking and the sale, trafficking, and possession of opium suitable for smoking were enacted. Since the 1870s, a campaign against opium smoking had been growing, and it was reinforced by opposition to Chinese immigration. The new Commonwealth of Australia acted quickly to control the habit. Prime Minister Alfred Deakin persuaded the states to accept a federal prohibition on the import of smokeable opium, and in 1905 a national ban was authorized. The states progressively tightened the restrictions on the personal use of opiates and other drugs, with Victoria leading the way. That state's Poisons Act of 1920 extended coverage to cocaine, synthetic cocaine, heroin, cannabis, morphine, and other opium derivatives. The

1925 Poisons Act made possession a crime (Parssinen, 1983, 204–6; Finch, 1999, 74–80; O'Callaghan, 2001, 21–26; Lewis, 2003b, 80–81).

Although uncertainty reigned into the nineteenth century about how opium (and derivatives) acted on the body, its use in medicine in Britain and other parts of the Anglo-Saxon world increased. The most fervent advocates saw it as a true panacea. In Jonathan Pereira's 1839 text on materia medica, opium was said to reduce pain, allay spasms, induce sleep, banish nervous restlessness, promote perspiration, and halt mucous discharge from the bronchial tubes and gastrointestinal tract (Berridge, 1999, 66).

Opium was widely employed in everyday practice. In London, of the prescriptions dispensed by an Islington pharmacist between the mid-1840s and the 1860s, 14–20 percent had opium as the base. The Ebert Prescription Survey of 1885, which included 15,700 prescriptions dispensed by nine pharmacies in Illinois, found that the most common ingredients were morphine and quinine. The Medical Act of 1858 brought into being the first British pharmacopoeia. It listed fourteen opium preparations, plus some preparations of poppy capsules and morphine. Thirty years later the same medical substances were still named, along with a much larger list of morphine preparations.

THE PROBLEM OF ADDICTION

The wide use of morphine in the U.S. Civil War seems to have promoted addiction. In Europe, too, iatrogenic addiction increased, and in the early1870s articles appeared in British and U.S. medical journals warning about addiction. In the United States, middle- and upper-class native-born women of middle age, addicted to morphine through its use in medical therapy, were the typical sufferers of morphinomania; male sufferers were mainly doctors. In Britain, addicts tended to be middle-class, middle-aged males working in the health professions The medical use of opiates in Britain and the United States probably reached a high point in the 1890s. In Britain, the Poisons and Pharmacy Acts of 1868 and 1908 introduced some requirements concerning the sales of opiates and cocaine, but legal restrictions came only in 1916 under Defence of the Realm regulations. In the United States, the Pure Food and Drug Act of 1906, by forcing producers of patent medicines containing opiates to state the contents on the label, had the effect of cutting sales considerably.

Between the 1890s and the 1920s, British consumption of patent medicines declined, though more slowly than the marked fall in the United States after the 1906 act. Under the Dangerous Drugs Act of 1920, a prescription (one time only) was required to obtain opium, cocaine, morphia, and heroin. Those dealing in drugs were required to keep records of the drugs they handled. In the United States, the Harrison Act of 1914 similarly required registration and detailed records, and opiates and other narcotics were available only by prescription. Medical maintenance of addicts was held to be illegal by the Supreme Court in 1919. It has been argued, however, that the act did not in fact improve the addiction situation because, since it criminalized addiction, it simply created the drug peddler, who in turn created addicts.

Another factor in the reduction of iatrogenic addiction after the 1890s was the declining use of narcotics in therapy. Public health advances reduced the huge burden of gastrointestinal illnesses, for which opium had traditionally been used. Moreover, safer substitutes for opiates (e.g., aspirin and Veronal) appeared in this period.

In 1930 the U.S. Federal Bureau of Narcotics was established. Harry J. Anslinger, the head of the bureau, publicly painted a picture of the addict as in many cases a criminal. Although in 1925 the Supreme Court reversed its position on medical maintenance of addicts, the bureau successfully pursued its established policy. In 1934 the diagnosis of drug addiction was listed in the handbook of the American Psychiatric Association for the first time.

The issue of addiction as vice and crime or as disease was also played out elsewhere in the English-speaking world. A key point made by the 1926 Rolleston report in Britain was that addiction should be regarded as a manifestation of disease. The British system, unlike that in the United States, allowed doctors to treat those addicted to morphine or heroin with maintenance doses of the drug. The system continued in its essentials until the 1960s, when, under pressure to deal with a growing problem of drug abuse, governments became more restrictive. Addicts now had to register for treatment at special clinics.

It needs to be said that Britain's recreational (as opposed to iatrogenic) drug culture developed two to three decades after that of U.S. cities in the 1890s, and its total addict population was always comparatively small. Furthermore, where British users (now mainly young male criminals and female prostitutes in London) used cocaine, Americans used heroin. When British police moved against cocaine in the 1920s, the small recreational market contracted quickly. This could not have happened so easily with heroin, which is more addictive. The aging population of morphine addicts was also shrinking; thus, by 1926, when the doctor-directed British system was officially sanctioned, both recreational and iatrogenic addiction were declining and therefore more manageable.

It might also be argued that drug addiction was more deeply entrenched in the United States because of the historical legacy of Prohibition. By 1920, when the Eighteenth Amendment made alcohol use illegal, prohibition already existed in a number of counties and states. The illegality and stigmatization of alcohol use would have made narcotics a more attractive alternative to more people than in Britain, where temperance had been the prevailing approach to control. Thus the British working class enjoyed easy access to cheap beer, while the more well-to-do had wine and spirits (Parssinen, 1983, 208–20; Manderson, 1993, 105–6; Porter, 1997, 664–66; Berridge, 1999, 62–72, 131).

In Australia, state regulations in the 1930s did not allow the medical maintenance of addicts. In practice, however, with the cooperation of state police and state and federal health authorities, doctors continued to provide maintenance. Most addicts, apart from some Chinese smokers of opium, were middle class (not infrequently doctors or nurses). This remained the case until well into the postwar era.

In Australia, heroin was extensively used in medical practice for chronic and acute pain. It was prescribed for the pains of terminal cancer and childbirth. Australian consumption was very large: 3.10 kilograms per one million persons; in total, more than the United States, Canada, or Germany; per head, second only to New Zealand.

Under pressure from the United States, the secretary general of the League of Nations sought the views of member states on the limiting of production. The conference on the 1931 Geneva Convention proposed that members look at the possibility of ending its use. Political and medical leaders in Australia differed over this. In 1935 Prime Minister Joseph Lyons, told the league's secretary general that the federal council of the Australian branch of the British Medical Association knew of no addiction problem, and, because of the clinical value of heroin, it did not support prohibition.

The 1936 Geneva Convention for the Suppression of the Illicit Traffic in Dangerous Drugs required signatories to enact laws to punish the manufacture, conversion, extraction, preparation, possession, and offering for sale of narcotic drugs. But the Commonwealth was not interested in expanding its role in the suppression of the drug trade, and the states were satisfied with the status quo. Western Australia considered addiction very uncommon. Victoria said it had very little; South Australia, a negligible amount; and Queensland, none at all. The Commonwealth did not ratify the 1936 Convention before World War II (Manderson, 1993, 101–13).

The linking of the problem of addiction with the use of opiates to control pain thus has a long history in these Anglo-Saxon countries. In the postwar era it was to continue to affect medical practice in relation to pain control in terminal disease, and in particular it reinforced a strong tendency to undertreat cancer pain.

LATER NINETEENTH-CENTURY MEDICAL DISCOURSES ON PAIN

Marcia Meldrum has identified within medicine three aspects of the focus on pain from about the 1850s: first, palliation of the pain of life-threatening diseases such as cancer; second, relief of acute pain; and third, relief of chronic pain from conditions that are not life threatening, such as rheumatoid arthritis. What seems clear is that the advocacy of the vigorous use of analgesics for the pain of dying patients was voiced by a minority. The conquest of surgical pain by anesthesia did not immediately translate into the wish to relieve pain caused by other conditions.

Pain continued to carry religious meaning and was also seen as a possible sign of pathology. Later in the century, confidence about the imminence of new cures for cancer distracted attention from pain control as a therapeutic end in itself. Also, concerns about iatrogenic drug addiction from use of the opiates increased. Moreover, the pain of terminal illness could be managed only more or less well, not totally banished. Undoubtedly, medicine's mind-body dualism promoted the view that only pain associated with a visible lesion was real. Nevertheless, a minor voice in Anglo-Saxon medicine did teach that the caring doctor always seeks to relieve suffering (Meldrum, 2003, xxx; Holmes, 2003, 24–25).

Three British doctors represent this minor strand: William Dale and John Kent Spender, both provincial doctors; and Herbert Snow, a London specialist. Dale published four papers on pain relief in the *Lancet* in 1871. In them he strongly urged the use of opiates to relieve the pains of the dying. Dale, like William Munk (known for *Euthanasia,* his 1887 text on care of the dying), was influenced by Thomas Watson's *Principles and Practice of Physic* (1836), which addressed the issue of pain in the context of the care of the dying.

As a Bath doctor, John Kent Spender saw many people who had come to the town's famous spa because of chronic illness. In 1874 he wrote that the relief of pain was the primary obligation of the true physician. However, as did Herbert Snow, Spender saw pain as more than a sign of disease; it was also able to destroy organic structures.

Herbert Snow, a surgeon for almost three decades at the London Cancer Hospital, was the inventor of the Brompton cocktail, the analgesic mixture later adopted by the modern hospice movement. In the 1890s he utterly condemned the failure to use opiates at the outset in cancer cases not amenable to surgery. Indeed, he even urged the induction of dependency as it allegedly halted progress of the disease by inhibiting cell metabolism (Snow, 1896, 718; Holmes, 2003, 22–33).

THE EMERGENCE OF PAIN MEDICINE

The specificity theory of pain tended to dominate medical teaching in the early twentieth century. People with chronic pain that could not be explained in terms of that model were dismissed as hypochondriacs or as manipulators seeking addictive drugs. In the United States, where official and professional concern about drug addiction was particularly strong, in the interwar period a quest began for a nonaddictive analgesic. Reid Hunt, a Harvard University pharmacologist, thought it might be possible to separate the analgesic from the addictive capacity of morphine. The Committee on Drug Addiction, which functioned under the auspices of the U.S. National Research Council in 1929, became responsible for a research program at the universities of Virginia and Michigan and later at the National Institutes of Health (NIH). While the program investigated new analgesics such as oxycodone and methadone, no derivative of morphine that was powerful and nonaddictive was found.

René Leriche treated many World War I cases of nerve injury by resecting the arteries near the injury and then injecting procaine. If pain relief was still inadequate, he would ligate the periarterial sympathetic nerve fibers or the sympathetic ganglia that supplied the limb. William Livingston, who established a pioneering pain clinic at the University of Oregon in 1947, used serial blockade, often successfully, to suppress pain. In 1902 Rudolf Schloesser used alcohol blocks for trigeminal neuralgia, which produces one of the severest pains known to medicine.

The work of Leriche and Livingston encouraged the practice of using an anesthetic instead of a neurolytic block. In 1936 Emery Rovenstine established a nerve-block pain relief clinic at Bellevue Hospital (Lipton, 1990b, 3; Meldrum,

2003, 2470). In the early 1930s Achile Dogliotti used alcohol intrathecally to relieve cancer pain. Because it is hypobaric, alcohol presents difficulties when injected into the cerebrospinal fluid (CSF). In the 1950s Robert Maher introduced the use of the more manageable phenol in glycerine (Lipton, 1990a, xxix; Brown and Fink, 1998, 21).

The great number of battle casualties in World War II meant clinicians had an unprecedented opportunity to expand their thinking about pain control. William Livingston published his classic, *Pain Mechanisms,* in 1943, and René Leriche published *The Surgery of Pain* in 1939. H. K. Beecher noted that military patients seemed to experience less pain than civilian patients and suggested that clinical pain had cognitive and emotional components. He developed scales that quantified a patient's subjective experience of pain and could be used with double-blind crossover trials to evaluate new pain control methods.

Another factor in the development of pain medicine was the state of anesthetics itself. The problem of pain in the postoperative period had required anesthesiologists to become expert in analgesia and pharmacodynamics. They also worked at refining locoregional anesthesia using temporary or permanent nerve blocking (Baszanger, 1998, 22; Meldrum, 2003, 2470–75).

In 1944 John Bonica (1917–1994), who was to become a great driving force behind the development of pain medicine, was appointed head of the anesthesia and surgery unit at Washington State's Madigan Army Hospital, a 7,700-bed facility that received wounded soldiers from the Pacific theater of war. Seeking diagnostic and therapeutic insights into cases of complex pain, he consulted with specialist colleagues—neurologists, neurosurgeons, psychiatrists, and orthopedists—and then established case meetings during which different specialists discussed problems until they reached agreement on diagnosis and treatment. Access to such a range of specialties on a collective basis was not the norm in civilian hospitals of the time.

On leaving the army, Bonica became head of the Department of Anesthesia at Tacoma General Hospital in Washington State in 1947. Importantly, he brought with him the conviction that complex pain had to be treated more effectively. His work over the next two decades or so may be divided into four areas: building an interdisciplinary team concerned with pain such as the one he had pioneered at Madigan Army Hospital; building a base in anesthesia; constructing a framework for pain medicine; and publicizing the need to improve the treatment of pain. Because of the fee-for-service nature of medical practice, it was no easy task to establish a collective evaluation of individual specialist practice. Nonetheless, Bonica brought together an anesthesiologist, a neurosurgeon, an orthopedist, a psychiatrist, an internist, and a radiologist in regular meetings.

In the immediate postwar years, other anesthesiologists were setting up pain clinics, but these were limited to the provision of analgesic blocks and did not reach out to other disciplines as Bonica's did. The exceptions that pursued a broad view of pain were Livingston's clinic and F. A. D. Alexander's clinic at the Veterans Administration Hospital in McKinney, Texas, which was also established in 1947.

By 1950 Bonica had accumulated information from more than 2,000 military and civilian cases that he had treated. He came to realize that many practitioners thought the primary therapeutic weapons were nerve blocks; many of them had little knowledge of pain mechanisms, symptomatology, and therapeutic modalities, and they were happy just to provide technical assistance to the referring doctor.

In *The Management of Pain* (1953), Bonica outlined a multidisciplinary approach to diagnosis and therapy. He pointed to the contrast between acute and chronic pain and called for more research on the subject. Absolutely central to his conception of pain is the notion of an overlap between physical and mental effects. The patient's perception of, and reaction to, pain are intimately related. He pointed out that, until only a decade earlier, medicine had focused on the laboratory study of pain and omitted the influence of the mind.

Soon after Bonica's appointment to the University of Washington in Seattle in 1960, he established a multidisciplinary pain clinic with the assistance of Lowell White, a neurosurgeon, and Dorothy Crowley of the Faculty of Nursing. Subsequently, staff from psychiatry, orthopedics, rehabilitation medicine, clinical psychology, oral surgery, general surgery, and radiation therapy joined the program. Benjamin Crue and colleagues also set up a multidisciplinary program at about this time at the City of Hope Medical Center in Duarte, California. However, it was Bonica's clinic that set the benchmark for the many multidisciplinary programs created in the United States and other parts of the world over the next few decades.

Although Bonica was to receive much recognition, for more than a decade his efforts to convince doctors that chronic pain was a disease condition and that pain management demanded a multidisciplinary approach seemed to be going nowhere (Bonica, 1988, 10–13; Liebeskind and Meldrum, 1997, 25–29; Baszanger, 1998, 21–27). In the early 1970s he believed the time was ripe to take another major step toward the creation of pain medicine. He himself identified a number of helpful factors, especially the intellectual ferment created by the publication of the Melzack-Wall gate theory of pain in 1965 and the widespread lay interest in Chinese medicine's analgesic acupuncture.

The gate theory's emphasis on the psychobiological unity of pain supported Bonica's call for a multifaceted approach to bring together neuroscience, psychology, and clinical medicine. It also supported the established clinical view that pain involved complex perceptions with no necessary connection with physical lesion. Like Bonica's vision, it served to promote cooperation between scientist and clinician, as well as between doctor and patient. The theory encouraged Bonica to create an international professional association devoted to pain, the International Association for the Study of Pain (IASP) in 1974 and then in 1975 to establish a new international journal, *Pain,* with Patrick Wall as editor in chief. Ulf Lindblom, founding editor of the *European Journal of Pain* (the journal of the European chapters of IASP), noted in 1990 that a majority of senior colleagues had identified the setting up of *Pain* as the most important initiative taken by Bonica and his associates.

In 1972 the National Institute of General Medical Sciences organized a symposium on trauma, to which Bonica contributed. He then suggested an interdisciplinary meeting on pain. The director promised funding, and Bonica organized a conference of clinicians and researchers from 13 countries. Problems with the funding almost killed off the project, but finally, in May 1973, the Seattle-Issaquah conference took place. Location in an isolated place probably promoted the participants' willingness to talk across their various disciplines, and Bonica networked to prepare for the implementation of his idea of an international association. Edward Perl formally called for the formation of an IASP and received unanimous support. Bonica's goals of national chapters, international congresses every three years, and a new journal were also endorsed.

As Liebeskind and Meldrum have observed, Bonica's professional world of pain medicine had the advantage of not having to grow from a fragmented base of national and disciplinary associations. By 1976, the IASP had a membership of almost 1,600 from 55 countries and 81 research fields and clinical disciplines (Bonica, 1988, 13; Liebeskind and Meldrum, 1997, 28–29; Baszanger, 1998, 63–80; Lindblom, 2001, 344).

The first World Congress took place in Florence in 1975. Denise Albe-Fessard, a distinguished French neurophysiologist, became the first president of the IASP, but Bonica was to occupy senior positions for almost the first decade and thus guide the body in its formative years. Bonica was eager to see a national pain association established in the United States because it was the country with the greatest biomedical resources. By 1976 there was an Eastern Pain Association and a Western Pain Society, which were chapters of the IASP. Some in the eastern group believed that Bonica was closer to the western group, but these differences were overcome, and in 1977 the American Pain Society came into being.

By the end of the twentieth century, the IASP had recruited 6,500 members representing 91 countries and 61 disciplines, and 54 countries had national chapters. The advance of pain medicine can also be seen in the speedy growth of pain clinics around the world. In 1977, of 327 pain clinics worldwide, 60 percent were in the United States; 20 percent in Europe; 7 percent in Canada; and 6 percent in Australia and New Zealand. In 1987 there were 1,800–2,000 pain clinics, of which 1,000–1,200 were situated in the United States, 200–225 in Western Europe, 75 in Canada, and 80 in Australasia and Asia. Other countries with clinics had 2–20 each (Bonica, 1988, 13–15; Liebeskind and Meldrum, 1997, 31; Meldrum, 1999, 94–95).

As mentioned earlier, Bonica himself identified the appearance of the gate control theory of pain and the community interest in acupuncture analgesia as factors that were significant in the launch of pain medicine in the 1970s. In addition, Liebeskind and Meldrum suggest that the considerable development of neuroscience at the same time and, in the United States at least, a professional belief that the success of research grant applications to the National Institutes of Health in part depended on showing the relevance to health of the proposed research. Another (but more distal) factor was the great significance, in economically advanced countries, of chronic diseases in morbidity and mortality after the 1940s (Liebeskind and Meldrum, 1997, 29–30; Baszanger, 1998, 13–14). With chronic diseases, not only is long-term pain common, but management of the illness— rather than cure—is usually the aim.

The story in Britain is somewhat different. A great deal of the early treatment of chronic pain there centered on the pain of terminal cancer. In 1936 W. Ritchie Russell reported a small number of cases he had treated by using intraspinal injections of alcohol. He suggested that, because of the high risk of side effects, such injections should be used only with terminal cases of cancer. J. R. J. Beddard tried alcohol spinal blocks for cancer pain sufferers when he read about the technique in a U.S. journal in 1950.

The first nerve block clinic was established in the United Kingdom in 1947, when B. G. B. Lucas opened a clinic at University College Hospital in London. In 1948 Eric Angel opened a nerve block clinic in Plymouth. In 1951 Douglas Wilson, a Londonderry anesthetist, reported on his work with autonomic nerve blocks and intrathecal alcohol for cancer pain. In 1954 H. C. J. Ball began a pain clinic at Southampton General Hospital, and the next year O. H. Bellam and G. H. Dobney opened a clinic at the Whittington Hospital.

An interdisciplinary clinic was established by Ritchie Russell at Churchill Hospital in Oxford in 1964. In late 1970 anesthetist John Lloyd opened the Oxford Regional Pain Clinic Unit. It seems that Lloyd was treating cancer patients so effectively with neurolytic nerve blocks that many were able to resume life at home. In the late 1980s about 200 pain clinics had been established, although a great many provided only outpatient care in two to three sessions per week (Beinart, 1987, 124–32; Beinart, 1988, 182–84).

In the 1960s, one of the pioneers of pain clinics in the United Kingdom, Mark Swerdlow, became interested in promoting a better exchange of information and in 1967 invited colleagues across the United Kingdom and Ireland to a meeting at Salford University. The next year the meeting was held in Cambridge and in 1969 in Bristol. At the 1971 Birmingham meeting, the group became the Intractable Pain Society of Great Britain and Ireland, with Swerdlow as chair. In 1977, 59 members responded to a society survey, and of these, 29 said their clinics had functioned for more than five years, while 17 said they had been open for one to five years (Swerdlow, 1992, 977–80; James, 1976, 56).

In Australia, pain clinics were established quite early. In 1962 a multidisciplinary clinic was set up at one of Sydney's teaching hospitals, Saint Vincent's in Darlinghurst. The consultants included a neurosurgeon, a psychiatrist, a radiotherapist, and an anesthetist.

In 1965 Russell Cole of the Royal Melbourne Hospital Pain Relief Clinic and the Peter MacCallum Cancer Clinic said that his policy was to send the few cancer patients seen in the pain clinic back to their attending doctors rather than have the clinic act as a terminal care unit (McEwen and deWilde, 1965, 676–82; Cole, 1965, 682–86).

Twenty years later Gordon Coates of the Pain Clinic at the Prince of Wales Hospital in Sydney stated that the idea was still common among both cancer patients and health professionals that pain was intractable. He believed this notion sprang from inadequate professional education, widespread taboos concerning drugs, and lack of experience in pain management. David Allbrook, of the Hospice Palliative Care Service of Western Australia, reported that, like Coates, he used a pain management model developed by Robert Twycross and Cicely Saunders. He agreed with Coates that standards of general practice in this area had to be raised (Coates, 1985, 30–34; Allbrook, 1985, 327).

In 1952 a Faculty of Anaesthetists with 69 foundation fellows was created within the Royal Australasian College of Surgeons. Forty years later, the Australian and New Zealand College of Anaesthetists (ANZCA) was established. With 2,100 fellows and 500 trainees, anesthetists were the third largest group of medical specialists in Australia. Worldwide, the college had 3,200 fellows and assisted with training in Singapore, Malaysia, and Hong Kong.

In 1992 the ANZCA established a working party on certification in pain management. Then, a joint advisory committee in pain medicine, including representatives of the Royal Australasian College of Surgeons, the Royal Australian and New Zealand College of Psychiatrists, the Royal Australasian College of Physicians (RACP), and the Australasian Faculty of Rehabilitation Medicine of the RACP, investigated training requirements in pain medicine in Australia and New Zealand. In 1998 the governing board of the ANZCA established a Faculty of Pain Medicine, and the first examinations for admission to the faculty took place in November of the following year. The faculty quickly established good working relations with the Chapter of Palliative Medicine of the RACP. The faculty's multidisciplinary medical representation enables it to provide for the management of acute, chronic nonmalignant, and cancer pain (Dwyer, 1998; http://www.anzca.edu.au/about/fpmhistory [retrieved March 5, 2006]).

Australian anesthetists were involved early on in the IASP, with Australia forming one of the first national chapters outside North America. Michael Cousins, head of the Pain Management and Research Center, Royal North Shore Hospital, Sydney, was the fifth IASP president (1987–1990). Cousins and Sir Sydney Sunderland organized the first small meeting of the Australasian Chapter of IASP (the Australian Pain Society) in 1976. Only Australians attended, but the second and third meetings drew New Zealanders as well. New Zealand later formed its own chapter.

Like Australians, Canadian health professionals were quick to become involved in the IASP. The Canadian Pain Society (CPS) was incorporated in 1982 as a chapter and by the end of the century consisted of about 1,000 members. In 1997 the CPS issued a position statement on pain relief. It said that almost all cancer and acute pain can be relieved, while many patients with chronic nonmalignant pain can be helped; patients have the right to the best relief possible; unrelieved pain complicates rehabilitation; patient self-reporting should be used as much as possible because pain is a subjective and very variable experience; and patients (and families) should be encouraged to reveal the true severity of their pain (Mendelson, 1990, 406; Lipton, 1990a, xxix; Gilbert, 1997, 17–18; http://www.canadian painsociety.ca/cont-ang/1apropos-politiques.htm [retrieved March 6, 2006]).

In the mid-1990s the CPS launched its own journal, *Pain Research and Management,* but by the fourth year, the president was expressing concern at a decrease in the number of articles submitted. In early 2000 the editor of the journal, Harold Merskey, said that more articles were needed on cancer pain, palliative care, pain in the aged, and arthritis. In late 2003 the Canadian Pain Coalition made plans for a national public awareness campaign about pain. The hope was that pain, like breast cancer or arthritis, would become a topic on the national health agenda so that more research funds and better clinical services might result and the public might become better informed. The coalition consisted mainly of patients and their families and members of the CPS. The inaugural meeting took place in Winnipeg in May 2002, and a second meeting was held in Ottawa in November, at which a Charter of Rights and Responsibilities was formulated (*Newsletter of the Canadian Pain Society,* 2000, 3–4; 2003b, 1; 2003a, 3–4).

The international pain medicine movement built by and around John Bonica in the early 1970s had always paid considerable attention to the problem of cancer pain relief, as well it might, because, although the five-year survival rate from cancer had increased from 20 percent in 1930 to 50 percent in 1980 (in the United States), due to better treatment, effective pain control reached only some cancer patients. At the first World Congress on Pain, Bonica presented the 1975 figures from England, the United States, and Italy, which showed that 50–85 percent of patients with advanced cancer had pain that was not properly treated. He painted the same dismal picture at the first International Symposium on the Pain of Advanced Cancer held in Venice in 1978. It had become clear that each cancer specialty pursued its own narrow end: oncologists, seeking to control the disease, saw that as the main analgesic intervention, whereas pain medicine practitioners were concerned exclusively with the pain.

I noted earlier that, in the first four decades of the twentieth century, concern increased about iatrogenic addiction and the diversion of drugs to illicit users. In the United States during the postwar era, doctors continued to be concerned about the association of the opiates with addiction.

In his 1953 work, Bonica acknowledged the danger of iatrogenic addition and said that the primary concern was always to titrate the dose to the pain's intensity; nonnarcotic analgesics were to be used before moving up to opiates; and the opiates were to be given (and given at regular intervals) in the smallest dose that controlled the pain. Marcia Meldrum concludes that, in U.S. hospitals between the 1950s and the 1970s, while the treatment remained curative, a sparing dose of only 15 mg of morphine was probably the standard one. However, once death was imminent, the dosage might be increased to quite high levels; as a result, shortly before death, the dying person might be heavily sedated (Donovan, 1989, 258; Swerdlow, 2003, 157; Meldrum, 2003, 193–99).

Studies in the United States and Britain in the 1970s showed that cancer pain was often undertreated in hospitals and even more so in the home. In the 1980s Bonica himself advanced various reasons for what he considered the continuing failure to apply existing medical knowledge: inadequate instruction of students and residents (in the United States) in management; very little published information (seven leading English-language texts on cancer devoted only 18 of 9,500 pages to the treatment of pain); and the attending doctor's inadequate knowledge of the mechanisms of pain and the associated complex of perceptual, sensory, and emotional factors. Inadequate knowledge of pharmacology was reinforced by misplaced concerns about the risks of addiction. Moreover, most doctors and, unfortunately, many oncologists lacked knowledge of treatment modalities other than drugs—nerve blocks, neurosurgical interventions, and psychological techniques.

The main federal institution in the United States supporting cancer research, the National Cancer Institute, expended $2.5 billion between 1971 and 1975, of which only $560,000 went to cancer pain research. Happily, in the late 1970s, it set up a pain control program. It was also funding hospice and rehabilitation programs involving pain treatment and began to support the study of multidisciplinary cancer pain treatment. In the late 1970s pharmacologist Raymond Houde noted the continuing fears about the induction of addiction by the use of the opiates. This issue remained a cultural obstacle to reform in the practice of cancer pain control for the next two decades (Bonica, 1981, 91–96; Meldrum, 2003, 194–201).

Pain Medicine and Palliative Care

Around 1950, two lines of clinical research and practice were developing—one at Memorial Sloan-Kettering in New York and the other at Saint Christopher's Hospice in London. By the 1980s they had changed the way English-language medical texts dealt with cancer pain management. They also influenced practices around the world through the cancer pain relief guidelines promoted by the World Health Organization (WHO).

I have already discussed the quest for an effective nonnarcotic analgesic conducted by the Committee on Drug Addiction of the U.S. National Research Council. For two decades beginning in 1951 at Memorial Sloan-Kettering, Raymond Houde and Ada Rogers (a research nurse) carried out trials of new analgesics in comparison with morphine or other established medications. They reported their results to the committee but received only limited exposure in the larger world of medicine. Houde and Rogers applied a patient-oriented approach in which the suffering of the particular individual was the focus. Dissemination of their approach was made easier when a pain service and a training fellowship were established at Memorial Sloan-Kettering in the early 1970s. Some outstanding contributors to pain medicine, such as Kathleen Foley, Ronald Kanner, Russell Portenoy, and Richard Payne, held fellowships in the 1970s and 1980s.

Palliative care and pain control were inextricably interconnected in the British hospice movement of the 1950s. Through Cicely Saunders's support for the Brompton cocktail—she endorsed it in her first published paper in 1958—the popularity of this analgesic mixture spread with the migration of the palliative care idea to the United States and Canada. As I pointed out earlier, the Brompton mix of morphine and cocaine was first advocated by Herbert Snow of the London Cancer Hospital. It was adopted by the nearby Brompton Hospital and by 1935 was being used to relieve pain at Saint Luke's Hospital in Bayswater, one of the homes for the dying set up in the late nineteenth century. In the 1950s it was being used in many English hospitals, and by 1976 it was listed in the British National Formulary.

In some formulations, heroin was substituted for morphine for its speed of effect; alternatively, cocaine might not be included, and heroin and morphine might be used together. There were questions about its use, first of all because it was believed to be used sometimes to hasten death and, second, because, as an oral analgesic, it might not be effective enough. On the other hand, its advantages were that it obviated painful injections and might be taken at home or self-administered on the ward as needed. Cicely Saunders's strong concern with effective pain relief meant the Brompton mixture was investigated quite early at Saint Christopher's.

Saunders invited Colin Murray Parkes to compare the hospice's terminal care with that of local hospitals. Parkes demonstrated that, where 20 percent of those dying in hospitals experienced pain and 29 percent of those at home did so, only 8 percent of hospice patients experienced it. In 1971 Robert Twycross began investigating the Brompton cocktail. He addressed issues such as the standardization of the mixture, the role of cocaine, and the relative advantages of heroin and morphine. Saunders did not see the giving of effective analgesia as just a response to the terminally ill patient's pain but as a measure to prevent the establishment of intractable pain. Chronic pain was not simply a problem of correct pharmacology. It was a problem of meaning that, unless controlled, threatened the patient with overwhelming despair. A willingness to listen to the patient's narrative was as integral to her approach to pain control as the analgesics.

Twycross found that both oral morphine and oral diamorphine were effective, although because it is more soluble, the latter might be preferred where high-dose injections are required. In a crossover trial he also investigated the question of whether the addition of cocaine to morphine and diamorphine elixirs made any difference to alertness or pain relief. At the standard dosage, cocaine provided no significant respite. Thus, practice at Saint Christopher's changed in 1977. Morphine in chloroform water became the routine, while the combined use of cocaine and diamorphine ceased.

The Brompton mixture traveled to where the hospice idea took root. In Montreal, Balfour Mount, director of the Palliative Care Unit at the Royal Victoria Hospital, and his colleagues wrote in 1976 that the mixture was a very effective, safe, and convenient way of managing the chronic pain of cancer. In 1976 Ronald Melzack, Balfour Mount, and J. G. Ofiesh reported on use of the mixture (plus a phenothiazine) with terminal patients in the Palliative Care Unit (PCM), general wards, and private rooms. The McGill-Melzack Pain Questionnaire was used to measure pain in 92 patients. The difference in pain scores between the PCM patients and the others was significant—pain control in 90 percent (as opposed to 75–80 percent in ward and private patients), with the mixture reducing pain in its three dimensions—sensory, affective, and evaluative. However, in 1979 Melzack, Mount, and J. M. Gordon, in a double-blind crossover trial, confirmed Twycross's findings of no significant difference between the Brompton mixture and oral morphine. Both provided effective pain relief in about 85 percent of patients (Mount, Ajemian, and Scott, 1976, 122; Melzack, Ofiesh, and Mount, 1976, 125; Melzack, Ofiesh, and Mount, 1979, 435).

Thus Twycross and the Canadians demonstrated that the mixture was pharmacologically a fancy means of achieving what oral morphine could do on its own. Yet, the use of the Brompton mixture did not disappear immediately. A British general practitioner who prescribed the mixture in the 1970s said he discontinued using it for a combination of reasons—patients objected to the particular alcoholic spirits (whether gin or brandy) included, Saint Christopher's opposed it, and the health department stated that mixtures could be dangerous if the dosage were increased because then all of the ingredients were increased. It continued to be used in some places in Britain and the United States in the 1980s. Indeed, supporters of a proposal for a compassionate pain relief act in the United States—the medical use of heroin would have become legal under the act—valued the Brompton mixture (Clark, 2000b, 1–4; Clark, 2003, 87–94).

Since the 1950s Saunders had been maintaining that managing pain offered an opportunity to help patients deal successfully with other personal and existential problems. Her concept of "total pain," first discussed in the 1960s and thenceforth central to hospice clinical practice, included the physical, psychological, social, emotional, and spiritual aspects of pain (Clark, 1999b, 727). The concept highlighted the significance of the caregiver's listening to the patient's story; moreover, she contended, the social, emotional, and spiritual needs of the person caught in the trap of chronic pain had to be met.

At the end of the 1970s, the leaders of the international pain medicine movement invited Saunders to contribute to a book on advances in pain research edited by John Bonica and Vittorio Ventafridda. Soon afterward, she contributed to a book (edited by Mark Swerdlow) on the therapy of pain, contrasting the picture of widespread unrelieved pain in nonhospice patients with the results at Saint Christopher's Hospice: from 1972 to 1977, of almost 3,400 patients (75 percent of whom entered with pain), only 1 percent had ongoing pain.

The groups at Saint Christopher's and Sloan-Kettering shared a concern with cancer pain control but had different perspectives on their results. Twycross questioned Houde's conclusions at the sessions on cancer pain at the First World Congress on Pain in 1975. Houde wanted to compare the effect of a single dose of oral morphine with that of a single dose when injected. He quantitatively established the degree of patient tolerance following extended use of each opiate. Because he wanted to compare pain before or after each dose in the same patient, the hospice approach of maintaining analgesia to sustain well-being was incompatible. In this approach, oral morphine was preferable on the grounds that it supported patient autonomy and maintained effective relief when taken on a predetermined schedule. In the unlikely event the patient developed tolerance, pain control would not be threatened by concern about keeping the dosage down.

Twycross warned against allowing pain to reappear before the next dose because that practice caused unnecessary suffering and promoted tolerance. Houde recognized that on-demand dosage reimposed pain before medication could suppress it, to the detriment of patient morale. The disadvantages, however, with regular dosage was the cloaking of new complications or a remission in the disease. The particular areas of common ground were preference for morphine as a reliable analgesic as opposed to diamorphine, meperidine, metapon, methadone, propoxyphene, and pentazocine, as well as titration of doses according to patient pain, not adherence to a set standard. Indeed, out of the testing of the Brompton mixture against oral morphine came recognition of the great significance of titration, although the hospice movement would say, always within a holistic approach to care of the patient. While not agreeing on the likelihood of tolerance and how to deal with it, both groups agreed it could be managed. Finally, the great majority of patients could enjoy effective pain relief, although the attending doctor had to be careful if adequate management were to be achieved (Meldrum, 2003, 201–5; Clark, 2003, 97).

The new knowledge generated by the London and New York groups supported the WHO guidelines on cancer pain control published in a booklet titled *Cancer Pain Relief* (1986) that Robert Twycross and Jan Stjernsward (a Swedish oncologist) copublished. Stjernsward, who had become head of the WHO cancer unit in 1981, was interested in developing a control program based on prevention, early detection and treatment, and pain relief.

It was clear that, although access to proper therapy for all of the world's cancer sufferers was an impossible dream, improvement in pain relief provision was feasible. Stjernsward and Swerdlow sent a questionnaire to cancer clinics in 11 countries. They also recruited experts to advise them on formulating a simple pain relief program: John Bonica; Kathleen Foley (Memorial Sloan-Kettering Cancer Center, New York); Robert Twycross (Sir Michael Sobell House, Oxford); Vittorio Ventofridda (National Cancer Institute, Milan); and Anders Rane (Huddinge University Hospital, Stockholm).

Responses to the questionnaire revealed that only 10 percent of patients enjoyed full relief, while 29 percent enjoyed little or no relief. If the program were to be applicable globally, it had to be simple enough to be used in resource-poor, third-world countries. The key idea was a progressive three-step ladder of analgesics from nonopioids to strong opioids. The drugs were to be administered orally (promoting patient autonomy), by the clock, not on an as-required basis, and the dose was to be titrated to meet the particular patient's needs. Five types of adjuvants were recommended to improve pain control and help combat associated illness; radiotherapy, chemotherapy, or palliative surgery would be used with persistent pain. The major analgesics were aspirin (or acetaminophen), codeine (or dextroproposyphene), and morphine (or methadone, meperidine or buprenorphine). The adjuvant drugs were anticonvulsants, neurolytics, anxiolytics, antidepressants, and corticosteroids.

It was realized that, for the program to have a real effect internationally, supporters would have to encourage wider access to drugs in underdeveloped countries. Almost all of Africa and the Indian subcontinent lacked access to oral morphine. They would have to educate underprescribing doctors, underdosing nurses, and reluctant pharmacists about opioids and modern pain control; moreover, they would have to find a way to help those professionals overcome fears of causing addiction, which also permeated the wider culture and influenced the policies of governments. Even in many Western countries the legal use of oral opiates was not widely allowed because of a wish to curb illicit drug use. Much liaison work with national health ministries in relation to the effects of narcotic drug controls was carried out, and the work was continued by David Joranson of the WHO Collaborating Center at the University of Wisconsin. Indeed, the establishment of WHO collaborating centers around the world did much to promote the WHO cancer pain relief program. The first were the Center for Palliative Cancer Care, Sir Michael Sobell House, Oxford; the Center for Symptom Evaluation in Cancer Care, Madison, Wisconsin; and the Center for Cancer Pain Relief, National Cancer Institute, Milan. Later, others were set up in Winnipeg, New York, and Saitama (Japan).

Cancer Pain Relief (1986) was quickly translated into 15 languages. In 1998 WHO published a monograph titled *Cancer Pain Relief and Palliative Care in Chil-*

dren, which stated that since most children suffering from cancer lived in developing countries, they did not receive curative treatment; thus, proper care would consist primarily of palliation of pain and other symptoms (Stjernsward and Teoh, 1990, 9–11; WHO, 1998, 1; Swerdlow, 2003, 157–71). A survey of British and Australian children (7–12 years of age) suffering from cancer found that about a third had been in pain during the previous two days. More than 50 percent of this group experienced medium to severe pain, while a third were in severe pain. A study of children with cancer (10–18 years of age) at the Memorial Sloan-Kettering Cancer Center found that 84 percent of inpatients experienced pain; 87 percent said it was moderate to severe, and 53 percent said it was severe. Among outpatients, 35 percent experienced pain; 75 percent rated it moderate to severe, while 26 percent said they were suffering quite a bit to very much.

Even in the 1990s, clinicians remained in conflict over opioid tolerance. One group represented by Twycross saw no great problem with long-term use, whereas the other was unwilling to prescribe until death was close for fear the drugs would decline in effectiveness. In the early 1990s there was evidence that oncologists continued to undertreat pain for that reason, and the position seemed to have garnered support from laboratory studies with animal models indicating that tolerance was inevitable. However, many cancer and noncancer patients showed no evidence of tolerance although they used the same dose for many years. Indeed, Katherine Foley and Robert Twycross separately argued that the increase in dosage arose from the advance of the cancer disease, not from growing tolerance of the drug. The escalation of doses itself promoted confusion of tolerance with physical dependence and addiction.

The work of Jane Porter and Herschel Jick (1980) showed that addiction (compulsive use, continued use, and use even in the face of harm) was rare where the opioids were being used medically: only 0.03 percent of 11,882 patients in pain who received narcotics at Boston University Hospital. In 1981 Ronald Kanner and Kathleen Foley reported a study of 103 patients who attended Sloan-Kettering Pain Clinic for two years. There was no evidence of abuse in 45 patients with cancer who continued on opiates after six months; only 2 of 17 noncancer patients on opiates took more than what was prescribed, and both presented with a long history of drug abuse.

Patients who need pain relief have to be differentiated from patients who have an addiction disorder. Further, the model of addiction originally developed in the 1920s in the United States saw the addict as having a severe personality disorder very difficult to overcome and as typically coming from a lower-class and/or nonwhite background. In the 1960s and 1970s, drug abuse spread widely in the white middle classes, and a new model appeared in the 1980s: genetic, psychological, and social factors interacted with learned behavior that could be modified. This fitted better with the idea of careful physician management of opiate use by the patient suffering pain.

In 1986 Russell Portenoy and Kathleen Foley published the results of a study of 38 patients with noncancer pain; only two were either dependent or using analgesics too much, but only 24 enjoyed satisfactory relief. While unable to specify patient psychological or social factors with a very strong correlation with satisfactory therapy, they did identify as significant the involvement of the attending physician. In this they were pinpointing the factor of physician involvement and concern with the patient that, earlier, Twycross and, separately, Houde and Rogers had found to be important. This was the sort of involvement that Cecily Saunders had proposed in response to the total pain of the terminally ill patient in the context of hospice palliative care.

In his 2003 address to the annual meeting of the American Pain Society, John Loeser argued that failure to see the limitations of the biomedical model had led to a dichotomous approach to chronic pain management in the United States—a divide between those who performed procedures and those who provided care for pain patients—a division Bonica had warned against half a century earlier. Loeser went on to point out that the emphasis on technical interventions was reinforced in the United States by a payment system in which financial rewards from fees, set by the government and the insurance agencies, were skewed toward interventions; as a result, clinics were under great pressure to do more procedures and increase revenue (Cleary and Backonja, 1996, 1–10; Meldrum, 2003, 207–8; Loeser, 2003, 5–6).

PAIN AND PUBLIC POLICY

WHO's global strategy of promoting the concept of the ladder of cancer pain relief in the mid-1980s has been discussed. Efforts were also made within countries to promote national and, where relevant, state policy to improve access to the management of cancer pain, drug availability, and the education of health professionals.

In 1984 the Compassionate Pain Relief Bill was introduced in the U.S. Congress. Members of Congress who had been deeply affected by seeing family and friends die in great pain wanted to promote pain relief throughout the country. The bill would have allowed doctors to use heroin with dying patients. Members of Congress, knowing that heroin was used in British hospices, erroneously concluded that it was the answer to the problem of cancer pain. June Dahl, chair of Wisconsin's Controlled Substances Board (WCSB), sought to explain to Wisconsin's congressional representatives that heroin was not the best way to provide patients with relief. Dahl and David Joranson lobbied congresspersons to oppose the bill, and the bill was not enacted.

The WCSB was committed to preventing prescription drugs from falling into the hands of those who would misuse them, but it did not want this objective to undermine efforts to improve management of cancer pain.

Dahl and colleagues, as the Wisconsin Initiative for Improving Cancer Pain Management (later the Wisconsin Cancer Pain Initiative), identified a number of key goals: effective pain relief treatments were available and simply needed to be applied more widely; not only terminal pain but also pain at any stage of the disease should be targeted; attitudes and behaviors of professionals, as well as knowledge, had to be addressed; and any program for Wisconsin should also be useful in other states. Clinicians, schools of medicine and nursing, professional societies, state agencies, and pharmacists were involved, and a major planning session was held at the end of 1986. Luminaries such as Jan Stjernsward, Kathleen Foley, and J. C. Duffy (Assistant U.S. Surgeon General) spoke to the participants, who included a representative of the National Institute of Drug Abuse and Mexican and Indian pain relief advocates. The Wisconsin Cancer Pain Initiative (WCPI) became a WHO demonstration project.

At the Second World Congress on Cancer Pain in New York in 1988, a workshop was held on the work of the WCPI. The following year, the WCPI sponsored a national meeting of those from other states who wanted to form their own initiatives, and in 1992, the Robert Wood Johnson Foundation funded the Resource Center for State Pain Initiatives. This assisted the establishment of initiatives in various states over the next decade. By 1996 the movement was ready to form a national body, the American Alliance of Cancer Pain Initiatives (AACPI).

At the seventh national meeting of State Cancer Pain Initiatives, attended by representatives of 30 states, as well as Australia, the American Alliance of Cancer Pain Initiatives was established. The AACPI was to devote its efforts to the goal of making effective management a top priority in all health care environments.

Public policy on pain control was being developed by the states themselves. In 1994 the Florida legislature created a state pain commission to address treatment issues not only in cancer pain but also in acute postoperative, acute medical, chronic, and acute and chronic pediatric pain. To the same ends the Michigan House of Representatives created the Michigan Council on Pain. In 1992 Gov. William Weld appointed a special task force on pain management in Massachusetts. The Ohio Health Department established a committee of experts to study the state of education about, and the resources devoted to, pain management.

Various professional efforts in the early 1990s helped advance recognition of the need for effective pain control. Position statements were issued by the Oncology Nursing Society and the American Society of Clinical Oncology, while the American Academy of Pain Medicine was formed for physicians, and the American Society of Pain Management Nurses for nurses. The pain management movement contributed to the defeat of a Drug Enforcement Administration (DEA) proposal for legislation requiring all U.S. physicians to use government-issued prescription forms for all controlled substances. The proposal would have ended oral prescriptions for schedule 3 analgesics such as codeine and hydrocone combinations. Earlier, members of the American Pain Society and professional associations lobbied successfully against a Maryland bill that would have introduced a triplicate prescription system. Cancer Care, a New York social service agency that supported cancer patients and their families, recommended that New York State replace the requirement that doctors use government-issued prescription forms for opioids and benzodiazepines with a less intrusive system; an electronic prescription monitoring system was proposed as a substitute (Dahl, 1996, 1–3; Joranson, 1996, 1–2; Angarola and Bormel, 1996, 1–5; Dahl, 2003, 63–66).

In mid-1998 the Southern California Cancer Pain Initiative (SCCPI) sponsored a pain summit to discuss regulatory issues and medical education as barriers to improvements in pain management. Participants reported that the California Bureau of Narcotic Enforcement and the Board of Pharmacy were now evaluating the system of triplicate prescriptions versus electronic monitoring to improve patients' access to controlled substances while preventing violations of prescribing privileges.

In 1998 the legislature of New York State ended the use of triplicate prescription forms, and the Ohio legislature enacted laws on the use of opioids in cancer pain and for nonterminal chronic pain. The Florida legislature and the Virginia Medical Society issued, respectively, practice guidelines for pain treatment and guidelines for use of opioids in chronic noncancer pain. The law in Massachusetts now allowed prescriptions to be sent electronically, schedule 2 prescriptions from any state to be filled, and the validity of such prescriptions to be extended from 5 to 30 days.

Not only legislators, bureaucrats, and health professionals were becoming more aware of the need to improve pain relief. The press was also educating the public about the matter. The *Wall Street Journal* published two editorials in mid-1998: "Treat the Pain" (July 27) and "Progress against Pain" (August 11). Moreover, lay advocacy and social service agencies were working to change public perceptions. In 1989 Cancer Care established the Cancer Pain Support and Education Initiative to bring about changes in public policy and perceptions. While recognizing that progress had been made over the decade of the initiative's work, Cancer Care also recognized that pain medication continued to be controversial, with disagreement among doctors about what level of relief to give and, too often, the needs of patients not being met (Hastie, Kovner, and Ferrell, 1998, 1–5; Strassels, 1998, 1–2; Blum, 1999, 1–5).

Lay advocacy groups were also working closely with specialist professional bodies. In 1997 the American Pain Society (APS) invited patient advocacy groups to join the society, establishing a patient organization liaison task force to facilitate communication. The hope was that the close relationship would educate APS members about patient needs, assist the APS in promoting its policy agenda, make APS expertise available to patient groups, and advance research by encouraging patient involvement in clinical trials and data collection.

In 2001 the AACPI and the American Cancer Society formally entered into a cooperative relationship. Each brought strengths—the first, its capacity to work at the state level when states present problems that cannot be addressed effectively from the national level, as well as its access to health care providers and to expertise on pain management; the second, its high reputation for service and its skills in advocacy, fund-raising, and organization of meetings.

The state initiatives addressed issues in professional education, patient education, and community education and sought to change the health care system itself in order to break down barriers to better pain management. The WCPI ran model programs for physicians and nurses in 26 states in the course of the 1990s, and the practice spread to other initiatives. Broad public education was pursued on television and through specific public relations campaigns.

In 2000 WCPI published *Building an Institutional Commitment to Pain Management* to assist health care institutions in making pain relief central to patient care. Then, in 1999 the APS cooperated with the Joint Commission on Accreditation of Healthcare Organizations (JCAHO) to produce new standards for pain assessment and treatment. At the beginning of 2001 these became part of the survey and accreditation process. Thus, the process of making satisfactory pain relief a patient right was greatly advanced because the JCAHO accredited 80 percent of U.S. hospitals (which have 96 percent of national inpatient admissions), as well as long-term care facilities, home health agencies, and behavioral health facilities. Accreditation was necessary to achieve the status that was required for Medicaid and Medicare funding.

As I mentioned earlier, state regulations on prescribing and dispensing controlled substances were significant obstacles to effective pain control, and the initiatives have therefore worked to have such regulatory barriers removed. In particular, they sought to have model guidelines, published by the Federation of State Medical Boards in 1998, followed. Against a background of concern expressed by the media and law enforcement agencies about growing diversion of the painkiller oxycontin into illicit drug circles, the AACPI contributed to a position statement issued in 2001 by the Drug Enforcement Administration (responsible for the Federal Controlled Substances Act) and 44 health bodies. The statement recognized as central the need to balance the use of opioids for effective pain relief with the need to ensure they were not abused.

State initiatives also attempted to deal with the barriers represented by the health care system itself since neither private health insurance nor Medicare covered many of the expensive newer drugs. Thus, the Virginia Cancer Pain Initiative helped to obtain legislation requiring health maintenance organizations to fund drugs and access to hospice services, as well as to pain medicine practitioners and oncologists, without requiring the patient to have a referral.

Much has been achieved in improving cancer pain relief since 1986, when the WCPI began its work. Some 15 state initiatives have now broadened the disease focus of their efforts to all forms of pain and, like the Wisconsin Pain Initiative, have deleted "cancer" from their names. The cultural focus has broadened, too, with the Unbroken Circle Initiative, a Native American cancer pain initiative, having become part of the AACPI. The latter has joined the Intercultural Cancer Council, an organization that works to reduce the disproportionate burden of cancers falling on racial and ethnic minorities (Glajchen and Calder, 1998, 1–2; Chapman, 2000, 1; Ashburn, 2001, 1; Dahl, 2003, 167–72).

The struggle to prevent reactions to opioid abuse from infringing the rights of those in severe pain to drug relief continued as the North Carolina Pain Initiative recognized in a 2001 statement on opioids for severe pain; any action to reduce drug-related crime (e.g., fingerprinting patients) should not create barriers that prevent people from using medications they need for pain.

In October 2000 the U.S. Congress proclaimed that the "Decade of Pain Control and Research" would begin on January 1, 2001. Originally proposed by Philipp Lippe, it was strongly promoted by the American Academy of Pain Medicine and the Pain Care Coalition, formed in 1998 by the Academy, the APS, and the American Headache Society. With the precedent of the Decade of Brain Research and Neuroscience in mind, proponents hoped that benefits such as more research funding and national legislation relating to better pain management might ensue.

One great achievement of the Decade of Pain Control and Research is the National Pain Care Policy bill of April 2003, sponsored by Rep. Mike Rogers from Michigan. The introduction followed several years of lobbying by the Pain Care Coalition and the AAPM. The bill authorized a White House Conference on Pain Care that would create an agenda for the Decade of Pain Control and Research and establish a National Center for Pain and Palliative Care Research at the National Institutes of Health. The center would support clinical and basic scientific research, begin a program of interdisciplinary research, coordinate all research on pain done at NIH, and report annually on public and private funding of pain care research. The legislation also provided for six regional pain research centers; for the Agency for Healthcare Research and Quality to disseminate protocols on pain and palliative care and to fund the education of health care professionals in pain and palliative care; for the U.S. Department of Health and Human Services to educate the public about pain as a national public health problem and about patients' rights to treatment; for the Secretary of Defense and the Secretary of the Department of Veterans Affairs to introduce pain care initiatives in their respective health care facilities; for requiring managed health care plans offering Medicare + Choice (now Medicare Advantage) plans to seniors to cover pain relief and to make a similar provision for military personnel and dependants under Tricare plans; and for the centers for Medicare and Medicaid services to report annually to Congress on Medicare spending on pain and palliative care (Lippe, 2000, 1; North Carolina Pain Initiative, 2001, 1; Gitlin, 2003, 1–3).

In 1997 the AAPM became concerned about the need to standardize medical school education about pain. The next year it established an undergraduate education committee. Frustrated by the failure to achieve improvement in medical education by voluntary means, some state legislatures such as that of California mandated medical student education in pain management. The medical school of the University of Texas in Houston introduced an elective course in end-of-life care and pain management in 1997. In mid-2000 a session on end-of-life care and pain management became part of the required internal medicine clinical rotation for senior medical students. Debra Weiner and Gregory Turner carried out the same sort of curricular innovation at the University of Pittsburgh.

In July 2000 the board of directors of the AAPM approved a position statement on undergraduate medical education on pain management, end-of-life care, and palliative care. The announcement states that one of the significant impediments to effective end-of-life care is lack of proper education. Although acknowledging that the Liaison Committee on Medical Education (the national accrediting body for MD programs in U.S. and Canadian medical schools) had just mandated education and clinical experience in end-of-life care for accreditation, it nevertheless called for education in the broader scope of pain medicine. The academy recommended the following:

1. The core curriculum of medical schools should include pain medicine, end-of-life care, and palliative care.
2. Integrated, multidisciplinary courses should be included rather than an isolated lecture or clinical time.

3. Such courses should be run by staff with specialist training in these three areas (AAPM, 2000; Gallagher, 2002, 1; Chang, 2002, 1–2).

Now that pain medicine was becoming better established, some practitioners began building more direct links with palliative care medicine. In 1998 the APS created a new palliative care special interest group, and 200 APS members indicated an interest in joining. The cochairs of the special interest group, Myra Glajchen and Donna Zhukovsky, pointed out the close parallels between pain medicine and palliative care; both involved an interdisciplinary model requiring team-based management of the physical, psychological, social, spiritual, and existential needs of patients; and both involved the question of generalist versus specialist practice.

At the same time, Maywin Liu of the Pain Management Center at the Hospital of the University of Pennsylvania called for more involvement of anesthesiologists in palliative care because of the prevalence of pain at the end of life. Palliative medicine, which was dominated by oncologists, did not appear to be providing adequate pain control for a sizeable number of patients. Despite WHO guidelines, the appropriate use of opioids was not widespread enough largely because physicians feared loss of license and patient addiction. Anesthesiologists needed to become more involved in palliative medicine, even though it was at that time a small and not very glamorous field (Liu, 1998, 1–2; Zhukovsky and Glajchen, 2001, 1).

Russell Portenoy, head of the Department of Pain Medicine and Palliative Care at the Beth Israel Medical Center in New York, pointed out in 1999 that pain specialists had a great opportunity to be among the leaders in the speedily evolving field of palliative care. Indeed, some pain specialists had already become palliative care practitioners. They faced a historical situation in which hospice based on the British model had been the center of palliative care in the United States for more than two decades. However, late referral to hospice was common, and only 40 percent of those dying of cancer (and about 15 percent of all others) entered a hospice program. Moreover, hospice could not always provide a specialist physician and could not make available expensive palliative treatments. The best development would be for interdisciplinary palliative care programs in institutional environments to link with existing hospice programs, as the Department of Pain Medicine and Palliative Care at the Beth Israel Medical Center had done in 1997 and 1998. The result would ideally be an integrated model of care whose practitioners could then obtain referrals from other hospital departments. The integrated model provided specialized palliative services at an earlier stage for patients for whom hospice was not yet appropriate, as well as more appropriate referrals to hospice. Moreover, there was also continuity of clinician care.

At Beth Israel, Portenoy had inherited an eight-bed hospice, the Jacob Perlow Hospice Program, and a hospice home care program. He set out to provide intensive medical care in the inpatient hospice unit and access for home care nurses to palliative care physicians. Like most U.S. hospices, the Perlow hospice had previously had little access to medical expertise. Portenoy planned to extend access to physicians to the home care patient by instituting home visits by doctors. He believed future development demanded that palliative care and hospice become part of mainstream health care. This would require educating staff members of other hospital departments, as well as individual practitioners, so that they would make referrals; as a result, palliative care would become just another specialty (Portenoy, 1999, 1–5; Portenoy, 2003, 1–13).

In the late 1970s Kathleen Foley established the first pain and palliative care service in a U.S. cancer hospital. The contributions of Foley and her colleagues at the Memorial Sloan-Kettering Cancer Center in New York to research into cancer pain management in the pioneering era of pain medicine have been discussed. In 1998 Richard Payne named Foley as head of the service. Payne, like Portenoy, had a vision of integrated palliative care and pain management, as well as a broad view of the palliative care of cancer patients.

I noted earlier that the Intractable Pain Society of Great Britain and Ireland was formed in 1971. The membership at that time consisted mainly of anesthetists who managed pain clinics. By the end of the century, the membership had become multidisciplinary and included nurses, physiotherapists, psychologists, psychiatrists, occupational therapists, and scientists, as well as medical practitioners. The Intractable Pain Society, which in 1988 changed its name to simply the Pain Society, was the British chapter of the International Association for the Study of Pain. Like the American Pain Society, it was reaching out to patients to ensure their views on policy were known (Pain Society, 2003, 1–2). Indeed, in 1997 the Pain Society, in issuing a document on desirable criteria for pain management programs, specifically stated that the document took a patient-centered approach.

The authors of the document addressed key issues such as patient referral, appropriate staffing, and training. Concerning the first, they pointed out that immediate expert assessment of new patients was needed to determine whether they were suitable for treatment because many health care professionals were ignorant of the range of therapies available. The second key issue was that, ideally, staff members would include a pain specialist physician, clinical psychologist, physiotherapist, occupational therapist, and nurse. However, the minimum should be a physician, a psychologist, and a physiotherapist. As to the third key topic, the Royal College of Anaesthetists was preparing a training document for doctors. Because no formal accreditation for pain programs existed, the institution of training programs for all of the relevant disciplines was essential.

A number of major problems beset pain centers in the United States, and many also applied in Britain and Ireland: inaccurate information on the costs of individual treatment components; lack of evaluation of outcomes; disagreement among practitioners about what constituted effective treatment; too many health care professionals and citizens who were unaware of chronic pain as a health problem; inadequate regulation of practice; and admission of patients for package treatment rather than individualized care (Memorial Sloan-Kettering Cancer Center, 1998, 1; Pain Society, 1997, 1–9).

In 1997 the Pain Society joined with the Association of Anaesthetists of Great Britain and Ireland to report on the provision of pain services. The report stated that people with cancer pain might present to the pain physician in a hospital, hospice, or home setting, and specialist techniques might be required to manage them. It also stated that chronic pain was a complex biopsychosocial problem and that a third of patients with chronic pain lacked objective signs of organic disease. Control of pain was a basic human right. Palliative care services dealt adequately with cancer pain in 90 percent of patients using simple drug therapy, but they should cooperate with pain services in the more difficult cases.

The Calman-Hine report on improvement of cancer services proposed that consultants establish close clinical and operational ties with local pain clinics and that pain management and palliative medicine be integrated managerially as well as clinically. The resources required for cancer pain therapy were similar to those required for chronic pain, and appropriately equipped facilities should be available within the hospice or elsewhere so that hospice or home care patients could be brought in for short-term care (Association of Anaesthetists of Great Britain and Ireland and Pain Society, 1997, 1–9).

At the turn of the twentieth century, about 200 of the 270 large hospitals in Britain offered chronic pain services. Coverage varied by region: London had 20 clinics but Northern Ireland only 6. Clinic facilities also varied, and some were described as crowded or inadequate. The most commonly offered chronic pain treatments were opioid medication (92 percent of services offered it); single epidural injection (95 percent); sympathectomy (local anesthetic) (95 percent); transcutaneous electrical neurostimulation (95 percent); and acupuncture (90 percent). Moreover, a low level of cooperation with other specialties existed. The specialties with which joint clinics were more often held were palliative medicine (15 percent of chronic pain services); rheumatology (8 percent); orthopedic surgery (7 percent); and psychiatry (6 percent). Those with which pain services least often held joint clinics were oncology (2 percent of chronic pain services); ENT surgery (2 percent); hematology (1 percent); and urology (1 percent) (Pain Society, 2003, 1–8).

In 1984 the advisory committee on the management of severe chronic pain in cancer patients reported on cancer pain treatment to the Canadian Minister of National Health and Welfare. It noted that cancer pain management, and in particular the reintroduction of the therapeutic use of heroin, had in recent years become controversial. It concluded that inadequate pain control resulted not from the failure to employ heroin but from the deficient use of oral morphine, which, when regularly used, was effective for 90 percent of patients with cancer pain. Among the reasons for poor pain management were failure to deal with psychological, social, and spiritual factors; inadequate application of adjuvants such as radiation and chemotherapy, nerve and spinal blocks, palliative surgery, transcutaneous electrical nerve stimulation, acupuncture, and relaxation techniques; entrenched professional attitudes such as unrealistic fear of inducing drug dependence; and pain clinics (which were available in major cities but were absent in the rest of the country). It therefore recommended better education of health professionals, plus greater federal support for the development of pain control services. In addition, it recommended the marketing of a highly concentrated form of hydromorphine, an injectable form of methadone, more concentrated formulations of morphine hydrochloride, and sublingual and rectal formulations of available potent analgesics (*Cancer Pain*, 1984, 5–7, 15–16).

In 1994 a survey of 14,628 Canadian physicians concerning cancer pain treatment practices yielded 2,686 responses; a little more than 18 percent of general practitioners and family physicians, slightly more than 39 percent of medical or radiation oncologists, and 17.5 percent of other specialties responded. The survey found that only 50 percent were ready to use strong opioids in the initial pain management regimen, although oncologists (53 percent) were more likely to prescribe them than general practitioners (37 percent) or palliative care specialists (38 percent); 76 percent of oncologists and 73 percent of palliative care specialists but only 54 percent of general practitioners recommended the use of palliative radiotherapy. Only 5 percent of physicians rated their medical school education in pain management as excellent, while 25 percent rated it good. Of the barriers to optimal pain management, physicians ranked highest, along with the issues of pain assessment and doctor-patient understanding of the use of analgesics. Of intermediate importance were patient access to pain control, reluctance of doctors to prescribe opioids, access to nonpharmacological pain management, and nurses' discomfort with opioid use. The authors of the survey proposed that inquiries into pain and other symptom control at the provincial and regional levels be carried out. They also pointed out that, in the United Kingdom and Australasia, recognition of palliative medicine as a specialty had resulted in the formal training of a group of well-qualified physicians who were able to act as consultants to oncology and family physician colleagues (MacDonald, Findlay, Bruera, Dudgeon, and Kramer, 1997, 332–41).

In 1998 the Canadian Pain Society announced that a working group had completed a consensus statement and guidelines on the use of opioid analgesics in the treatment of chronic noncancer pain. In mid-2001 the society drew up a patient pain manifesto, which was intended to be a bill of rights for patients in pain. The president of the society, Celeste Johnson, observed that half of hospital patients unnecessarily experience moderate to severe pain. The professional use of pain-rating scales had to become as common as the taking of blood pressure and body temperature.

In mid-2002 the Canadian Pain Coalition was launched. Composed of patients and their families and CPS members, the coalition stated that its main aims were to raise public awareness of the extent of the problem and to lobby governments to fund better services. It proclaimed the first week of November to be National Pain Awareness Week. It noted that the costs of pain (due to lost productivity and treatment) were estimated to be billions of dollars (Clark, 1998, 1–2; Pinker, 2001, 1; Letter from the President, 2003, 1; *Canada NewsWire,* 2004, 1–2).

While anesthetists in New Zealand had for many years used nerve blocks to relieve chronic cancer pain, specialist pain clinics date only from the 1970s. An example is the work of anesthetist R. E. Rawstron, who in 1977 studied in clinics in England, Germany, and the United States in preparation for opening a weekly clinic at Palmerston North Hospital; the clinic began operating in 1978. A decade and a half later, the medical director of Arohura Hospice, Dr. A. Farnell, was conducting two clinics a week in the hospital (Rawstron, 2002, 37–45). The New Zealand Pain Society was formed in 1983, and its first president was Michael Roberts. The 1990s saw the further growth of pain treatment facilities and professional organizations.

Soon after its inauguration in 1992, the Australian and New Zealand College of Anaesthetists established a working party on certification for pain management. An advisory committee on pain medicine, with representatives of the Royal Australasian College of Surgeons, the Royal Australian and New Zealand College of Psychiatrists, the Royal Australasian College of Physicians, and the Australasian Faculty of Rehabilitation Medicine, drew up training requirements for a certificate. In 1998 the governing board of the College of Anaesthetists approved the establishment of a Faculty of Pain Medicine, and the first membership examination took place in November 1999. Good working relations were quickly established with the Chapter of Palliative Medicine of the Royal Australasian College of Physicians (ANZCA, 2003, 1; Anesthesia, 2003, 1; New Zealand Pain Society, 2003, 1).

Historically, Australia and New Zealand have been large consumers of opioids. In 1934 the *Medical Journal of Australia* pointed out that New Zealand used 3.36 kilograms of heroin per million population, and Australia used 3.10 kilograms, but Canada used only 1.75 kilograms; the United Kingdom, 1.09 kilograms; and the United States, 0.06 kilograms. Twenty years later, Australia and New Zealand were substantial consumers of morphine and pethidine (Table 5.1).

From 1986 to 1995 Australian consumption of oral morphine increased markedly. Methadone syrup (used in heroin addiction therapy) increased at the same rate, while other schedule 8 opioids increased only slightly. The number of injectable opioids used annually increased over the same period from 4.1 to 7.1 million ampoules. Annual consumption of oral morphine rose from 117 to 578 kilograms between 1986 and 1995. All other oral schedule 8 opioids in total rose from 93 to 149 kilograms in the same period. It seems likely that prescribing patterns were influenced by the availability of slow-release morphine in 1990 since the rate of increase in morphine prescriptions clearly increased from that time. Figures from the drug utilization subcommittee of the Commonwealth Pharmaceutical Benefits Advisory Committee indicated that the use of panadeine forte increased from 1.9 million prescriptions in 1991 to 3.7 million in 1995.

The Commonwealth director general of health, A. J. Metcalfe, told the UN Expert Committee on Drugs in 1950 that addiction was rare in Australia. Sensitive to its international reputation, the federal government nevertheless prohibited the importation of heroin in 1953, and the states soon fell into line by prohibiting its

Table 5.1. Consumption of Morphine and Pethidine per Million Population in 1953

Morphine		Pethidine	
Country	Kilograms per Million	Country	Kilograms per Million
United Kingdom	15.84	Australia	53.53
Australia	15.49	New Zealand	51.13
New Zealand	8.52	United States	41.81
United States	7.32	Canada	20.65
Canada	5.34	United Kingdom	19.34

Source: Medical Journal of Australia, 1957, 120.

manufacture. The legal use of heroin thus effectively ended, although in some states it could still be legally prescribed (*Medical Journal of Australia,* 1934, 487; Manderson, 1993, 125–29).

In 1980 the relative merits of heroin and morphine for relief for terminal cancer pain were debated in the *Medical Journal of Australia.* The chair of the standing committee on anticancer medications of the Clinical Oncological Society, Martin Tattersall, listed the conclusions reached by the committee:

1. The efficacy of morphine, when used appropriately, was not less than that of heroin.
2. Clinical studies revealed a similar incidence of side effects.
3. Chronic patients have no preference, but former addicts prefer morphine.
4. The key issue is the correct administration of oral morphine, which should be given in doses large enough to suppress pain, frequently enough to prevent pain recurring; cocaine admixed is unnecessary, although phenothiazines may enhance the analgesia.
5. Because it is more soluble than morphine, heroin permits smaller amounts to be injected; thus, with large-dose injections, heroin is more advantageous, but this does not outweigh the problems arising from the widespread use of heroin.
6. The committee does not endorse the use of heroin in therapy.

Soon thereafter, Alan Lane, a Tasmanian doctor, called for heroin to again be made available for terminal patients, pointing out the comforting euphoria it gave the patient. Sydney palliative care expert Gordon Coates responded, saying that morphine, when used correctly, produced the same result as heroin (Tattersall, 1981b, 492; Lane, 1986, 334; Coates, 1985, 59–60).

A decade later Jim Siderov and J. R. Zalcberg, Repatriation Hospital, Melbourne, stated that opioids were still being underused for cancer pain partly due to doctors' conservative attitudes. However, they argued, this was also due to restrictive policies under which the states required prescribers to obtain Health Department permits for drug treatment beyond a certain period. Moreover, the Commonwealth Pharmaceutical Benefits Scheme, under which citizens obtained government-subsidized access to prescribed medications, tightly controlled the amount that could be prescribed.

In 1989 the National Health and Medical Research Council (NHMRC) issued a report on the management of severe pain. The NHMRC called for changes in the training, attitudes, and practices of medical, nursing, and related professionals and for greater community awareness of the need to treat pain. It pointed out that, in Western countries such as Australia, 40–80 percent of severe cancer pain was not alleviated. However, this could be reduced to 5 percent with good management. The correct management required repeated assessment; round-the-clock dosage; adjuvant treatment; time to listen to the patient; and empathy from caregivers, family, and friends. Unfortunately, some doctors saw heroin as the answer to terminal pain when it had no benefits that were not attainable from other analgesic regimens (NHMRC, 1989, vii, 6; Siderov and Zalcberg, 1994, 515–16).

Eleven years later, palliative medicine specialists Kiran Virik and Paul Glare stated that unfounded fears still led to suboptimal use of morphine. Where the adverse effects of morphine were greater than the analgesic effect, opioid substitution should be pursued. The choices included sustained-release oxycodone; fentanyl (a full opioid agonist available in transdermal patches); methadone; hydromorphone (five times more potent and six times more soluble than morphine; it was popular in the United States and had become available in Britain); and tramadol (it had been used in Europe for two decades but had only recently been adopted in English-speaking countries). Norelle Lickiss, pioneer palliative medicine specialist, wrote that morphine was still the gold standard in the treatment of cancer pain, but it had to be appropriately used: careful calibration of the dose and counseling of the patient about myths concerning addiction or tolerance were requisite. The relief of cancer pain was both an ethical imperative and an exercise of compassion. The Sydney Institute of Palliative Medicine (of which Lickiss was the founder) advised four treatment steps:

Step 1. Assess and reduce the noxious stimulus.
Step 2. Raise the patient's pain threshold.
Step 3. Exploit the opioid receptor system.
Step 4. Recognize and treat neuropathic pain.
(Virik and Glare, 2000, 1167–71; Lickiss, 2001, 5–14)

In New Zealand, the first hospices had been set up in 1979: Mary Potter within Calvary Hospital, Wellington; Saint Joseph's within Mercy Hospital, Auckland; and Te Omanga, Lower Hutt, an independent, inpatient institution. The next year, acting on the finding of a report by the Department of Radiotherapy and Oncology, Wellington Hospital, that a comprehensive regional policy on the care of the terminally ill was needed, the medical superintendent of the hospital, Caleb Tucker, asked the Wellington Health Services Advisory Committee (WHSAC) to establish a working party on the matter. In its December 1981 report, WHSAC pointed out that 50 percent of deaths in the region were from cancer and that 28 percent of those took place in a hospice. However, it also stated that physical problems were often poorly controlled for long periods of time. Pain relief was more effectively delivered in a hospice context, and hospices should be seen as resource centers whose staff members have special skills in the care of the dying. In 1991 the impact of hospice care was assessed by R. Dunlop for a seminar in Wellington. He concluded that hospice services had significantly contributed to the care of the terminally ill; moreover, a high degree of symptom control had been attained and the psychosocial needs of patients and families had also been met (*Care of the Terminally Ill,* 1981, 1, 4, 9; Barnett and Smith, 1992, 12).

PAIN AND HIV/AIDS

In 1991, about a decade into the HIV/AIDS epidemic, Roger Cole, Department of Palliative Care, Prince Henry and Prince of Wales Hospitals, Sydney, stated that care of patients with AIDS was a controversial challenge to palliative care because it had evolved to care for terminal cancer patients. The controversy is illustrated in the differing responses of Elisabeth Kübler-Ross and Cicely Saunders. The former asserted that any hospice refusing to take AIDS patients should not be called a hospice, while the latter argued for the establishment of special AIDS hospice facilities.

Cole further pointed out that pain was experienced in 53 of 100 consecutive patients in the San Francisco AIDS Home Care and Hospice Program. The most widely experienced pain was that due to peripheral neuropathy; next was abdominal pain and, in descending order, headache, skin pain, oropharyngeal pain, and chest pain. Opiates, paracetamol, and nonsteroidal anti-inflammatory drugs were all useful (Cole, 1991, 96–111).

The prevalence of pain among people with HIV is high, with estimates ranging from 30 to more than 90 percent depending on the stage of the disease, the care setting, and the study methodology. About 25–30 percent of ambulatory patients with early HIV disease have clinically significant pain.

In a prospective study of ambulatory patients, participants reported they had two to three pains at a time, thus experiencing a pain burden similar to that of cancer patients. A 1989 study of hospital patients found that pain was the presenting condition in 30 percent, and more than 50 percent needed therapy for pain. A 1993 study of ambulatory men found that 80 percent had one or more painful symptoms during a period of six months. A 1990 study of hospice patients reported 53 percent in pain, and a 1996 hospice study reported that 93 percent experienced at least one 48-hour period of pain over the final two weeks of life. A study by William Breitbart of the Memorial Sloan-Kettering Cancer Center and colleagues revealed that men and women had comparable pain prevalence rates, although women experienced higher average intensity levels.

Pain in HIV/AIDS may result from the effect of HIV on the central or peripheral nervous system, from immunosuppression (enabling opportunistic infections or cancers to develop), from the side effects of medications, or from etiologies not connected with HIV or its treatment. Peripheral neuropathy (the most common neurological complication) is both painful and relatively frequent, being experienced by as many as 30 percent of patients. A not uncommon side effect of medication is abdominal pain. A sample of 156 ambulatory patients in the late 1990s revealed that about 50 percent of pain syndromes were the direct result of immunosuppression, 30 percent were connected to therapy, and 20 percent were due to other causes.

Breitbart and others suggested that almost 85 percent of HIV/AIDS sufferers in their sample who reported pain did not receive adequate relief, based on WHO guidelines. This was well beyond the figure for the undertreatment of cancer pain. This was the case despite the publication by the U.S. Agency for Health Care Policy and Research of federal guidelines for the management of pain in patients with cancer and with HIV disease. Breitbart and colleagues investigated pain, psychological distress, and other factors in quality of life for ambulatory HIV patients. They established that pain and its intensity were significantly associated with measures of distress, depression, hopelessness, and quality of life. Functional disability correlated significantly with pain intensity and depression, and those in pain were more functionally impaired than those without pain.

Patients, physicians, and healthcare institutional factors all contributed to the problem of undertreatment of patients' pain. Fears that pain indicated disease progression or that pain would complicate diagnosis or treatment or involve unwelcome interventions could all lie behind patients' reticence to report pain. Recovered injecting drug users (who constitute a notable percentage of patients) feared they might become addicted to analgesics. Some patients believed they might be seen as difficult or might overburden their doctors. Medical practitioners might have unrealistic fears about inducing addiction, be ignorant of how to provide effective pain management, or be unable to consult with pain specialists. Furthermore, limited time for consultations might also push pain into the background. Low-income patients might simply lack access to treatment, and the managed health care organizations in the United States rendered it difficult to include treatment of pain. Many patients saw different practitioners for different aspects of their condition, and pain treatment fell through the cracks in the absence of communication between practitioners.

A particularly problematic area was pain management for patients who abused drugs. Such patients were much more likely to be undertreated for pain. Clinicians, fearing promotion of addiction, often tried not to prescribe opioids. Yet, long experience with cancer pain in drug abusers shows that opioids may be used responsibly when certain management principles are followed:

1. Tolerance and physical dependence must be distinguished from psychological dependence.
2. Active abusers, people on methadone maintenance, and those recovering must be distinguished from one another.
3. Pain treatment must be tailored to the individual patient.
4. The WHO ladder should be followed.
5. Pharmacologic and nonpharmacologic interventions (for example, cognitive-behavioral therapy), attention to psychosocial concerns, and a team involvement should be part of any pain management plan.

In the late 1990s, after highly active antiretroviral therapy (HAART) turned HIV/AIDS into a chronic illness, the locus of treatment shifted from specialty programs in hospitals to primary care settings. However, primary care practitioners might lack knowledge of management guidelines and access to pain specialists (Breitbart, Rosenfeld, Pasick, McDonald, Thaler, and Portenoy, 1996, 243–48; Breitbart, 1997, 63–91; Marcus, Stein, Kerns, Rosenfeld, and Breitbart, 2000, 260–81).

The staff of the special unit at London's Mildmay Hospital (which opened in the late 1980s as Europe's first specialized HIV/AIDS hospice) saw the admission picture alter as HIV disease changed: where in 1987, 50 percent of patients died at their first admission, in 1999, only 3 percent did so. The introduction of HAART brought about remission of Kaposi's sarcoma, refractory cryptosporidiosis, and progressive, multifocal leukoencephalopathy, as well as improvement in common symptoms such as night sweats, fatigue, weight loss, and seborrheic dermatitis. Although the new treatment had had these successes, new diagnoses of HIV in the

United Kingdom continued to increase. Moreover, HAART's viral suppression does not work in the long run; 40–50 percent of patients endure virological failure 12–24 months after the commencement of HAART.

The change in cancer care from active to palliative management used to happen at a particular point but is now introduced progressively as the disease advances. In contrast, HIV/AIDS disease displays an episodic quality with a period of extensive management in which to establish symptom control, which gives way to times when little if any has to be provided. Indeed, a patient considered terminal may then return to a good quality of life.

The percentage of patients—about 60 percent—who die in hospitals in Britain has remained more or less stable since the late 1980s, and their palliative care may vary in quality. People in the advanced stages of the disease commonly want to die at home, but many lack a general practitioner and will not establish a relationship with one because they fear discrimination or lack of confidentiality (Taylor-Thompson, 1992, 35–39; Easterbrook and Meadway, 2001, 442–49).

New HIV infections in Australia reached a peak in 1984 and fell thereafter, mainly because of primary preventive strategies. Diagnoses of AIDS peaked in 1994. The subsequent downward trend in these diagnoses was more precipitous than anticipated because of the impact of HAART. While there were 2,000 Australian people living with AIDS in 2000, there were as few as 100 deaths a year.

There are significant differences between pain in cancer and in HIV/AIDS. Psychiatric comorbidity, dementia, and drug dependence are encountered more often in advanced HIV patients. Polypharmacy, greater sensitivity to drug side effects, and drug interactions are more common. Little access to pain specialists and limited evidence for the efficacy of analgesics and coanalgesics such as antidepressants are also problems. The WHO ladder approach to analgesia looks less appropriate now that HIV/AIDS has changed from a progressive fatal illness to a chronic disease.

An Australian study of pain control in a group of predominantly young, educated, white, homosexual males set out to establish how somatic treatments (mainly analgesics) influenced pain in these ambulatory patients suffering from HIV disease. Abdominal pain was common. The pain on average had lasted for more than six months and was mild to moderate. The HIV infection on average had been present for eight years. The men were both moderately depressed and anxious. For 73 percent of the group, physical therapies (mostly pharmacotherapy) for the pain were provided. Scores for pain intensity, anxiety, or disability had not changed after four weeks, although depression scores had fallen somewhat (Glare, 2001, 43–48).

Pain control in terminal HIV/AIDS patients has become caught up in the controversy over the acceptability of euthanasia or physician-assisted suicide of dying patients. Arguments for and against—respect for the autonomy of suffering patients versus sanctity of life and the alleged inevitable slide into abuse of legalized euthanasia—seem irreconcilable. In any case, as Roger Magnusson states in his study of the euthanasia underground among HIV/AIDS patients in Sydney, euthanasia has been practiced to a significant extent not only in Sydney but also on the West Coast of the United States and in Vancouver, Canada, and the Netherlands.

A 1993 Sydney study found overwhelming support for the right to access euthanasia: of men with AIDS, 90 percent said they wanted to exercise this option should they receive a life-threatening diagnosis. While only 19 percent (of the 105 subjects) feared death, 86 percent feared the suffering of dying. A Sydney physician (anonymous to protect him from legal action), working in a hospital unit, told Magnusson that over a decade the staff at the unit had changed their approach. The intention to hasten death had become more widely accepted. The narcotic drip would be documented, for legal reasons, in the patient's chart as pain control, not euthanasia. The physician would only assist and then only after the patient requested euthanasia or the next of kin or someone with power of attorney did so. The physician believed the attitudes and values of the staff mirrored those of the gay community, which they saw as a historically disenfranchised group that had always had to establish its own standards of moral practice.

In 2002, People Living with AIDS and the AIDS Council of New South Wales assisted in the drafting of legislation that sought, unsuccessfully, to legalize euthanasia in New South Wales. They had supported similar bills in other states in the 1990s. Magnusson found in his interviews with HIV/AIDS patients that other factors than pain and suffering also fueled requests for assisted suicide. Thus, fear of future deterioration (and a need to regain a sense of control), rather than current factors, may lie behind talk of suicide. The same may be said of treatable depression (which, when eliminated, was replaced by a new sense of meaning) and, in some cases, a feeling of needing to honor past commitments that now no longer seemed right (Magnusson, 2002, 83–92, 195, 250–51; Sendzuik, 2003, 220–21).

A Canadian study in the late 1990s provided more data from patients in what has been a much underresearched area. Loss of self rather than pain, depression, or a high need for control emerged as the motivation for seeking assisted suicide. A sense of personal disintegration may be the result of disabled function but may also result from loss of community, and this may follow from the individual patient's sense of incapacity to sustain personal relationships.

Focus on the issue of intolerable suffering rather than loss of community would miss the great importance of the social context of dying shown by this study. The availability of good palliative care is by implication, therefore, an important clinical and policy matter. Another important question to be decided by further inquiries is whether the Canadian findings reflect the situation for patients with other illnesses and in other countries. As the authors of the Canadian study noted, loss of self is based as much in individuals' perception of their loss of integration in a community as in bodily disintegration. The authors suggested that their findings are supported by the philosophical, psychological, and sociological insights of Daniel Callahan, Aaron Antonovsky, and Irvin D. Yalom.

Callahan has claimed that loss of self has not been widely enough recognized as an explanation for the dying patient's wish for assisted suicide or euthanasia. Antonovsky has written of the need for a sense of coherence that allows the individual, facing stressors, to experience life as meaningful (the wish to cope), comprehensible (belief that the challenge is understandable), and manageable (belief that resources that enable coping are at hand). The strength of one's sense of coherence is a significant facilitator of the tendency toward health. Yalom has maintained that suffering is inevitable in relation to ultimate concerns such as death, freedom, existential isolation, and meaninglessness (Antonovsky, 1996, 15; Lavery, Boyle, Dickens, Maclean, and Singer, 2001, 362–67; Back and Pearlman, 2001, 344–45).

OBSERVATIONS

Modern pain control measures, when properly applied, have given the physician a hitherto unknown capacity to significantly reduce the suffering of many (but not all) of those who are facing death. This is essential to the doctor's role in the management of the dying in late modern society. Yet, voluntary euthanasia and physician-assisted suicide have in recent years acquired substantial levels of popular support. Indeed, for many citizens and some doctors, euthanasia is the next logical step in the expansion of patient autonomy and the doctor's role in the management of death. Nonetheless, for many others it is a step across a critical line in the sand that must not be taken if medicine is to maintain its moral integrity and society its claim to being civilized.

6   MEDICINE AND EUTHANASIA

In the Western cultural tradition, four meanings of euthanasia may be identified. The first is inducing death in those who are suffering; in the last 50 years this has often been called physician-assisted suicide or voluntary, active euthanasia. The second is terminating the lives of the socially unwanted—involuntary euthanasia. The third is caring for the dying in the best possible way—Francis Bacon's good or comfortable death. The fourth is allowing people to die, known since the mid-twentieth century as passive euthanasia.

The Greeks and Romans allowed both involuntary and voluntary euthanasia. Socrates and Plato saw the termination of the lives of defective people as justifiable. The Stoics from Zeno to Seneca saw the choosing of suicide as a responsible act, to be preferred to the passive acceptance of the cruel outcomes meted out by disease or human beings. The physician promoted health through a healthful regimen of food, drink, exercise, personal hygiene, and sleep. The art of medicine was limited to such unheroic interventions. Patients with poor prognoses might seek religious healing in the temple of Asclepius. However, the physician desisted from attempts to cure them and might even assist in their suicide. Yet, some, like the Pythagoreans, opposed the induction of death in the incurable, as did Aristotle, although he supported the killing of defective children (Gourevitch, 1969, 502–3, 508–10; Griffin, 1994, 109–10, 117; Momeyer, 1995, 500; Vanderpool, 1995, 555–56).

THE ATTITUDE OF CHRISTIANITY IN THE PREMODERN ERA

By the fourth century, the church had developed a powerful critique of certain features of Greco-Roman culture, condemning infanticide, abortions, gladiatorial contests, various sexual behaviors, and suicide. While the Bible does not condemn suicide, it was seen to be at odds with central Christian virtues such as faith, hope, patience, and acceptance of God's supremacy. Moreover, Christ's passion exemplified the redemptive capacity of suffering, while his ministrations to the sick and dying became the model for a compassionate response. Saint Augustine (354–430

A.D.) saw suicide as breaking the Sixth Commandment (not to kill). Saint Aquinas (1225–1274) extended the argument against suicide (and active euthanasia), establishing the objections the Catholic Church still clings to: it is contrary to Christian tradition, to natural law, to the welfare of civil society, to Christian compassion, and especially to God's sovereignty over human beings. By the High Middle Ages (1200–1500), to die with your sins forgiven meant salvation; to die in a state of sin meant consignment to hell. So important had become the spiritual conditions under which the Christian died that manuals on dying—the *Ars Moriendi* (the Art of Dying)—were produced to instruct the dying person on how to behave. Spiritual matters took clear precedence over medical treatment. Indeed, in the thirteenth century Pope Innocent III decreed that, until the spiritual needs of the dying person had been met, no medical attention was to be given. In the post-Reformation era, both the Catholic and Protestant churches continued to encourage the idea of a good Christian death (Vanderpool, 1995, 556–57; Copenhaver, 1995, 549–51; Battin, 1995, 2446; Kliever, 1995, 510).

Philosophical Arguments for Euthanasia

Between the sixteenth and the nineteenth centuries, there emerged in Europe a line of thought that justified the voluntary induction of death in terminally ill and injured people. In his *Utopia* (1516), Thomas More, a faithful son of the church, related that, in his ideal society, if life for the incurable became unbearable, the magistrates might prescribe euthanasia, and they would end their lives by starvation or drugs. However, Bacon supported euthanasia in the sense of a painless, comfortable, noninduced dying. Michel de Montaigne (1533–1592), a professing Catholic, wrote that, if living is worse than dying, God gives us permission to take our lives.

The coming of the Enlightenment gave greater scope to such dissenting views on euthanasia and suicide. Poet (and dean of Saint Paul's, London) John Donne (1572–1631) used Christ's own example of choosing death before his natural time to justify "self-homicide." Playwright John Dryden (1631–1700) and deist Charles Blount (1654–1693) supported suicide in cases of suffering. David Hume (1711–1776) attacked the traditional Christian arguments against suicide and voluntary euthanasia. If suffering negated one's capacity to meet one's social duties, one might exercise one's "native liberty" to induce death. However, Immanuel Kant (1724–1824) rejected suicide, arguing that, if seen as a universal course of action, it would destroy the underpinnings of morality itself (Webling, 1993, 795–96; Emanuel, 1994, 793–94; Battin, 1995, 2446; Vanderpool, 1995, 557–58).

The Debate about Euthanasia Goes Public

In the later nineteenth century, arguments for euthanasia ceased to be confined to philosophical and literary circles. The emergence of euthanasia as a topic of public discussion owed something to the declining intellectual and social influence of religion. It also owed something to the rising cultural and social influence of medicine. Physicians had become the key attendants in the care of the dying. The 1847 Code of Ethics of the American Medical Association stated that doctors should not abandon a patient because the case was deemed incurable; their attendance would continue to be highly useful since they might alleviate pain and other symptoms and soothe mental anguish.

Nineteenth-century physicians commonly refused to end the lives of incurable or dying patients. Composer Hector Berlioz angrily denounced the doctors who were attending his sister, who refused to speed her death with chloroform; she had suffered six months of intense pain from breast cancer. However, in 1873 Hon. Lionel Tollemache advocated active euthanasia for the suffering incurable. Three years earlier, schoolmaster S. D. Williams proposed that anesthetics be used to end life in cases of hopeless illness. Leading journals of opinion said his arguments were plausible (Reiser, 1975, 27–28; Van der Sluis, 1979, 132; Emanuel, 1994, 794; Vanderpool, 1995, 558–59).

Williams rejected traditional religious notions about the intrinsic value of human life. His address was given a decade after Darwin's *Origin of Species* was published. Darwinian images were now beginning to permeate educated discourse, and by the 1880s they formed part of the prevailing intellectual paradigm. Williams argued that, if medicine encouraged the survival of the unfit, the doctor should be allowed to end the life of the suffering patient. Tollemache also saw euthanasia as a humane way to balance medicine's working against the effects of natural selection. In 1875 Annie Besant, socialist and birth control advocate, published an essay on euthanasia, proposing that the painless, voluntary death of the suffering person was an act of devotion to the general welfare; an outworn notion of the sanctity of life should not be allowed to stand in the way of a practice that lifted the burden from the suffering person and society alike.

Euthanasia began to be discussed in medical circles in the United States and Britain. In 1873 the Philadelphia-based *Medical and Surgical Reporter* said that the patient often beseeched the physician to end the terrible struggle. Refusing to answer, the physician would administer a narcotic dose large enough to induce a deep sleep from which the patient might not awaken. One of the first groups of doctors to discuss the issue publicly was the South Carolina Medical Association, a committee of which examined active euthanasia from medical, religious, ethical, and legal viewpoints in 1879. The committee concluded that legalization would give rise to large-scale abuse, and while it remained illegal, its practice amounted to murder. The few articles on the subject published in the more prestigious U.S. medical journals in the 1880s tended to focus on the legal aspects. In 1884 an editorial in the Boston *Medical and Surgical Journal* made a case for passive euthanasia.

In the 1890s lawyers and social scientists entered the debate. Then as now, the lawyers called for reduction of the physician's authority in the name of patients' rights. In 1895 Albert Bach, a New York lawyer, argued in favor of euthanasia on the grounds that patients had the right to end their own life. At the 1899 meeting of the American Social Science Association, S. E. Baldwin (later president of the American Bar Association) criticized the pride of many physicians in prolonging lives at any cost. In early 1906 the *New York Times* reported a speech by Charles Eliot Norton, a well-known Harvard professor, advocating euthanasia. Norton's advocacy caught the imagination of Anna Hill (whose own mother had cancer), who lobbied to have active euthanasia made legal in Ohio. The *New York Times* attacked the bill, which in any event was defeated 79 to 23. The *British Medical Journal* denounced the attempted legalization and the intellectuals who, frightened by pain, had inspired it.

In the United States as in Britain, Darwinian ideas had a profound effect on thinking about society. Lawyer, advocate of birth control, feminism, and racial tolerance, and campaigner against traditional Christian morality, Robert Ingersoll placed his faith in evolutionary theory and in modern science's promise of material (and moral) progress. In 1894 Ingersoll said that suicide was a rational response for sufferers of incurable cancer who were burdens to themselves and others. Three years earlier, Felix Adler had publicly supported suicide of the incurable. Adler's Ethical Culture attracted people from reform Judaism and liberal Christianity. Like Ingersoll and later proponents of euthanasia, he did not see human life as sacred and argued that some lives were more valuable than others.

In the early twentieth century, eugenics—the "science" of breeding superior humans—influenced biology, medicine, and public health, as well as public policy on marriage, immigration, and social welfare throughout the Western world. The term was introduced in the 1880s by Francis Galton, a cousin of Charles Darwin. At a time of mounting social and economic tensions, eugenics seemed to offer scientific answers free of traditional ethical concerns about the weak and vulnerable. The culling of unworthy life through birth control, sterilization, and mercy killing seemed an efficient (and sufficiently humane) way to promote the health and well-being of the great majority of the people. It is no coincidence that, until Nazi policies discredited eugenics, many advocates of euthanasia were also advocates of eugenics. The American Eugenics Society was established in 1923; teaching in schools, colleges, and universities was influenced by eugenic ideas; and national immigration quotas were introduced in part because of eugenic thinking. The 1930s saw 41 states outlaw marriage for those with mental illness and intellectual handicaps, while 30 states introduced the sterilization of eugenically unacceptable people.

The *British Medical Journal* published seven editorials on euthanasia between 1901 and 1915. The editors expressed satisfaction at the findings of an inquiry carried out by the *Daily Mail,* which showed that all of the doctors that were questioned had opposed euthanasia. In that same period the *Journal of the American Medical Association* ran six editorials on euthanasia, all of which condemned mercy killing. From 1901 to 1909 the *New York Medical Journal* published four editorial articles that criticized the use of the term "euthanasia" for mercy killing, correctly pointing out that this was not the long-established meaning of the term. In this era, the editors of leading medical journals were clearly at odds with lay advocates of active euthanasia (Fye, 1978, 500–2; Van der Sluis, 1979, 132–37; Emanuel, 1994, 795–96; Kemp, 2002, 19–26; Dowbiggin, 2003, 6–15).

MEDICINE AND AN EASY DEATH

In Victorian Britain, physicians attending the social elite often practiced supportive management of the dying. A medical text that had a large impact was William Munk's *Euthanasia: or Medical Treatment in Aid of an Easy Death,* published in 1887. Munk saw opium as the key to pain relief, but sherry and port, given in small, frequent doses, were also valuable because they were quickly absorbed.

His advice derived to a large extent from the practice of Sir Henry Halford, long-time president of the Royal College of Physicians and physician to royalty, and that of Prof. James Young Simpson. For Munk, Halford's bedside manner—his sympathy and gentleness—was particularly important, often helping the patient more than drugs. Munk's text continued to be the standard reference for three decades. Others, such as Oswald Browne, who in 1894 composed a pamphlet for nurses, followed Munk. Browne believed that care of the dying was the supreme privilege of the health care professional's working life.

Euthanasia as mercy killing was first seriously advocated by a member of the British medical profession in 1901. C. E. Goddard, a public health doctor, not a clinician, identified two classes of sufferer for whom termination of life was desirable: the hopelessly diseased and the hereditarily defective, whose useless lives would be compulsorily terminated. A few years later, when philosopher Maurice Maeterlinck criticized doctors for seeking to prolong life at any cost, Dr. Robert Mac-Kenna responded: drugs could relieve most pain; abstract arguments for mercy killing of incurables were easy to formulate when one did not have personal responsibility for such acts; medicine was the art of healing, not dealing death; finally, the call for mercy killing was ultimately selfish because it was intolerance of personal distress that made people shrink from death-bed suffering (Porter, 1989a, 77–94; Jalland, 1996, 86–96; Kemp, 2002, 34–35, 44–46).

AUSTRALIAN DOCTORS AND CARE OF THE DYING

There is no direct evidence that Munk's 1887 text, although influential in Britain, was widely read in Australia, and in any case the number of consultants attending to the class of patient Munk was discussing was very small because of the comparatively small size of the colonial elite. Medical journals in the nineteenth and early twentieth century did occasionally discuss the issue of death, but there was no direct consideration of euthanasia. Leading Sydney surgeon Robert Scot Skirving said that, of the many deaths he had observed between 1880 and 1920, they were rarely the dramatic ones described by some religious writers. He was critical of the evangelical concern with terminal utterances because the capacity to reason often disappeared in the last stages of life. He later criticized the ineptitude of the average clergyperson, who delivered death-bed rites in a meaningless mumble. However, in 1945, H. M. Moran, a Sydney specialist in cancer medicine who was himself in the late stage of cancer, berated his own profession for its absurd promises concerning the efficacy of treatment. His attitude toward death was one of stoicism and redemption through suffering (Moran, 1946, 286, 289; Cannon, 1998, 733; O'Callaghan, 2001; 21–22; Jalland, 2002, 95–99).

In 1934 Guy Griffiths, a Sydney physician, directly addressed the issue of euthanasia at the Australasian Medical Congress. In lingering deaths such as those from certain cancers, opium, morphine, and cocaine were available to relieve suffering. The only ground for active euthanasia as such was great suffering from an incurable disease. Under any legalized system, incurability and severity of pain would have to be certified independently by two senior physicians, and permission given only after an official inquiry. The killing would be carried out by the patient or a family member or, failing all else, by a state official. Medical practitioners ought never to be required to perform the act because it was their duty to preserve life and such action would undermine public confidence in doctors (Griffiths, 1934, 161–62).

EUTHANASIA AND CARE OF THE DYING IN THE 1930S

In the first five to six decades of the twentieth century, the capacity to prolong life became greater and greater. The early 1900s saw the introduction of cardiac massage and injections of epinephrine into the heart. By the 1930s mechanical respirators were available. The polio epidemics of the 1950s saw the widespread employment of the iron lung respirator to sustain breathing. Endotracheal and masked ventilators were developed in the 1950s, while blood oxygenators were used in surgical operations at that time. By the 1960s, cardiopulmonary shock devices were in use.

In the United States, Alfred Worcester was criticizing colleagues in the 1930s for excessive resort to resuscitation and for neglecting the art of caring for the dying. He had a life-long concern with quality of care in nursing as well as medicine. At Harvard, he wanted the title professor of the care of patients, but the faculty would not grant this, and he had to settle for professor of hygiene. At the age of 80, he published *The Care of the Aged, the Dying, and the Dead* (1935). At the start of the chapter on the care of the dying, Worcester pointed out that, while midwifery (or assistance for those coming into the world) had vastly improved over the previous 50 years, the art of caring for the dying (or assistance for those leaving) had deteriorated. He stated that the bodily discomforts and pain of dying could almost always be relieved. He recognized the value of the doctor's attention to the emotional needs of the dying patient and foreshadowed the modern emphasis on truth telling (Worcester, 1977, 33–49, 57; Kerr, 1992, 14, 37; Vanderpool, 1995, 559).

In Germany the notion of euthanasia had expanded to include involuntary death for the unfit. In the 1900s Ernst Haeckel, employing social Darwinist and eugenic arguments, noted the gains for the collective from disposing of the physically and mentally incurable. His ideas were influential wherever German science was valued.

Das Monistische Jahrhundert, the Monist League's journal—monists were social Darwinists—hosted a debate on euthanasia initiated by a dying member, Roland Gerkan, who wanted the league to campaign for legalization. The journal's editor, Wilhelm Ostwald, a Nobel laureate in chemistry, supported Gerkan in the name of social utility. Some participants were wary of state abuse if euthanasia were made legal, whereas others favored legalization to promote the biological fitness of the collective. The advent of World War I stopped further discussion, and the medical press remained silent in the decade and a half before the war began.

In 1920 legal philosopher Karl Binding and eminent psychiatrist Alfred Hoche produced a pamphlet on destruction of life that is not worth living. Binding argued that some lives were not only worthless but also burdensome to the individuals concerned; those who were mentally sound but who wished to die; idiots and those with senile dementia; and those in an unconscious, vegetative state. The mercy killings would be carried out by some state body. He did not think the intellectually handicapped should be killed at this stage because public opinion would not yet accept it. Like Haeckel, he noted the insignificance of the individual life compared with the interests of the whole (the state). However, at the 1921 annual meeting of German physicians, the views of Binding and Hoche were rejected.

In England, the 1930s saw an upsurge of public discussion of euthanasia, which was begun by public health doctor Charles Killick Millard. Well known for his support for a eugenic approach to birth control, he also advocated sterilization of the feebleminded. In 1931 Millard, who was a Unitarian in religion, like so many euthanasia proponents in the United States, called for the legalization of euthanasia. His draft bill provided for a court to review a euthanasia permit filed by a dying person for whom two doctors certified that the person was suffering a fatal disease likely to be both painful and protracted; relatives were to be interviewed by a referee, and a magistrate was to attest to the application. Having reviewed the application, certificates, and referee's evidence, the court could issue a permit to the applicant and to the doctor or "euthanizer."

Millard, whose position was supported by the eminent physician Sir Arbuthnot Lane, encountered considerable opposition in the British Medical Association (BMA). However, there was enough support among professional elites for the Voluntary Euthanasia Legalisation Society (VELS) to be formed (specifically to press for enactment of Millard's bill) in 1935. Anglican Church luminaries R. W. Inge and the dean of Saint Paul's Cathedral, W. R. Mathews, supported the society. The president was Lord Moynihan of Leeds, a past president of the Royal College of Surgeons, England, and one of the two medical vice presidents was Sir Humphrey Rolleston, past president of the Royal College of Physicians, London. A key figure on the executive committee of the society was consulting surgeon C. J. Bond, who was also a vice president of the Eugenics Society.

The society convened a public meeting in December 1935, at which a motion calling for legalization was passed. Lord Moynihan assured the attendees there was no wish to legalize the killing of those with mental handicaps or those with senile dementia. However, the chair of the executive committee was reported as saying that, when public opinion accepted euthanasia, further progress along such lines would be possible.

When the bill was introduced into the House of Lords in late 1936, it was vigorously debated. Viscount Dawson and Lord Horder, medical peers, expressed opposition, the first because he rejected the bureaucratic process envisaged by the bill (not because he rejected euthanasia), and the second because he doubted whether a seriously ill person had the requisite mental stability to make a reasonable decision. The archbishop of Canterbury was concerned that, acting from motives other than compassion, the relatives would pressure the patient to request euthanasia. The bill was defeated by 35 votes to 14.

At its first annual meeting in February 1937, society membership was 268, of whom 70 were doctors. Millard remained convinced that legal access to voluntary euthanasia would come to be seen as one of the great reforms of the age. In early 1940 he claimed that only the advent of World War II had prevented reintroduction of the bill (Van der Sluis, 1979, 138–54; Humphry and Wickett, 1990, 13–14; Kemp, 2002, 84–86).

In the United States, bills to legalize voluntary euthanasia were introduced in the legislatures of Ohio and Iowa in 1906 and Nebraska in 1937. The work of the British Society inspired a group to come together in 1938 to form the Euthanasia Society of America. Within the society opinion differed as to the target population. Dr. Foster Kennedy, the second president, focused on the congenitally unfit, while Dr. Alexis Carrel wanted painless disposal of incurables, criminals, and lunatics.

The most prominent pro-euthanasia figure in the United States in the interwar years was Charles Francis Potter. Originally a Baptist minister, he became a Unitarian pastor in 1913. Nationally known for his endorsement of progressive causes such as feminism, birth control, and abolition of capital punishment, Potter was religious adviser to defense lawyer Clarence Darrow in the famous 1925 trial of John Scopes, a Tennessee teacher who broke the state law against the teaching of the theory of evolution. In 1929 Potter resigned from the Unitarian Church and founded the First Humanist Society of New York. An outgrowth of liberal Unitarianism, humanism was a naturalistic religion, denying the divinity of Christ and the existence of God. For him, euthanasia was one of the key causes for the humanists. He supported not only voluntary killing of the suffering terminally ill but also the mandatory disposal of defective babies and the incurably insane.

For Dr. Inez Philbrick, birth control, eugenics, and euthanasia were interconnected issues, just as they were for Potter. Her 1937 Nebraska bill allowed both voluntary and involuntary euthanasia. The bill was opposed by the state medical association, the University of Nebraska School of Pharmacy, the editor of the *Journal of the American Medical Association,* and most clergy.

The cofounder with Potter of the Euthanasia Society was Ann Mitchell, a wealthy New York woman who was hospitalized for mental illness from 1934 to 1936. She emerged from this difficult period believing that cure of such hereditary disease was not possible and that involuntary killing of psychiatric patients (and handicapped babies) was the only solution. Learning of the initiatives of Millard and VELS in England, she approached Potter about founding a similar society in the United States. Millard quickly recruited a number of prominent people, including Robert Frost, Somerset Maugham, and Max Eastman, as well as distinguished physician Walter Alvarez and physiologist Walter Cannon. Launched as the

National Society for the Legalization of Euthanasia in January 1938, it soon became the Euthanasia Society of America (ESA).

Like VELS, ESA drew its membership—only about 200 by the end of the 1930s—from the educated elite. More than 70 percent of its founding members were eugenists. Eugenist members of VELS who also became members of ESA were Millard, Fabian socialist H. G. Wells, sexologist Havelock Ellis, and biologist Julian Huxley. The executive officers and board of ESA were replete with eugenists: Clarence Cook Little, president of the University of Michigan and the American Society for the Control of Cancer; Robert Latou Dickinson, gynecologist and birth control campaigner; Frank H. Hankins, Clark University and Smith College sociologist; Stephen S. Visher, Indiana University geographer; Walter F. Willcox, Cornell University professor of economics and statistics; and Wyllistine Goodsell, Columbia University professor of education.

Promoting public awareness of the euthanasia issue was the increasing number of cases of mercy killing and assisted suicide. Juries often refused to find the perpetrator guilty, or they recommended mercy in sentencing. Some examples are the 1925 case of Harold Blazer of Colorado, who killed his incurable daughter after more than 30 years of caring for her. In 1934 May Brownhill, an Englishwoman, killed her 31-year-old intellectually retarded son because she was to undergo major surgery and feared that no one would take care of him. In 1939 *Time* magazine reported that one mercy killing a week was taking place in the United States.

In 1937 a *Fortune* magazine survey revealed that 40.5 percent of respondents opposed euthanasia for defective babies under any conditions; 14.5 percent were undecided; and 45 percent approved. It also revealed that 47.5 percent unconditionally opposed euthanasia for the incurable; 15.2 percent were undecided; and 37.3 percent agreed.

The American Institute of Public Opinion in 1936 and again in 1939 asked people whether they approved of mercy killing, under official supervision, for incurable invalids. The responses were as follows: in 1936, 38.6 percent approved; 45.4 did not; and 16 percent did not express an opinion; and in 1939, 41.4 percent, 48.6 percent, and 10 percent, respectively. A separate survey of doctors found 53 percent in favor and 47 percent against. When the British Institute of Public Opinion carried out a poll, 69 percent supported the principle of euthanasia.

Thus, in Britain and the United States, in the first four decades of the twentieth century, despite a significant proportion of citizens favoring mercy killing and strenuous lobbying by euthanasia societies, attempts to legalize euthanasia failed. The story was different in Germany. There, the government endorsed the idea of "life not worthy of life." The Nazi program of killing thousands of mentally and physically defective people, labeled as euthanasia, was to blacken the cause of mercy killing in the immediate postwar era (Humphry and Wickett, 1990, 14–19; Vanderpool, 1995, 560; Dowbiggen, 2003, 36–55).

In 1933 the National Socialists passed a law for the compulsory sterilization of people suffering from hereditary diseases. The "Volk," composed of Aryan Germans, would not permit "life unworthy of life" (the incurable and defective) to block their way to world domination. The National Socialists introduced a new term, "unnütze Esser" (useless mouths), to describe the same people, and this description had a strong resonance in wartime conditions. The sterilization program was pursued openly, but the compulsory euthanasia program proceeded in a climate of secrecy. In some 30 pediatric departments throughout Germany, defective children were euthanized—about 5,000 in all. The program was then extended to psychiatrically ill adolescents and adults; 80,000–100,000 were killed in gas chambers disguised as showers. This physician-supervised program became the model for the subsequent destruction of millions of Jews, Gypsies, homosexuals, and others.

A few Catholic and Protestant clergy publicly denounced the program. In 1935 Catholic theologian Franz Walter stated that the universality of Christ's teaching of love was being attacked by rabid nationalism. At Easter of 1934, Cardinal Faulhaber of Munich and Freising condemned euthanasia of the incurable insane. Archbishop Gruber of Freiburg, an honorary member of the *Schutzstaffel* (SS) until the late 1930s, also protested.

People heard rumors that the aged would be the next category to be included, and even badly wounded soldiers might be euthanized. In 1941 Pastor Gerhard Braune of the German Protestant Church said the program should be ended immediately since it threatened the moral foundations of the nation. However, Protestant opponents were hampered by their habit of subservience to the state. In August 1941 Hitler issued a verbal order for the program to be halted; whether he did so because he was concerned about national morale or because all those to have been killed had already been killed is unclear. Yet, compulsory euthanasia continued until 1945.

It seems likely that any individual doctor who protested against the program would have been killed. The medical profession chose to turn a collective blind eye. Some analysts have subsequently explained this moral bankruptcy by pointing to a gradual slide down a slippery slope (Van der Sluis, 1979, 155–58; Humphry and Wickett, 1990, 21–27; Burleigh, 1991, 326; Vanderpool, 1995, 560).

The war crimes trials widely publicized the Nazi euthanasia program, and the revelations discredited the euthanasia movement for two decades. Nevertheless, individual cases of mercy killing received much publicity. Carol Paight, a 21-year-old college student from Connecticut, shot her father, who was suffering from end-stage cancer. She was acquitted of second-degree murder because she was found to be temporarily insane from "cancer phobia." New Hampshire doctor H. N. Sander injected an incurably ill woman with air. Sander was acquitted on the grounds of lack of causation, with the defense arguing that the patient was already dead when injected. The Euthanasia Society said that such action should be made legal, but evangelist Rev. Billy Graham called for Sander to be punished in order to deter others.

In England, the clergy were on both sides of the fence. The dean of Saint Paul's Cathedral, W. R. Matthews, expressed support for voluntary euthanasia at the same time as the archbishop of Canterbury was voicing opposition. The Anglican Hospital Chaplains' Fellowship opposed euthanasia when the bishop of Birmingham was endorsing it. In November 1950 the House of Lords discussed a motion in favor of euthanasia. Both the archbishop of York and medical peer Lord Horder opposed the motion, maintaining that it put pressure on the aged to end their dependence on others. The five medical peers who spoke on the motion opposed it. The motion was ultimately withdrawn.

Some support continued to surface. Joseph Fletcher drew a distinction between murder and mercy killing in terms of intent and contended that qualities such as freedom and autonomy justified euthanasia. Fletcher, an Episcopal minister and social reformer—Sen. Joseph McCarthy called him the "Red Churchman"—was important in the right-to-die movement in the United States because he moved away from the established eugenically oriented rationale for euthanasia to one based mainly on the autonomy of the patient. He also supported involuntary sterilization of criminals and those with mental handicaps.

In 1951 the general council of the Presbyterian Church condemned euthanasia as contrary to the Sixth Commandment. The next year the general convention of the Protestant Episcopal Church of America rejected legalization under any conditions. In 1957 the archbishop of Canterbury equated mercy killing with murder. The Roman Catholic position was made clear by Pius XII in statements of 1957 and 1958: control of pain was in accord with God's intentions, and drug-induced pain relief was best even if the unintended result was to shorten life (the double-effect principle).

In the course of the 1960s euthanasia began to gain a respectable face. In Britain, the Euthanasia Society in 1961 proposed amending the suicide bill to decriminalize the assisting of a suicide by a compassionate doctor acting in good faith. The bill was enacted without this amendment (Van der Sluis, 1979, 161–64; Humphry and Wickett, 1990, 49–60; Dowbiggen, 2003, 100–3).

However, medical, psychological, and social researchers were starting to become interested in understanding how the aged and the dying felt about death. In 1958 Mayo Clinic psychologist Wendell Swenson carried out a study of the attitudes of 210 nonterminal people over the age of 60 years. He found that those in homes for the elderly were more anxious about death than those living in the community; those who were religious were more positive about death; and few overall would say they feared death. In 1960 Canadian psychiatrist Daniel Cappon studied attitudes of dying and of healthy people: 90 percent of the dying wanted a quick death, and a majority of all those involved in the study supported euthanasia (73 percent of the dying did so). The next year in England, A. N. Exton Smith, a physician, studied the pain experienced by 220 terminally ill people; 20 percent of those with cardiovascular, respiratory, or nervous system disease had moderate to severe pain; in those with a cancer, pain was controlled by drugs. However, those with locomotor disease experienced severe and protracted pain, and their sense of lack of control was heightened by the fact that they remained alert mentally.

In 1962 psychiatrist J. M. Hinton compared the suffering of terminal and seriously ill patients. He discovered that the terminally ill patients experienced more physical distress; for 33–50 percent this distress was alleviated, but nausea, breathlessness, and exhaustion were often persistent. While 50 percent of the terminally ill could acknowledge the fact that they were dying, almost that same number were very depressed. The most religious were the least anxious about dying. Hinton highlighted the fear in the dying patient generated by growing loss of control and loneliness. However, he did not support euthanasia, pointing out that many religions rejected it and that there was a problem of deciding when it was suitable. In their 1960s study, sociologists B. G. Glaser and A. L. Strauss pointed to the conspiracy of silence commonly found among health professionals, which prevented dying patients from facing the truth about their future. However, the most influential work of this era, both among health professionals and in the community, was Elisabeth Kübler-Ross's *On Death and Dying* (1969). By 1976 one million copies had been sold.

The demystification of death at the hands of professionals such as Kübler-Ross may be viewed as part of a larger cultural and social phenomenon of the 1960s and 1970s; the rise of new social movements devoted to the rights of women, homosexuals, African Americans, and Native Americans; and the counterculture and environmental and antiwar movements. The counterculture stressed both individual liberation and collectivism in communal lifestyles. The environmental movement focused on ending population growth to halt increasing global pollution. The antiwar movement called for the United States to pull out of its "unjust" war in Vietnam and, more broadly, for reduction in the power of the military-industrial complex, which promoted such actions.

There was a widespread crisis of confidence in the beneficence of science, and nowhere was this clearer than in relation to medicine. Between 1965 and 1973, public esteem for doctors declined from 72 to 57 percent of those polled. Hospitals, which had been the pride of local communities, came to be seen as cheerless places where the dying died lonely, often painful, deaths. Life-sustaining technologies, along with heroic therapeutic interventions, came to be seen as unnecessarily prolonging suffering. Many citizens now wanted the patient's right to refuse treatment to be recognized. In 1973 the American Medical Association endorsed a patient's bill of rights that did just that, among other things.

Public disenchantment with modern medicine was evident in attitudes to cancer. Although five-year survival rates had improved from one in five to one in three between 1930 and 1960, public optimism about major therapeutic breakthroughs dissipated in the 1970s. Moreover, quality of life was becoming an important issue.

A locus of strong criticism of medicine was the women's movement, which urged women to reduce their dependence on expertise by learning more about the functioning of their own bodies. The movement sought to overcome medical paternalism and reduce the dominance of male practitioners within medicine. Feminists progressed from the demystification of sexual and reproductive matters to breaking the silence about death and dying. Moreover, the gendered division of labor in health meant that most nurses were female and that women commonly attended the sick and dying in the home. With longer life expectancy than men, women were more likely to be dependent on people outside the family in the terminal stage of their own lives. The majority of members of right-to-die organizations were women, although they were usually not social radicals.

In England, medical opinion about euthanasia was assessed in the mid-1960s, when 2,000 randomly selected general practitioners were surveyed. Their responses were similar to those in the United States: almost 49 percent reported having had a request from a terminal patient; 36 percent would carry out active euthanasia if it were legal; 76 percent believed that some practitioners gave treatment that hastened death; and they were equally divided in their response to the question of whether workable safeguards could be enacted in law. In a survey of members of the American Association of Professors of Medicine and the Association of American Physicians, 80 percent of 333 physicians responding said they had carried out passive euthanasia; 10–15 percent of Protestant and Jewish physicians approved of active euthanasia; but almost all Catholics disapproved.

In 1968 the World Medical Association affirmed its rejection of euthanasia. In 1969 the annual meeting of the British Medical Association overwhelmingly endorsed its council's opposition to the practice.

In that year the Euthanasia Society sponsored another attempt to legalize euthanasia. A Labor peer, Lord Raglan, introduced a bill that was defeated by 61 votes to 40, with only one medical peer, Lord Platt, supporting it. The proposed legislation included provision for an advance declaration under which a person could make known a desire for euthanasia prior to experiencing a terminal illness. Passionate partisanship marked public discussion of the 1969 bill. A Human Rights Society was established by a Conservative member of Parliament to lobby against the bill. The Catholic auxiliary bishop of Westminster stated that it was always wrong to take a person's life. A rabbi expressed opposition to the bill, saying that since human life has infinite value, even a small fraction of additional life lived was as valuable as all of life. Cicely Saunders said there were few forms of physical distress that could not be dealt with by skilled palliative care (Van der Sluis, 1979, 165–68; Humphry and Wickett, 1990, 65–89; Dowbiggen, 2003, 110–15).

In the United States, after the first modern hospice was created in New Haven, Connecticut, in 1974, hospices were soon being established throughout the nation. Almost 200 courses involving death studies had been introduced at colleges and universities by the mid-1970s, and many medical schools now included such material in their curricula. The numbers joining the Euthanasia Educational Council rose almost exponentially—from a membership of 600 in 1969 to more than 300,000 by 1975. Wider public acceptance of voluntary euthanasia seemed to be developing.

In a randomly selected population of 3,000 U.S. doctors in 1974, 82 percent said that passive euthanasia for their family members was acceptable, and 86 percent, for themselves. Fifty-nine percent of doctors in Seattle hospitals reported that, if they possessed an agreement signed by a patient or family, they would facilitate passive euthanasia, and 27 percent would perform active euthanasia if a more accepting climate prevailed. Ninety percent of medical students in their fourth year of study at Washington University and 69 percent of first-year students were willing, if they had signed agreements, to practice passive euthanasia; 46 percent of both groups supported the legalization of active euthanasia. Nurses in the same survey revealed similar sentiments.

Polling of citizens showed comparable support for euthanasia. Fifty-three percent in a Gallup poll agreed that doctors should be allowed to carry out mercy killing if the patient or family wished it. A Louis Harris poll carried out about the same time found that 62 percent of respondents supported passive, and 37 percent active, euthanasia.

In the 1970s there was a spate of attempts to legalize euthanasia. A bill on termination of treatment was unsuccessful in the Florida legislature. Death-with-dignity bills were introduced but not passed in the Wisconsin and Washington state senates. A voluntary euthanasia bill was introduced in the Oregon legislature in 1973, but its progress was halted. Attempts to make legal living wills failed in the Massachusetts and Delaware legislatures in 1973 and in the Maryland senate in 1974. Failure to obtain committee support for a death-with-dignity bill in the Virginia legislature in 1975 ended the bill's progress. Six other states also saw bills proposed, but only in California was a bill to legalize living wills passed. The Natural Death Act became law in late 1976.

The Euthanasia Educational Council and its political partner, the Euthanasia Society of America (in 1975 its name was changed to the Society for the Right to Die), campaigned for the legalization of passive euthanasia. The New York State Medical Society agreed in 1973 that the patient and/or the family, on the advice of the family physician, should be able to decide to stop extraordinary life-support measures if death was inevitable. The American Medical Association opposed mercy killing but adopted a report that endorsed the right of the patient and family to have extraordinary means of life support suspended.

The British Medical Association rejected euthanasia in 1971, instead calling for more resources to be put into care for elderly people. The Council of Social Services in 1972 and the Royal Society of Health in 1973 sponsored a conference on euthanasia. In Britain the idea of hospice as an alternative to euthanasia was strong. The general council of the Canadian Medical Association decided in a close vote (76 to 66) that it was ethical in some instances for a doctor to prescribe that a dying patient not be resuscitated.

In 1974 South Africa acquired its own euthanasia society. At the same time, societies were established in two Australian states—the Voluntary Euthanasia Society of Victoria and the Voluntary Euthanasia Society of New South Wales. In 1976 a euthanasia society was established in Japan. In the mid-1980s, the international movement had expanded to include 27 societies in 16 countries.

The case of Karen Quinlan, a 21-year-old New Jersey woman who in April 1975 went into a coma but was kept alive on a respirator, greatly influenced opinion in the United States. Three months later, her father and mother, both Catholics, decided to have her taken off the respirator. The state supreme court endorsed this decision in the face of the hospital's opposition, which was based on the fact that Karen was not brain dead. She survived removal from the respirator and remained alive but in a coma until mid-1985, when she finally died. In 1977, 50 bills that recognized people's right to include in an advance declaration their wish that, if terminal, they should not be subject to life-prolonging measures, were introduced in the legislatures of 38 states. The bills became law in Arkansas, California, Idaho, Nevada, New Mexico, North Carolina, Oregon, and Texas. By 1985, a total of 36 states had enacted such right-to-die legislation.

Between 1979 and 1980, a split occurred between the Society for the Right to Die and the Euthanasia Education Council. The council, which now became Concern for Dying, disapproved of the society's activist pursuit of legislation. Meanwhile, in 1979, the English Voluntary Euthanasia Society (now known as EXIT) faced an internal division over the proposed publication of a guide to suicide for the dying. The recently established Scottish EXIT went ahead, however, and published such a guide. Derek Humphry proposed bringing out a similar manual in the United States. He was eager to go beyond passive euthanasia, the long-held position of the right-to-die organizations in the United States, and in 1980, with his second wife, Ann Wickett, established the Hemlock Society. Humphry became very well known as the author of *Final Exit,* which made popular the plastic bag as a means of suicide.

By 1981, four guides to suicide for the terminally ill had been published—Scottish EXIT's *How to Die with Dignity;* the Hemlock Society's *Let Me Die before I Wake;* the Dutch *Justifiable Euthanasia;* and the English EXIT's *Guide to Self-Deliverance.* In 1985 the U.S. organization Concern for Dying again stated its opposition to such publications, although it admitted it had no answer for a dying patient whose family, friends, or professional attendants refused to assist with suicide.

By the 1990s the Netherlands was widely if mistakenly believed to have legalized euthanasia. In 1973 the Royal Dutch Medical Association and the Royal Dutch Nursing Association published guidelines that made active euthanasia or physician-assisted suicide legitimate under certain conditions: if it was carried out by a doctor on a competent patient who was suffering unbearably and who had repeatedly and voluntarily requested relief; if a second doctor had been consulted; and if no other means acceptable to the patient existed to alleviate suffering. The guidelines provided a framework for discussion of euthanasia in Europe and the United States. A survey, the results of which were published in the early 1990s, showed that 54 percent of Dutch doctors had carried out euthanasia. Although the law had not been changed at this stage, doctors who followed the guidelines and the criteria developed in case law were not prosecuted (Humphry and Wickett, 1990, 91–117; Baker, 1993, 880–81; Vanderpool, 1995, 561; Smith, 1995, 4).

Catholic opposition to abortion prompted the creation of the right-to-life movement in the 1960s. In 1973 in the United States, the National Right to Life Committee was formed to act as a political lobbying group. The pro-life movement saw legalization of involuntary euthanasia of the sick and aged as the next battleground. In the 1970s the movement campaigned against right-to-die legislation. The Christian fundamentalist group called the Moral Majority, which Jerry Falwell founded in 1979, was concerned with opposing abortion, not euthanasia, and was not ready to condemn advance directives. The pro-life group in Minnesota, the Human Life Alliance, was, however, highly critical of euthanasia. Its president, Mary Senander, criticized right-to-die laws for promoting the view that the aged and the sick were financial and emotional burdens.

In January 1985 the Supreme Court of New Jersey ruled in the Claire Conroy case that the removal of feeding tubes was lawful. The pro-life movement was taken aback by the results of a Gallup poll on attitudes toward the outcome of the case; the poll found that 81 percent of citizens approved of the court's ruling and that 77 percent of Catholics, compared with 80 percent of Protestants, endorsed this position.

C. Everett Koop, surgeon general of the United States in 1981, was an outspoken critic of abortion and euthanasia. He believed that sanctity of life took precedence over quality of life and was a cornerstone of day-to-day medical practice. He told the National Right to Life Convention in mid-1985 to accept some minor reverses in order to maintain the legal ban on active euthanasia.

In Britain, the Festival of Light was the public voice of the right-to-life movement. Journalist Malcolm Muggeridge was an articulate spokesperson, opposing euthanasia and abortion with traditional Christian arguments about life's sacredness as God's creation and pain and suffering as a source of moral growth. The movement looked to the modern hospice as the alternative to legalized euthanasia.

In 1988, the right-to-die movement in the United States believed that public opinion had shifted sufficiently to seek legalization of euthanasia in California. However, supporters could not obtain the required number of voter signatures on a petition for the proposal to be placed on a ballot. The next effort was mounted in Washington State. Here Initiative 119 qualified for a place on the ballot in 1991, but the proposal was defeated 54 to 46 percent. In California, Proposition 61 qualified to proceed to a ballot, but, again, as the potential problems with the law were made clear, public support declined. It was defeated by 54 to 46 percent.

The pro-euthanasia lobby now focused on Oregon, which had a reputation for political libertarianism. Also, the national office of the Hemlock Society was located there. The lobby's measure required that a dying person be a competent adult with a terminal disease defined as incurable and such as to lead to death within six months. The safeguards included obtaining a second opinion on diagnosis, disclosure of alternatives to induced death, and vetting of the request to ensure it was voluntary. Where the patient was thought to be depressed, referral for counseling was required, as was a "cooling off" period of 15 days. The family could be kept ignorant of the patient's request. Measure 16 was passed, and in 1994 physician-assisted suicide for terminal patients became legal in Oregon. However, a decision by the federal government to ban the use of federally controlled drugs for physician-assisted suicides threatened the viability of the procedure (Humphry and Wickett, 1990, 163–69; Smith, 1995, 27–40).

In Australia, there was little public discussion of euthanasia in the 1950s and 1960s. K. S. Jones, in his 1962 presidential address to the New South Wales branch of the Australian Medical Association, discussed the care of dying patients and euthanasia. He stated that, when he first began to practice medicine, he had no idea how to care for dying patients, and he recommended that students be instructed in hospice settings. With regard to euthanasia, he discussed two types of cases. The first were those in which the patient was enduring considerable pain and death was imminent, and the second concerned patients who felt powerless but for whom death was nevertheless fairly distant. In the first, drugs administered without fear of shortening life were the answer. The second scenario appeared to suggest a situation in which mercy killing might be appropriate. However, doctors were reluctant to be state executioners, especially with the memories of Nazi concentrations camps still so fresh; moreover, patients rarely demanded it, and the trust of the dying person should not be betrayed.

In 1969 the editor of the *Medical Journal of Australia* pointed out that the question of legalizing euthanasia had not been vigorously explored in Australia and that most Australian doctors did not favor it. However, the practice of passive euthanasia and the double effect were generally not condemned (Jones, 1962, 332–33; *Medical Journal of Australia*, 1969, 987–88).

By the mid-1970s there was sufficient interest in the needs of the dying for a conference to be held at the Concord Repatriation Hospital in Sydney. The gathering agreed that, apart from provision of physical comfort, those who were dying needed to be accompanied on their emotional journey. In 1976 the *Medical Journal of Australia* identified three reasons that legalization of active euthanasia had failed in Britain and the United States: the majority of citizens did not support the idea; doctors were unwilling to become involved; and the problems of devising legislative provisions were as yet insurmountable. The real alternative to active euthanasia was the best possible care of dying patients. A. L. Saclier, secretary of the Voluntary Euthanasia Society, replied that the editorial was misleading because the bill did not propose legalizing the active taking of life; rather, it allowed for passive euthanasia. Moreover, opinion polls revealed that a growing majority of citizens accepted the right to seek an induced death (*Medical Journal of Australia,* 1975a, 897; 1976, 667–68, 963).

In 1979 Justice Michael Kirby, chair of the Australian Law Reform Commission, addressed the Clinical Oncological Society of Australia on the rights of the dying. He made the general point that citizens would no longer tolerate paternalistic professionalism, whether medical or legal. He pointed out that the right to die had been recognized in statute law in the United States and that such statutes did not seem to conflict with Christian or Jewish doctrine. Kirby also maintained that there was little agitation for such legislation in Australia but that the time would come when lawmakers would have to deal with this issue. Indeed, in South Australia, legislation was proposed in 1980 that allowed an adult to decline the use of extraordinary life-sustaining measures in some future terminal illness. Two correspondents writing to the *Medical Journal of Australia* said that circumstances in Australia were different from those in the United States. There, the medicolegal climate was such that hospital staff relentlessly applied supportive technology. Australian patients already had substantial legal rights to decline treatment; thus, special legislation like that proposed in South Australia did not seem needed (Kirby, 1980, 252–55; Gilligan and Linn, 1980, 473).

In the United States in 1982, the "Baby Doe" case, in which a newborn baby with Down's syndrome and requiring serious corrective surgery, was allowed to die because the parents refused permission despite the hospital's court challenges to their decision, prompted the president of the United States to threaten to withdraw federal funding from any of the 5,800 hospitals in the country that refused to treat (or feed) a handicapped baby. The medical profession was outraged at this intervention into a matter traditionally settled between parents and their doctors. Two similar cases in the United Kingdom also received much publicity.

The Australian College of Paediatrics drew up guidelines for its members and submitted them to the Human Rights Commission. Sydney pediatrician Douglas Cohen called for a law to recognize that the withholding or withdrawal of treatment where success was impossible was sound medical practice and that control of pain was mandatory even where this was likely to shorten life. The problem was that the two Hippocratic injunctions—to preserve life and to relieve suffering—were not always compatible (Cohen, 1984, 59–61).

At a 1984 Royal Australasian College of Physicians meeting on euthanasia, Harry Lander, professor of medicine at Adelaide University, argued that compassion was a compelling reason for passive and even active euthanasia. Another reason was the financial cost of caring for aging "dements" and the very handicapped. Paul Gerber, honorary lecturer in legal medicine and ethics at the University of Queensland, was critical of Lander's utilitarianism and his inability to see the difference between omission and commission—between allowing to die and killing. Roger Woodruff of the medical oncology unit, Austin Hospital, Melbourne, pointed out that the practice of medicine had improved in recent years and that, as a result, with adequate attention to physical and psychological symptoms, most terminal patients could live the last period of life with dignity; he also stated that requests for euthanasia were rare and arose from fear or depression. La Trobe University philosopher Robert Young criticized Woodruff, saying that patients had a right to choose euthanasia, that physicians other than Woodruff had not found pain relief to be effective for all patients, and that requests for euthanasia were more common than Woodruff asserted (Lander, 1984, 174–77; Woodruff, 1984, 548–49; Gerber, 1984, 142–43; Young, 1985, 166).

Philosopher Helga Kuhse, Peter Singer's colleague at Monash University, introduced new issues: a fruitful approach would be to focus on the best interests of the patient. Then, painless death by lethal injection might be seen as the best course of action. Brian Pollard, head of the Palliative Care Service, Concord Repatriation Hospital, Sydney, said the dying have a right to die, but this should not simply entail a right to be killed because the latter involved a duty to kill on somebody's part. Kuhse replied that doctors had a duty to act in the patient's best interests and, on occasion, active euthanasia would be the correct action to take (Kuhse, 1985a, 610–13; Kuhse, 1985b, 170–71; Pollard, 1985, 48).

In the early 1980s, some state legislatures considered bills about the withholding of treatment. In 1980 the Refusal of Medical Treatment Bill was introduced in the Victorian parliament but was not enacted. In South Australia, the Natural Death Act was passed in 1983. This recognized the power of an advance declaration directing that life-sustaining measures be withheld in the event of terminal illness or injury.

In 1985 the social development committee of the Victorian legislature was asked to report on a range of issues related to dying with dignity. The committee heard evidence from a range of groups, organizations, and individuals. The Catholic Bishops of Victoria welcomed the inquiry because so many of the aged faced difficulties arising from the lack of clarity in the various legal and ethical situations. The Anglican Church also welcomed the inquiry, as did the moderator of the Uniting Church. The patron of the Voluntary Euthanasia Society of Victoria, R. A. Mackenzie, a member of the upper house of the state parliament, also welcomed the opportunity for a range of viewpoints to be publicly stated, while the president of the Humanist Society urged parliament to pass legislation so that citizens would know where they stood.

It was the first inquiry of this kind in Australia, and it concluded that legislation establishing a right to die was neither desirable nor practicable but that legislation clarifying the existing common law right to refuse medical treatment was to be welcomed. Such legislation should include protection for the doctor who in good faith followed a patient's wishes. Moreover, the state health department should ensure that all institutions educating health professionals and all health care institutions should understand the law allowing the patient to refuse or discontinue treatment and that all health care professionals possess current knowledge about palliative care. It concluded that a coordinator of palliative care education should be appointed to each medical school in Victoria and that such education should be ongoing in professional development programs. Furthermore, major teaching hospitals should be required to establish bioethics committees to offer advice on ethical and social issues, and both legislation and the practice of medicine should be changed to ensure that all terminally ill people were provided with effective pain control. While unwilling to propose new legislation creating a right to die, the committee wanted to clarify the patient's legal right to decline treatment and to improve the conditions under which dying took place by encouraging the spread of good palliative care (Social Development Committee, 1987, v–xiii, 1, 12–15, 48).

Pollard pointed out that Kuhse had had her call for legalization of euthanasia rejected by the Victorian inquiry. Now she was calling for the introduction of the questionable Dutch practice of active euthanasia. Kuhse replied that the Dutch practice should not be dismissed out of hand since there was much to learn from it about the doctor-patient relationship. Palliative care physician Roger Woodruff said that, if the practice of euthanasia was indeed growing in Holland, then this was the result of social pressure on dying people. Evidence in favor of euthanasia from newspaper polls or the number of advance directives in Australia was not enough to demonstrate a significant desire for the measure. Kuhse would have to spend some time talking to terminally ill patients and their families to come up with real evidence (Pollard, 1988, 147–49,159; Kuhse, 1988, 159; Woodruff, 1988, 540).

In 1988 Kuhse and Singer published the results of a survey of doctors' attitudes. There was much criticism of their work. Melbourne practitioner Eugen Koh noted that, with a response rate of less than 50 percent, there had to be doubt about its significance; active and passive euthanasia were not distinguished; thus active euthanasia practice appeared greater than it really was. They could not argue that, since 65 percent indicated that illegality was a factor in their unwillingness to carry out active euthanasia, a majority supported legalization. Dr. Rodney Syme of East Melbourne defended Kuhse and Singer: even if only 1 percent of dying patients wanted euthanasia, their wishes should be respected. Kuhse and Singer replied to their critics: a 46 percent response rate to a mail survey was a high number, and there was no good reason to think that nonrespondents were greatly different in attitude from respondents; the claim that 60 percent of respondents supported legalization was not based on an interpretation of the percentage of doctors indicating that illegality was a factor influencing their involvement in active euthanasia; rather, it was based on answers to a straightforward question about whether they thought the law should be changed to permit active euthanasia. The percentage of doctors who helped a patient die was not expressed as a proportion of all respondents because the population surveyed was a random sample; thus many would have been practicing in fields such as dermatology, where a request for aid to die was very unlikely. Therefore, the percentage was calculated as a proportion of those who had received requests for aid (Koh, 1988, 276; Syme, 1988, 280; Kuhse and Singer, 1988, 280–81).

RECENT DEVELOPMENTS IN THE
UNITED STATES AND BRITAIN

By the late 1990s more than forty jurisdictions in the United States had legalized advance directives. In 1983 California passed the first legislation enabling the appointment of an agent with enduring power of attorney to make decisions about medical care. In 1990 the Patient Self-Determination Act was passed by the U.S. Congress, requiring all health care institutions that received federal funds to inform adult patients, upon admission, about their right under state law to execute an advance directive.

Late in 1994 Oregon enacted legislation decriminalizing physician-assisted suicide (PAS). Unlike earlier Washington State and California bills, this measure was concerned with PAS, not voluntary euthanasia. The challenges to its constitutional validity failed but delayed implementation of the law until October 1997. Meantime, anti-euthanasia groups persuaded the Oregon senate to hold a referendum on repeal of the law. However, voters supported the act a second time in November 1997. The Oregon measure was opposed at the federal level. The House of Representatives passed the Pain Relief Promotion Bill in 1999, which made it illegal for a doctor to prescribe federally controlled drugs in PAS. The bill was halted in the senate because of fears that such constraint would discourage doctors from providing adequate pain relief.

Eight other states considered decriminalization of PAS. In Washington State, Proposition 119, put to electors in late 1991, was defeated 55 percent to 45. In late 1992 Proposition 161 was put on the ballot in California and was defeated 53 percent to 47. In Iowa, the Assistance in Dying Act would have allowed voluntary euthanasia through a written declaration. In Maine, 1992 legislation would have done the same. A New Hampshire bill would have permitted terminally ill persons, including minors, to petition a probate court for PAS. A 1994 New York measure allowed for requests for aid in dying. In 1994 a state task force reported on euthanasia and assisted suicide, unanimously proposing no change in policy. Michigan's 1992 Death with Dignity Bill would have permitted competent adults to be helped to die. In 1994 the state's supreme court ruled that the state constitution did not support a right to assistance to die (New York State Task Force on Life and the Law, 1994, ix; *Report of the inquiry by the Select Committee on Euthanasia,* 1995, 44–47; Griffith and Swain, 1995, A-156; Cica, 1997a, 87–88; Magnusson, 2002, 64).

Two attempts were made in Britain during this period to legalize advance directives. Both failed. In 1976 Baroness Wootton of Abinger introduced the Incurable Patient's Bill, which declared the patient's right to be freed from incurable suffering. The bill made provision for a limited form of advance directive. By 85 votes to 23, the measure was defeated, however. In 1993, with the support of the Voluntary Euthanasia Society, Lord Allen of Abbeydale introduced a bill to legalize advance directives and health care proxies. The Medical Treatment (Advance Directives) Bill was read a first time but subsequently lapsed. The select committee that followed decided that advance directives already had binding force and that the

British Medical Association had publicly accepted the idea of advance directives since 1992.

In 1988 the authors of the BMA's guidelines said there was a tension between medical technology's capacity to prolong life and the right of patients to decide what will be done to them. The working party came to a number of conclusions: active euthanasia should remain illegal; however, a doctor should accede to a request not to prolong life; patient autonomy was to be respected, but the patient should not be able to require a doctor to terminate life; good care and communication between doctor and patient might be expected to dissipate pressure on doctors to carry out euthanasia; counseling was essential for young, severely disabled people requesting active euthanasia; discontinuing treatment of a severely malformed baby might be correct, but liberalization of active termination would amount to a basic change in the ethos of medicine; people who seriously attempted suicide but survived did not always, on reflection, want such a fate, but under the Dutch system of active termination, the chance to reflect was absent; advance declarations should receive respectful attention but should not be seen as immutable; the long-standing concern of the law with intent rather than consequence alone deserves regard, and any risk to the life of the patient from drugs is acceptable if the intent is to relieve pain or suffering; and the deliberate terminating of human life should remain a crime, thus affirming the absolute value of the individual (British Medical Association, 1988, 3–4, 67–69; Kemp, 2002, 219–22).

The cases of both Cox and Bland led to the establishment of a House of Lords select committee on medical ethics. Nigel Cox was a doctor who admitted administering potassium chloride to a patient to end her suffering. Tony Bland was a teenager in a persistent vegetative state for three years. His doctors were authorized to withdraw parenteral nutrition. The committee presented its report in 1994. The great majority of those giving evidence opposed euthanasia, but the Voluntary Euthanasia Society claimed that 79 percent of people in a national opinion poll favored it, although the general nature of the question asked undermined the society's claim.

The committee rejected the idea of creating a legal right to request aid in dying. Legalization of euthanasia would put undue pressure on vulnerable and disadvantaged people. For incompetent patients, the committee endorsed the creation of a new judicial forum empowered to authorize withdrawal of treatment. It recommended wider acceptance of advance directives but proposed this be pursued through professional codes of practice rather than changes in the law. The committee noted the current deficiencies in palliative medicine, proposing more research into pain relief, improvement of training in palliation, and encouragement of the development of hospice facilities. The committee did not resolve the question of whether parenteral feeding and hydration constituted treatment that may sometimes be legitimately withdrawn or withheld. The government said it agreed with the endorsement of a competent patient's right to refuse treatment, with its support for advance directives, and with the idea of the development of a professional code on advance directives.

The Law Commission of England and Wales and that of Scotland were considering the issue of advance directives. In early 1995 the former recommended that a directive should be presumed valid if it was in writing, signed, and witnessed. The directive did not apply where caregivers believed that advance refusal of treatment endangered a person's life or, in the case of a pregnant woman, the fetus's life. Advance refusal precluded neither basic care nor any action to prevent death pending a court decision on the validity of the refusal, and caregivers were not liable for the consequences when they believed an advance refusal applied or for any procedure refused unless they believed the advance refusal applied. The government announced it would not legislate on any of the Law Commission's proposals concerning mental incapacity, including those on advance directives, until the public had been consulted because the ethical issues involved were of great importance to many citizens (*Lancet,* 1994, 430–31; Cica, 1997a, 88–92).

LEGISLATION IN AUSTRALIA

In South Australia, a parliamentary select committee on the law and practice relating to death and dying was established in December 1990. It was to determine the extent to which the law and the health services offered adequate choices; whether public and professional knowledge of pain relief and palliative care and provision of services were adequate; whether the Natural Death Act was understood; how much community attitudes to death and dying were changing; and whether the law needed to be amended. In 1991 and 1992 the committee produced three reports in which the salient recommendations were the provision of medical powers of attorney and further development of palliative care. Euthanasia was little discussed.

A 1991 survey of South Australian doctors, involving 300 respondents, found that 33 percent had been asked by a patient to carry out active euthanasia, while 22 percent had been asked by the family; 47 percent had been asked by a patient to hasten death by withdrawal of treatment, and the same percentage had been asked by the family; intractable pain, terminal illness, and an incurable condition were the reasons most often given for the requests; 90 percent of doctors believed the request to be rational; 18 percent believed active euthanasia was acceptable; a further 46 percent believed it right if requested by the patient; and 45 percent favored legalization of active euthanasia under certain conditions.

In March 1995 Hon. John Quirke introduced in the parliament the Voluntary Euthanasia Bill. Under the proposed legislation, anyone over 18 years of age, competent to decide, terminally ill, and likely to die within 12 months, could request euthanasia. In July the bill was defeated in the assembly by 30 votes to 12.

In 1993, in the Australian Capital Territory (ACT), Michael Moore introduced the Voluntary and Natural Death Bill. This permitted a person of at least 18 years who was of sound mind and suffering from a terminal illness to request that extraordinary life-sustaining measures not be applied or that death be induced by the administration of a drug. The bill prescribed conditions similar to those embodied in other bills. A select committee proposed its progress be halted but that a bill on withdrawing or withholding treatment be introduced. In August 1995 Moore introduced the Medical Treatment (amendment) Bill. It was defeated by 10 votes to 7.

As I have noted, the report of the Victorian parliament's 1987 social development committee was largely devoted to passive euthanasia and the right to refuse medical treatment. In 1988 the Medical Treatment Act clarified the law on the patient's right to refuse treatment, while it also enabled an agent to decide about treatment on behalf of an incompetent person. This last matter was taken further in the Medical Treatment (Enduring Power of Attorney) Act of 1990 and the Medical Treatment (Agents) Act of 1992, which set down the powers of the agent and safeguards concerning the exercise of enduring power of attorney (Griffith and Swain, 1995, A-163–64; *Report of the Inquiry by the Select Committee on Euthanasia,* 1995, 55–57).

In March 1995 seven Melbourne doctors (including Rodney Syme, a supporter of euthanasia) had an open letter to the premier of Victoria published in the *Age,* a leading newspaper in Victoria. They said they had carried out euthanasia in their practices and urged the introduction of the assisted suicide legislation that the Voluntary Euthanasia Society was advocating. They were investigated by the Victoria police and the Medical Practitioners' Board, but, because of lack of evidence, no one was prosecuted. Where in the United States PAS has been at the heart of the debate, in Australia it has been active, voluntary euthanasia (AVE), and with AVE, it is the doctor who, of course, carries out the procedure.

Early in 1995, the chief minister of the Northern Territory, Marshall Perron, tabled the Rights of the Terminally Ill Bill. Perron has stated that he was moved to draft legislation by arguments in papers presented at a 1994 conference on the dying patient sponsored by the Australian Medical Association (AMA), papers by David Kelly and Roger Hunt and especially one by Helga Kuhse. At the time he had no knowledge of the international right-to-die movement, although he did know of the Voluntary Euthanasia Society of Victoria. A draft bill was released for public comment, the content of which relied heavily on the society's advice. There was also input from Syme, Kuhse, Kelly, Max Charlesworth of Victoria, and Hunt of South Australia.

When the bill was reintroduced, a package of information was widely distributed so that commentators would be fully informed. Perron agreed to a select committee review if it reported to parliament on its findings within three months. He did not think any of the members had changed their mind on the issue because of evidence, believing that opposition to AVE was always religiously motivated. During passage of the bill, a group led by Lynda Cracknell campaigned on its behalf in Operation TIAP (Terminally Ill Act Petition). The group became the Northern Territory Voluntary Euthanasia Society with Cracknell as president. After a marathon debate in which every member of the legislative assembly spoke, in a conscience vote the bill was passed by 15 votes to 10.

The Rights of the Terminally Ill Act of 1995 legalized both assisted suicide and AVE. The legislation attracted great attention both nationally and internationally. Margaret Tighe, head of Right-to-Life Australia, claimed that one-way tourism to the Territory would greatly increase. Churches and the AMA were opposed to the measure. Early in 1996 the act was amended to require two doctors (one of whom had to be a psychiatrist and the other a specialist in the patient's illness) assess the patient requesting assistance in dying.

The validity of the act was challenged in the Northern Territory Supreme

Court by the president of the Northern Territory branch of the AMA, Chris Wake, and aboriginal leader Rev. Dr. Djiniyini Gondarra. By two to one, the judges rejected the claim that the legislation was beyond the scope of the legal authority of the Territory parliament.

Several patients went to Darwin from other parts of the country to take advantage of the act. Marta Alfonse-Bowes, a retired Melbourne academic with colon cancer, who was in severe pain, arrived before the act was operational. She suicided alone in a hotel room. The first person to undergo euthanasia under the act was Robert Dent, a 66-year-old with prostate cancer, who was in constant pain, was unable to urinate, and was losing control of his bowels. Using Philip Nitschke's computer-controlled device, he self-administered a lethal injection of drugs. Kevin Andrews, a Catholic and Liberal Party backbencher, introduced a bill into the federal parliament that, relying on the Commonwealth's constitutional power to legislate for the Northern Territory and the ACT, sought to overturn the Territory act. The bill was endorsed by the prime minister, John Howard, although he allowed Liberals a conscience vote. Tim Fischer, leader of the National Party (the Liberals' partner in government), and the leader of the Labor opposition, Kim Beazley, also allowed a conscience vote (Griffith and Swain, 1995, 28; Perron, 1996, 1–5; Cica, 1997b, 112; Magnusson, 2002, 61–63).

A group called Euthanasia No, which had Catholic connections, lobbied federal members of parliament, while members of churches and of the right-to-life movement sent anti-euthanasia submissions to the senate committee deliberating Andrews's bill. When the bill passed by a majority of five votes in the senate in March 1997, the Catholic and Anglican churches expressed satisfaction.

Other attempts to have euthanasia bills enacted in state legislatures have not succeeded. Clearly, the churches and medical-professional organizations that are opposed to legalization are more formidable than a diffuse voter majority expressing support in what are often vaguely worded poll questions. When a conscience vote is allowed, lobbying of parliamentarians and the nature of their religious beliefs become significant. The major parties, knowing the subject is highly contentious, try to avoid having a high public profile on the issue.

Philip Nitschke, who has in recent years assumed the same prominence in the right-to-die movement in Australia as Jack Kervorkian in the United States, paid for a full-page advertisement in the local press, along with a number of other doctors in support of Perron's legislation. He was eager to develop an alternative machine using carbon monoxide and an oxygen mask to help patients to die. He was also interested in making available a suicide pill composed of materials that could be bought over the counter (Griffith and Swain, 1995, 34–37; Woodman, 1998, 76–77, 127–31).

HIV/AIDS and Euthanasia

Virtually from the beginning of the AIDS epidemic in the early 1980s, attempts were made to adapt the hospice approach to patients suffering from a disease with a progression different from that of the terminal cancers suffered by the occupants of established hospices. In the United States, the National Hospice Organization cosponsored a 1987 North American conference, which was held in Ottawa, on caring for terminally ill people with AIDS. A year later it was sponsoring regional conferences. In 1994 it sponsored an AIDS summit that enabled leading figures in the hospice movement to discuss with representatives of AIDS service organizations ways of adapting hospice to the care of AIDS sufferers. By the late 1990s, as new drug treatments turned HIV/AIDS into a chronic condition with much longer life expectancy, some early programs such as Hospice at Mission Hill (Boston) and Chris Brownlie Hospice (Los Angeles) had to close because the need for terminal care had declined so much.

By 1980 San Francisco, with a community of perhaps 100,000 mainly young homosexual men, was regarded as the gay capital of the United States. In 1981 clinicians there, as in New York and Los Angeles, had begun seeing a few cases of Kaposi's sarcoma (KS), a rare cancer, in young men. By 1982 links between the gay lifestyle, anal sex, KS, and opportunistic infections were being established, and from epidemiological, clinical, and scientific evidence a new immune deficiency disease, AIDS, was being identified.

As the cases mounted, San Francisco General Hospital (SFGH) set up a Division of AIDS Activities in 1983. In mid-year, Ward 5B, a 12-room facility for those sick with and dying of AIDS, was opened. Staff members worked in teams of physicians, nurses, social workers, nutritionists, and mental health workers. The more egalitarian organization freed nurses from their usual subordination to doctors and allowed them to work more at the bedside. Ward 5B, functioning as a combined hospital ward and hospice, gave impetus to the local hospice movement, which was then just beginning to emerge. At the end of 1983, the Hospice of San Francisco accepted a contract from the Department of Public Health to provide for AIDS patients, and others, such as the city's Laguna Honda Hospice, also accommodated such patients. San Francisco quickly became a model for other U.S. cities for community care of people with HIV/AIDS. In the course of the first decade of the epidemic in the United States, the proportion of AIDS patients (especially gay white men) dying in hospitals declined notably as more died at home, in a hospice, or in a nursing home: in 1983, 92 percent died in hospitals; in 1988, 79 percent; and in 1991, 57 percent (Kelly, Chu, Buehler, and the AIDS Mortality Project Group, 1993, 1433–37; Beresford and Connor, 1999, 26–27; Risse, 1999, 621–39, 658–62).

In Britain, the years 1987and 1988 saw the first funding by local authorities for AIDS work, and it went mostly to London local councils for social work positions and home care teams. Government spending increased markedly from about £2 million in 1986 to £200 million in 1991. In 1986 the national hospice organization, Help the Hospices, convened a conference on AIDS. Many existing hospices, although set up for cancer sufferers, also accommodated people dying of AIDS. Certainly, the Westminster government believed the existing hospice movement, with its mixture of voluntary effort and statutory involvement, was integral to the national strategy.

However, one strand of influential opinion within the movement was wary of opening the established hospices to young gay men with AIDS because they had been set up to accommodate largely older cancer sufferers of both sexes and because housing such a stigmatized group might reduce the flow of public funds. In fact, the latter did not happen, but the exclusionary attitude encouraged efforts to develop special AIDS hospice facilities (as well as clinics), one of the best known of which was the Lighthouse in Notting Hill, which opened in 1988. Mildmay, an AIDS hospice that accepted patients from all over London, also opened in 1988.

In the early 1980s in Britain, too, almost all HIV/AIDS patients died in hospitals, but in the late 1980s deaths at home and in hospices increased substantially. The experience of Saint Stephen's Clinic in central London (responsible for almost 20 percent of all British cases of AIDS) in the first decade of the epidemic was similar to that of other central London hospitals. In 1994, of all deaths of patients under the care of Saint Stephen's Clinic, 46 percent were in hospitals, 31 percent at home, 20 percent in hospices, and 2 percent abroad (Berridge, 1996, 167–70; Guthrie, Nelson, and Gazzard, 1996, 709–11).

The Canadian equivalent of London's Mildmay hospice was Toronto's Casey House. Opened at the beginning of March 1988, it claimed to be the first hospice in the world devoted exclusively to the care of people with AIDS. The background was that, after retired teacher Margaret Fraser was diagnosed with terminal cancer, a number of friends stepped in to care for her at home. One was June Callwood, who gave half the royalties from her book about the experience as seed funding for a hospice for AIDS patients. In the early days, residents were mostly younger gay men, but as the epidemic spread, women, those infected through contaminated blood transfusions, and injecting drug users were also accommodated. In 1993 a home hospice program was introduced, doubling the numbers cared for. By 1998 more than 11,000 people had been cared for at Casey House.

Toronto lay volunteers were pioneers in other ways as well. The Toronto AIDS Committee and Project Access, supported by Health Canada's HIV/AIDS Care, Treatment, and Support Program, developed a resource manual for people living with AIDS who wished to die at home, *Living with Dying, Dying at Home*. Available in 1994 at no charge, the manual was employed in the training of care providers throughout the country (Buckley, 1998; Supporting Self-Care: The Contribution of Nurses and Physicians, 1997).

Sydney is Australia's gay capital, and Saint Vincent's Hospital in inner-city Darlinghurst is the Australian equivalent of SFGH. In 1983 the first AIDS patients in Australia were treated at Saint Vincent's. By 1990, 40 percent of Australia's AIDS patients were being treated at Saint Vincent's, and in 1995 a refurbished ward of 24 dedicated beds was opened. In 1998 the National Center in HIV Epidemiology and Clinical Research reported that, from 1994 to 1997, deaths were 80 percent fewer and AIDS cases 43 percent fewer among a cohort of people with advanced HIV than in a matched cohort from 1990 to 1993.

In 1997 Paul van Reyk, former policy officer with the AIDS Council of New South Wales, said the council estimated that 12 attempts at euthanasia per year were made among people with HIV/AIDS in Sydney. About half of those were not successful, mostly because of ignorance of effective means and lack of medical assistance. AIDS patients constituted about 5 percent of referrals to urban palliative care services, but in inner-city Sydney the figure was as high as 25 percent.

By 1997, close cooperation between the general practitioner, the HIV treatment team, and the palliative care service was allowing many to realize their wish to die at home. Sydney palliative care physicians Paul Glare and Neil Cooney pointed out that feelings of hopelessness among AIDS patients commonly led to requests for physician-assisted suicide. However, most doctors found it difficult to fulfill such requests; moreover, when the patients' feelings were addressed, the interest in euthanasia usually disappeared. They believed palliative care could play a significant part in providing such a constructive response (van Reyk, 1997, 161; Glare and Cooney, 1997, 119–22; Cooper and Hickie, 2000, 377–87).

Legal academic Roger Magnusson has investigated illegal euthanasia among AIDS patients in Sydney (Magnusson, 2002). One counselor, who had moved from working in cancer to AIDS, said that almost everyone with an HIV/ AIDS diagnosis talked about euthanasia. A palliative care nurse pointed out that, unlike AIDS patients, cancer patients in the palliative phase had their symptoms managed, but AIDS patients generally continued to undergo dignity-denying treatments to control opportunistic infections; further, HIV/AIDS was still stigmatized, and many gay men feared abandonment when they approached death.

Somewhat paradoxically, it seems that doctors and nurses who do not try to discourage patients from seeing euthanasia as an option may help them regain a sense of control, and this in turn extinguishes the desire to suicide. Many gay men highly value control in their lives. Hedonism is also highly valued as is a secular world-view, and there is clearly much concern with personal identity and body image.

Physician-induced death was sometimes achieved indirectly through pain relief and sedation. Another procedure was to use increasing doses of morphine once the patient reached the stage of transition from oral morphine to syringe-driven, subcutaneous administration of the drug. Yet another common procedure was the use of breakthrough doses of analgesics if the established dosage was not controlling the pain. Existential fatigue and lack of dignity seem to be at least as significant as pain for gay men in the last stages of AIDS. While AIDS health care workers often saw pain and suffering as justifiable reasons for euthanasia, they accepted that it was important to ensure the patient was not suffering from treatable depression.

With greater life expectancy resulting from more effective therapy, AIDS-related dementia has become more common, and along with it there may be a greater risk of suicide. HIV dementia frequently seems to produce mood swings. Moreover, at least early on, the patient may remain insightful, so the role of cognitive decline in encouraging thoughts of suicide may be overlooked. Some doctors thought the dementia patient should be given the option of euthanasia before rational decision making became impossible. Magnusson stated that an illegal AIDS euthanasia underground has existed for some time in Sydney and Melbourne. Gay health professionals were the core personnel, and ties of friendship, professional connections, and common values held the networks together. Any one member of the underground had only partial knowledge of the whole underground, although the knowledge of some was greater. The first stage of the process leading to euthanasia, when it took place in the community, was commonly initiated by referral of a patient to a participating doctor. The other stages were obtaining drugs, carrying out euthanasia, debriefing, and the concealing of any evidence likely to be incriminating. Although factors such as the need to justify actions to colleagues discouraged euthanasia in an institutional setting, it did on occasion take place in hospitals.

Magnusson suggested that the existence of the underground proved that prohibition had failed. Even if it was largely restricted to AIDS patients, the underground practice of euthanasia indicated a policy crisis.

Further suggesting that it was a matter of whether to keep the euthanasia hidden or bring it into the open, he advanced various possible responses. The first was to maintain prohibition. A second was to say that regulation would not prevent some doctors from performing illegal euthanasia, but this could be decided only after legalization. A third was to advocate vigorous prosecution of doctors acting illicitly, but authorities had already been reluctant to prosecute. The fourth was to make it legal. This would reduce harm by bringing medical practice into line with the law.

Along with the legalization of assisted suicide would inevitably come the legalization of active voluntary euthanasia. In Australia both have been on the reform agenda. Legislation involving a statutory protocol was to be preferred over the establishment of a right to die through decisions of the courts because the likelihood of public accountability is greater and specific safeguards can be built into the protocol. The fifth response would involve doing something to overcome the unacceptable underground practices. An informal set of guidelines was needed, and a model existed in the policy of harm minimization applied to people injecting illegal drugs in order to reduce spread of HIV and other infections. Through needle distribution and exchange programs, the aim of educating users about safe behaviors in relation to injecting and sexual relations could also be pursued.

A basic question to be answered is whether euthanasia is to be restricted to competent adults having a terminal condition and experiencing excessive pain or suffering. Some people may wish to extend the reach, but such a proposal would have to be subject to public debate. In any case, Magnusson believed the medical profession and governments were obliged to minimize the harm that illicit euthanasia, a current reality, produced (Magnusson, 2002, 68–99, 174–202, 263–81).

Other research indicates that euthanasia has also been practiced in other parts of the world. A Dutch study found that assisted suicide or euthanasia was responsible for the death of 22 percent of gay men with AIDS; this was 12 times the national euthanasia rate. A 1998 study of a sample of San Francisco AIDS deaths found that patients or informal caregivers intentionally hastened death in 12 percent of cases. One commentator suggested that physician-assisted suicide was so common in West Coast gay communities that it was virtually legal. A similar conclusion was reached by the authors of a 1994 study of euthanasia in the gay community in Vancouver (discussed in Magnusson, 2002).

Magnusson noted some differences between Sydney and San Francisco. In the United States, AIDS health care professionals assisted in the patient's suicide or in the informal caregiver's euthanizing of the patient, where Australian health care professionals were ready to give drug overdoses themselves. The illicit distribution of euthanasia drugs was more often discussed in the United States than in Australia. Americans were more concerned about the dangers of legalization because, in the absence of universal health insurance coverage, many citizens lacked access to proper health care. Australians, working under a national health insurance program, were concerned with the more limited issue of access to proper palliative care.

Pointing to the potential for abuse in the euthanasia underground, Magnusson has argued that legalization will remove that potential. However, others have pointed to the impossibility of building guarantees against abuse into legislation. Brian Pollard has noted that five official inquiries, carried out in four different countries, concluded that legal guidelines allowing voluntary euthanasia could not be constructed so as to block the practice of involuntary euthanasia. The inquiries were those carried out by the select committee on medical ethics, the House of Lords (1994); the New York Task Force on Life and the Law (1994); the Senate of Canada (1995); the community development committee, the parliament of Tasmania (1998); and the social development committee of the parliament of South Australia (1999). The New York inquiry stated that, irrespective of how carefully guidelines were framed, the practice of euthanasia would be influenced by social inequalities, and those at most risk of abuse were the poor, the aged, minorities, and those without access to proper health care.

There is clear evidence that involuntary euthanasia is practiced in various settings. A 1994 survey of 1 in 10 doctors in south Australia revealed that 19 percent had practiced euthanasia, and in 49 percent of the euthanasia cases, the procedure had been carried out without the consent of the patient. A 1998 national survey of doctors in the United States showed that 54 percent of mercy killings were cases of involuntary euthanasia. In 1999 an anonymous survey of surgeons in Australia (683 of 992 responded) found that 36 percent had administered drug doses larger than needed with the intention of hastening death; 20 percent reported they had not received an unambiguous request for a lethal dose; only 5 percent reported they had administered a bolus lethal injection or made available the means to suicide following an unambiguous request (Pollard, 2001, 62–65; Douglas, Kerridge, Rainbird, McPhee, Hancock, and Spigelman, 2001, 511–15; Magnusson, 2002, 51–52, 140–41).

Commentators in Canada and the United States have raised the issue of the effect on the disadvantaged. Oncologist and bioethicist E. J. Emanuel has noted that the push to legalize euthanasia and PAS originated with educated, well-off, politically literate people who were used to having control of their lives. Further, they had good health insurance coverage, supportive family networks, and the skills to successfully negotiate a more and more bureaucratized health care system. They were therefore less likely to suffer any harmful consequences of legalization. However, this was not the case for the less well-to-do, who either lacked health insurance or had too little. They were more likely to be coerced into euthanasia by lack of financial means and had no access to good palliative care. If it is assumed that preferences in opinion polls reflect self-interest, then it is noteworthy that the poor, African Americans, and older people all oppose legalization.

Canadian ethicist Michael Stingl is likewise eager to situate the question of legalization in the context of the health care system. Emphasis there on more economically efficient services has seen a shift of focus from hospital and curative care to community-based care and health promotion. However, unless the move from hospital-based to home-based services is carried out in an equitable way, legalization of euthanasia will see some terminal patients put under great pressure because of the poor quality of home care available to them (Emanuel, 1999, 1–11; Stingl, 1998, 348–55).

As the right-to-die movement grows in strength, the disabled, the chronically ill, and relatives of patients in vegetative states are becoming more and more concerned about what legalized euthanasia might mean for them. A survey of 168 frail elderly people (who averaged 76 years in age), carried out by Duke University Medical Center investigators, revealed that 40 percent supported physician-assisted death for the terminally ill, but almost 60 percent of their spouses, siblings, and children supported it. The senior investigator stated that, if euthanasia were to be legalized, the frail aged, poorly educated, and demented might need to be specially protected by law.

In North America people with disabilities have publicly expressed concern that legalized euthanasia will mean that others will decide for them whether they have lives worth living. Diane Coleman, speaking for Not Dead Yet, an activist group that began its campaign in mid-1996 by protesting outside the Michigan home of Jack Kevorkian over his involvement in the death of Bette Lou Hamilton, claimed the views of the disabled were always ignored.

A disabled rights activist, Earl Appleby, who founded "Citizens United to Resist Euthanasia," has asserted that the right-to-die movement is largely about containment of the huge and growing cost of health care. Herbert Hendin, executive director of the National Suicide Foundation, who opposes euthanasia, has suggested that, in a very litigious society, under a regime of legalized euthanasia, doctors may well face a plethora of lawsuits.

As I observed earlier, the early twentieth-century debate about euthanasia included eugenics-based arguments. In Nazi Germany, this led to the state-sanctioned killing of 100,000 "defectives." However, it is worth noting that eugenics programs, albeit less drastic, were pursued in other European countries as well. In Sweden, even as recently as 1976, people were being sterilized—more than 60,000 in 40 years—to reduce the national welfare bill and to improve the "race." Dutchman Pieter Admiraal, a supporter of euthanasia legalization, believes that, in two decades, European countries may see euthanasia as an answer to the problem of the rising cost of caring for a ballooning population of aged people. Steven Drake, a member of Not Dead Yet, has pointed to the fact that contemporary supporters of euthanasia take offense when the earlier connection between eugenics and euthanasia is raised. However, Hitler took most of his ideas on eugenics from publications that originated in the United States.

The disability rights movement in Australia has also been concerned about the implications of legalization. A leading activist, who himself has a disability, Christopher Newell, has argued that both the consequentialist argument (seen in the approach of Singer and Kuhse) and the libertarian argument (freedom of the individual to choose death) for euthanasia ignore the marginalization of the powerless, including people with disabilities. Both Singer and Kuhse have dismissed the idea of the sanctity of life as impracticable and unrealistic. Newell suggests that there are some unhappy similarities between today's "social Darwinist" position and the Nazi idea of "life unworthy of life," although contemporary attitudes are more subtly oppressive. He concludes that medical killing is an attempted technical fix for illness and disability, which are an inevitable part of the human condition (Newell, 1996, 48–56; Woodman, 1998, 205–22).

OBSERVATIONS

The contemporary debate about euthanasia is of great moment, but it may not be solvable at the level of either values or empirical evidence. The issues go as deep as the meaning of human life and the very principles on which contemporary society is, or should be, based. In the long-term perspective, the debate has been taking place since the Enlightenment, and it began to spread beyond rarefied philosophical circles in the late nineteenth century. However, it is only in the last three to four decades that the pro-euthanasia movement appears to have gained the upper hand, although the not informidable forces of organized religion—the Catholic Church, evangelical Christians, Orthodox Judaism, and Islam—strongly oppose it.

According to Margaret Somerville, the current debate about euthanasia may usefully be viewed as a surrogate for a deeper conflict in Western society between exponents of two different worldviews. Those who hold the first, as materialists and reductionists, see humans as no more than very complex biological machines, the best feature of which is the capacity to reason. Those who hold the second see humans as being more than their biology, whether that extra dimension is termed spirituality or simply propensity to find meaning in the world. Historically, this second view has usually been expressed by and through Christianity, but in contemporary society Somerville suggests that a "secular sacred" approach may be a more appropriate expression for many: death is part of the mystery of life; respect for life entails respect for death; thus, while the artificial prolongation of life is not obligatory, it is obligatory not to shorten it deliberately.

Nick Bostrom sees the conflict of worldviews somewhat differently. On one side is the most recent manifestation of Enlightenment optimism about the perfectibility of humankind—transhumanism. Transhumanists see enhancement technologies such as genetic engineering and nanotechnology providing access to goods such as healthy life spans of indefinite duration, greater intellectual capacity, and better control over emotions. On the other side are the bioconservatives (some of whom are religious). They oppose the use of such interventions to change our species-specific nature. The transhumanists claim that bioconservatives groundlessly fear that posthumans will threaten the well-being of ordinary humans. They point out that we are not simply a product of our DNA but also of our technological and social contexts. We are therefore partly human made and thus open to improvement.

The Enlightenment philosophers promised that society would progress to the point where humanity would be liberated from the constraints of nature; in effect, social history would supersede natural history. The modern transhumanists claim that, with the advent of biomedical interventions based on molecular biology, we are near to the collapse of the traditional dichotomy between biology and culture. Social history will not so much supersede as alter natural history—in this case, our genetics. Thanks to biomedicine, our "natural" genetic condition becomes a social construct, and ontologically the "natural" and the "social" cease to be different (Somerville, 1996, 1–12; Rheinberger, 2000, 19, 29; Bostrom, 2003, 1–12).

7 Observations and Conclusions

The Anglo-Saxon countries, among the richest in the world, all manifest features typical of late-modern secular society. They were also the first countries in the world to provide hospice and palliative care services. Indeed, the hospice and palliative care movement began in Britain and quickly spread to the United States, Australia, Canada, and New Zealand in an immediate sense because of personal and professional connections among health care people. In a larger sense, it also spread because of their shared cultural, social, demographic, political, and economic heritage.

I have tried to deepen the understanding of the relationship between medicine and care of the dying in the five countries in the last two centuries by analyzing not only the internal history of medicine but also the history of the cultural, social, and other larger contexts within which medicine functions.

From one perspective, the modern hospice and palliative care movement was a reaction, originating to a large extent but not exclusively within medicine, to the failure of many practitioners of scientific medicine to offer a compassionate response to the needs of dying people and to help provide as comfortable a death as possible. Critics, both medical and lay, have in the last three to four decades pointed to the nature of scientific medicine and its key institutional locus, the hospital, as the cause of this failure. They have also decried the excessive concern with greater knowledge of disease and capacity to cure at the cost of care of the patient as a person. Some have mentioned the metaphysical supports of scientific medicine—its mind/body dualism, its reductionism, and its materialism—as the main source of the problem. Others have alluded to the failure to recognize that medicine is a deeply moral enterprise that greatly values the individual human life as well as an applied science. Descartes himself believed that medicine was the premier applied science and looked to it not only to cure and prevent disease but even to retard aging. Although they differed methodologically, both Descartes and Bacon saw science as enabling humankind to dominate nature, thereby advancing its material welfare.

I have suggested that this internalist analysis is helpful as far as it goes. Nevertheless, medicine has been influenced by the larger context in which it is located, whether cultural, social, demographic, political, or economic. Thus, a strong tradi-

tion of individualism—the great respect for personal autonomy—flowing historically from the strength of Protestantism, liberalism, and the market economy in the
Anglo-Saxon countries has helped promote both modern palliative care and voluntary euthanasia to a degree not found in other Western countries such as Italy,
where the importance of the family still challenges that of the individual. Furthermore, even health care chaplains in these Anglo-Saxon countries see their role
more and more as facilitators of the individual patient's own inner search for spirituality and existential meaning rather than as exponents of the teachings of their
particular denominations.

Demographic and epidemiological change has meant that typical deaths in late-
modern societies are slow ones due to cancer, dementia, or AIDS. They are not the
deaths of relatively short duration due to infection or trauma for which the ars
moriendi texts of the medieval and early-modern eras were appropriate guides to
behavior.

While secularization has proceeded in these five countries further than any-
where else, it is worth noting that 40 percent of Europeans and 75 percent of
Americans still believe in a spiritual afterlife, and in the 2001 census 68 percent of
Australians stated that they were Christian, whereas only 16 percent stated that
they belonged to no religion. Further, the multicultural nature of these Anglo-
Saxon countries means that many members of ethnic minorities have a strong traditional sense of community and hold strong religious beliefs (Gruman, 1966,
77–78; Walter, 2003, 218–19; Leet, 2005, 1–2).

Early in the book I note that sociologists have developed a typology of forms of
death characteristic, respectively, of traditional (or premodern), modern, and late-
modern society. In traditional society, representatives of religion, not medicine, deal
with death and dying and are assisted by the family of the dying person and other
members of the local community. In modern and late-modern society, doctors, not
priests, oversee the process, which commonly occurs in a health care institution,
not the home, but the autonomous late-modern patient may override the authority of medicine in the dying process by seeking euthanasia and that of religion
by arranging for funerary rituals cast in personal terms and symbols.

Zygmunt Bauman has offered his own version of the typology: in premodern
society the religion-based meanings of life are satisfactory because the timelessness
of the way of life fits the idea of the immortality of the soul. In modern society
there is a medical war on death, with a series of campaigns against particular diseases, turning death, at least in principle, into individually solvable problems (into
health hazards). In postmodern society the strategy is to "deconstruct" death—to
stop seeing it as a single, unique, irreversible event by turning life's significant
events into a series of bridge crossings in which no crossing is irreversible, so that
the distinction between what is transient and what durable is erased. However,
warns Bauman, real life today, as lived, for example, in these Anglo-Saxon countries, lacks the coherence of the abstract societies in the typology (Bauman, 1992,
10–11, 91–92, 173–74). Indeed, it presents, as I have suggested, such incoherences
as premodern, religion-based beliefs and practices concerning death and dying
existing alongside a modern, medicine-led war on death and alongside the late-
modern aspirations of the transhumanists, who look to gene therapy, nanotech-

nology, and other enhancement technologies to provide, in the not-too-distant future, healthy, Methuselah-like life spans for those able to afford the "treatments." There may be typical forms of death and dying in each abstract society constructed by the sociologists, but the real-life contemporary societies of our five countries contain beliefs and practices concerning death and dying drawn from each model. Reality is more untidy and incoherent than any abstract scheme.

If those sociologists concerned with identifying typical forms of death in successive types of society simply construct models without passing judgment, sociologist John Carroll is quite willing to pass judgment on what he sees as the profound costs (as well as the great benefits) of the rise to dominance of a secular/humanist culture in Western countries. Although Carroll is not directly concerned with the problem of providing compassionate end-of-life care in a health care system buttressed by scientific medicine and with the problem of resolving the deep divide over the legalization of euthanasia, these may be seen as subsets of his larger concern about the excessive individualism and rationalism that have developed out of the West's 500-year pursuit of secular humanism.

Carroll maintains that humanism's essential project was to put the individual person at the center of the universe instead of God and to create an earthly order of freedom and happiness not needing divine, transcendental supports. To do so it had to find a rock as strong as Christianity's faith on which to build this order, and it found it in the human will, especially that of the great individual as both creator and creature, an earthly equivalent of Christ as creator and creature. Without the will, humanity was at the mercy of the forces of necessity—birth, death, disease, want, war, and fate—as the tragic side of Greek culture recognized so well. The will to know and to bend nature to human purposes produced science and technology, the industrial economy, and unprecedented levels of health and material comfort for most citizens of modern Western countries.

Preparing the way for the Enlightenment, Descartes identified the rationalism of the individual as the deity of the new secular culture. The Enlightenment rationalists not only derided religion as the product of ignorance but also believed that rationalism would banish wrongdoing and injustice, also the products of ignorance. Thus, Adam Smith could claim that the rationality of the free market would of itself correct economic inequities. For Jeremy Bentham and the utilitarians, the moral law was reduced to a technical reckoning of units of pleasure—a calculus of happiness. With morality a mere category of happiness, the test of what was right and wrong became simply the greatest happiness of the greatest number.

Kant, reacting to the moral shallowness of these Enlightenment concepts, sought to provide humanism with a rationalist ethics centering on the moral law and the honorable individual who followed it. Practical reason enables us to know the moral law that replaces God as the center of the system. Free human beings apply their will to act on what their reason has revealed to them about the moral law, itself a sacred universal for all humankind. They act from shame and duty, not pursuit of happiness. Yet, Kant's key axiom that the rational individual will act according to the moral law is very questionable. The weight placed on reason runs counter to historical and contemporary experience. It simply does not allow for the power of the demonic in human affairs, against which only something as strong as faith has the force to act, Carroll believes. Reason supported by will cannot ensure that humans follow the moral law.

Indeed, it might be argued that sociological theory has not progressed beyond the great pioneers Weber and Durkheim, who identified significant consequences of this ultimate moral failure of secular humanism. Weber traced the central role of the secularization of the Protestant ethic in the rise of capitalism in the modern West and the accompanying "disenchantment" of a rationalized world, which by the late nineteenth century, was lacking the unifying ethical force of a shared sacred belief or myth. All that Weber could salvage of moral authority in this disenchanted world was a few individuals who act from the integrity that comes from their secular-vocational commitment and from the professional commitment, for example, of doctors. This is not enough to produce a unifying social ethic. Durkheim produced an equally pessimistic analysis of the state of modern society: the growth of individualism and loss of community meant that the shared core of religious-moral beliefs, considered sacred in premodern societies, was breaking down, leading to egoism and anomie as pervasive dysfunctions of modern Western life (Carroll, 2004, 3–7, 137–43, 148–52, 232–33, 251–53).

Echoing what is stated at the beginning of Chapter 1 about a Durkheimian perspective on the continuation of the sacred in new forms in secular society, Carroll asserts that piety is a universal human impulse; thus, even the most secular society will have its "pieties." Contemporary examples from these Anglo-Saxon countries might be "the natural environment" or "multiculturalism" or "art." However, for Carroll they are in fact pseudopieties since they lack a truly sublime dimension. In the secular present, only in circumstances of great stress such as severe illness or the process of dying may the individual experience a sense of a higher order or pattern behind the ordinary flow of events. Carroll states that Durkheim saw this as the experience of a sacred force, the core of every religion.

What is Carroll's answer to the problem he identifies of reinvigorating the true sources of the sacred in Western culture and society (which must mean the reinvigoration of Christianity)? As a traditionalist, he will have nothing to do with notions of the sacred secular (in the form of the environmental movement, for example) that Margaret Somerville says is appropriate to our secular times. As I have observed, this is one of Carroll's pseudopieties. He is cautiously optimistic about the chances of a religious restoration, pointing out at the beginning of the modern era, when the vitality of the Catholic Church was at a very low ebb, that the Reformation and Counter-Reformation breathed new life into Christianity. He believes that two doctrinal shifts are also needed: the first is a shift of the focus of Christian piety from an overly abstract and "lifeless" God to the more humanly accessible figure of Christ; the second is a shift from a guilt-producing Pauline emphasis on the sinfulness of the flesh to a sense of the unavoidability of guilt (in the sense of responsibility) arising from all human actions in the world (Carroll, 1986, 8–13; Somerville, 1996, 5–6).

Whether Carroll is right about the possibility of a reinvigoration of Christianity in the late-modern West (it is certainly flourishing in Africa and Latin America, which have not yet fully embraced modernity) is really an issue only for those who see the spiritual in religious terms and, more specifically, in Christian terms. It does nothing for humanists who do not accept the reality of a divine world.

As I noted earlier, Cicely Saunders had from the outset envisaged a significant role for the spiritual, in her case seen in Christian terms, in hospice and palliative care. Integral to her central concept of total pain was a spiritual dimension. Realizing the importance of this dimension, soon after the hospice movement reached the United States, Florence Wald organized a conference to try to reconcile the views of those who saw the spiritual in Saunders's religious way and those who wanted to reduce it to the psychosocial. However, unable to bridge the gap and even to use the same language, the participants just went ahead with establishing and running hospices.

In recent times, renewed effort has been put into exploring the meaning of the spiritual in the care of the sick and the dying. One approach has been to move away from the identification of spirituality with belief in a divine, supernatural reality. Accepting philosophy's focus on subjective experience since Descartes rather than an objective, metaphysical world of meaning (whether Plato's the Good or Christianity's God), exponents have focused on self-transcendence, the encountering of the mystery of the other person's subjectivity, and ethical, interpersonal relations.

A contemporary theorist of this process of encounter is Emmanuel Levinas, who talks of the ontological nature of the interpersonal relationship—the irreducible mystery of the other—since, if knowledge comes from appropriation of the object of knowing, knowledge of the other's subjectivity is not ultimately possible. I may choose to relate to the other in a pragmatic way as just another item in my world. Or I may choose to relate in an ethical way, in which the other is a source of mystery and an end in itself. If I follow the ethical way, the care and concern I extend to my own subjectivity I also extend to the other's. In the vulnerability of the other, I see my own vulnerability, and this calls forth my caring just as for Plato the transcendent reality of the Form of Goodness called forth a virtuous response. Caring, then, flows from a nonmetaphysical spirituality that nevertheless allows me to escape the prison of my own subjectivity.

This deep caring arising from an ontological relationship between two subjectivities should form the basis of the professional caregiver's humanistic response to the vulnerability of the ill or dying person. Caregivers respond to the vulnerability and uncertainty they share with the other rather than to a metaphysical world of divinity and certainty. Thus, Levinas offers us a coherent basis for a this-worldly spirituality out of which we may pursue an ethics of care toward the sick and the dying and explore contentious issues such as voluntary euthanasia (van Hooft, 2002, 43–50).

The matter of the contemporary meaning of spirituality in palliative care has been debated without much progress; models have been either exclusively secular or ecclesial. In contrast, Allan Kellehear has offered a multidimensional model of needs in an attempt to clarify the different dimensions of spirituality involved. Starting from the fact that humans desire to transcend suffering, he points out that they seek meaning in their current situation, in moral and biographical contexts, and/or in religious beliefs. These different sets of needs may manifest sequentially or in parallel.

The first, and for some commentators the most basic, need is to make sense of the immediate, sometimes very frightening, situation through a search for hope and companionship in order to cope with the new world of developing symptoms, treatments, and side effects and the alien environments of hospital or hospice.

The second set consists of moral and biographical needs that may be expressed in traditional religious terms. Often emerging from a review of the person's life, a desire may be expressed for reconciliation with alienated others and resolution of current or historical personal conflicts—putting one's house in order before death.

The third set is composed of religious needs that still remain common among the dying in our late-modern society. Redemption, divine grace, strength, and the support that comes from religious rituals may become unusually important to the dying person. Thus, spirituality in palliative care is a complex, multidimensional phenomenon, and it should not be seen as reducible to psychological and social needs (Kellehear, 2000, 150–54).

It is not simply a question of alternatives—either the spiritual or psychosocial in late-modern palliative care—just as it is not a question of either the secular or religious in real-life, late-modern societies. In both cases, both may exist. Moreover, the spiritual is not always the equivalent of the religious. As I have already suggested, we may have a spirituality that is based on Levinas's interpersonal relations and on the mystery of the other person's subjectivity, not the mystery of the Godhead. Similarly, while the hospice and palliative care movement began as a reaction against the inhumane conditions faced by the dying, which were a by-product of technologically driven medicine's headlong rush to know and to intervene aggressively, palliative medicine remains vitally dependent on modern technology. It is not a question of compassion or technology. Palliative care employs a multiplicity of technologies—laparoscopy, CT and MRI scanning, palliative radiography, relief of obstructing lesions by surgically and endoscopically inserted stents, serotonin antagonists, and somastatin analogues in the management of intractable nausea and bowel obstruction, not to mention the whole technology of pain relief ranging from biphosphonates for bone pain to portable, battery-driven pumps that allow ongoing, subcutaneous administration of analgesics, to objective assessment scales permitting quantification of pain and other symptoms and evaluation of outcomes (Seely and Mount, 1999, 1120–21).

The dichotomies and conflicts of late-modern society and culture such as individualism and communitarianism, humanism and religion, and naturalism and spirituality are unlikely to be resolved in some generally accepted higher synthesis. Rather, they will continue to coexist untidily (unless religious or political fundamentalists are able to impose ideological uniformity and social conformity on everybody else). Similarly, in the practice of palliative care, sophisticated technologies will have to coexist, sometimes not easily, with compassionate responses to perennial human needs for caring and solidarity in the face of death.

Intergenerationally and interpersonally, caring binds people together. In everyday life, it is a basic social glue. So, too, in the clinical encounter and especially in the care of the dying, caring as the physician's quintessentially human response to the extreme vulnerability of the patient must complement technical expertise.

According to the first modern theorist of medical ethics, eighteenth-century physician-philosopher John Gregory, that paragon of the humanistic physician may be distinguished from mere medical tradespersons by the "sympathy" (the "sensibility of heart") that motivates them to relieve the distress of a fellow creature. Yet, whether the ideal of humanistic physicians can prevail—whether they can straddle the plunging steed of technology and the steady horse of caring—is uncertain as the latest technological challenges to death itself loom beguilingly near. Over the next 20–30 years, powerful new technologies arising from the interaction of biology, information science, and nanotechnology will allow medicine to slow aging and degenerative-disease processes: the engineering of tissue (regrowing cells, tissues, and organs), the reprogramming of our genetic code, very precisely targeted drugs having virtually no side effects, and nanobots (robots comparable in size to blood cells that will permit us to rebuild our bodies and brains at the molecular level from within the body).

How will our ethical compasses, not to mention our societies, economies, and polities, cope when death at threescore years and ten or so itself is kept at bay for a great number of additional healthy years—when the "natural" time limit to the individual life (at least for the minority of humankind who can afford the new technologies) is stretched so far beyond what we have come to expect? Some look to nanomedicine not only to halt aging but also to reduce the individual's biological age by using three types of procedures: a cell maintenance machine to remove metabolic toxins and undegradable material from each cell; chromosome replacement therapy to correct genetic damage and mutations; and cellular repair devices to correct structural damage at the cellular level, such as disabled mitochondria. They then see life expectancy increasing to 700–900 years (barring accidents or violence).

These latest fruits of reductionist medical science open up the tantalizing prospect of extreme longevity for some people. As the contemporary standard-bearers for Enlightenment optimism, the transhumanists, point out, when the biological evolution of our bodies ceased tens of thousands of years ago, species survival decreed that we live on average not much longer than the period needed for our reproductive and child-rearing commitments—two to three decades. However, in the few thousand years since cities and civilization began, culture and socioeconomic organization have come to work on biology, and the scientific-industrial economy has enabled the last two generations who live in the richest countries to anticipate average life expectancies triple those that have prevailed for most of human history. Now, the transhumanists point out, in an age of material abundance, the limits set for the individual by scarcity no longer apply, and this just when medical science and technology begin to offer people a godlike level of control over their health and mortality.

The struggle in contemporary medicine identified by Daniel Callahan as one between a research imperative (with an implicit goal of overcoming death) and a very old clinical imperative to lighten the burden of dying (with an implicit view of death as an integral part of the life cycle) will no doubt continue. The hope must be that a more consciously humane medicine with genuine respect for the patient's perceptions and experience will be able to contain the deleterious effects of the research imperative while gratefully applying the undoubted benefits it offers.

Nevertheless, this will be a process whose outcome will not be decided solely within medicine itself. In the larger culture and society, religion and humanism will continue to struggle over the nature of the human spirit and the best way to ensure that civilized values and conduct prevail.

In Neanderthal graves, weapons, tools, and bones of sacrificed animals have been found, suggesting a belief even then in a world similar to the visible, material one and to which the spirits of the dead migrated. Indeed, anthropologists of an earlier generation, such as Bronislaw Malinowski, said that religion's core belief in a spirit that survived the death of the body was an ancient cultural invention to enable humans to come to terms with the immutable fact of death. More recent cultural inventions—reductionist science and medical technology—promise to soon move us much closer to fulfilling the modern humanist dream of banishing that need for a supernatural world of the spirit. But will we then perish morally and psychologically for want of a shared sacred myth, as Carroll would argue?

According to Karen Armstrong, myth has five important aspects: first, it is usually rooted in the fear of death; second, it is usually bound up with ritual; third, it is about the unknown—what is beyond our experience and what initially we lack words to describe; fourth, it is not just a story, for it shows us how to behave in very important situations; and fifth, it points to another, more powerful, divine reality that permits humans to attain their full potential through participation. In all premodern societies, mythology was a sine qua non of individual and collective life. In trading the power of myth for the power of science, have we lost access to the archetypal realm that seems vital to the long-term health and integrity of a culture? Or will we be able to make a this-worldly, Levinas-style "story" of ethical, interpersonal relations carry the daunting weight of our moral concerns, especially in the face of the well-demonstrated human capacity for barbarous, even demonic, acts (Goody, 1975, 1; Baker, 1993, 862–63; Reich, 1995a, 327–28; Callahan, 2000, 654–55; Kurzweil and Grossman, 2004, iv, 15–32, 377–78; Armstrong, 2005, 3–5; Hall, 2005, 252–53)?

References

Abel, Emily K. 1986. The hospice movement: Institutionalizing innovation. *International Journal of Health Services* 16(1): 71–85.

Abel-Smith, Brian. 1964. *The hospitals 1800–1948: A study in social administration in England and Wales.* London: Heinemann.

Abrahams, E. W. 1991. Tuberculosis control in Queensland. In *History of tuberculosis in Australia, New Zealand, and Papua New Guinea,* ed. A. J. Proust, 46–51. Canberra: Brolga Press.

Abu-Saad, H. Huijer, and A. Courtens. 1999. *Palliative care across the life span: A state of the art.* Maastricht, the Netherlands: Department of Nursing Service, Maastricht University and Pain Expertise Centre, University Hospital Maastricht.

Ackerknecht, Erwin H. 1958. Historical notes on cancer. *Medical History* 2 (January): 114–19.

———. 1982. *A short history of medicine.* Baltimore: Johns Hopkins University Press.

Addington-Hall, Julia M., J. Simon, and R. Gibbs. 2000. Heart failure now on the palliative care agenda. *Palliative Medicine* 14: 361–62.

Agnew, G. Harvey. 1974. *Canadian hospitals, 1920 to 1970: A dramatic half century.* Toronto: University of Toronto Press.

Alexander, Jeffrey C., and Piotr Sztompka. 1990. Introduction. In *Rethinking progress: Movements, forces, and ideas at the end of the twentieth century,* ed. Jeffrey C. Alexander and Piotr Sztompka, 2–9. Boston: Unwin Hyman.

Allbrook, David. 1982. Doctor's role in the Australian hospice movement. *Medical Journal of Australia* 2 (November): 502.

———. 1985. Management of cancer pain. *Medical Journal of Australia* 142 (March): 327.

American Academy of Pain Medicine. 2000. *Undergraduate medical education on pain management, end-of-life care, and palliative care.* [Position statement]. Glenview, IL: Author.

Anaesthesia. 2003. Retrieved February 15, 2006, from http://www.anaesthesia.org.nz

Anderson, Gerard F., Jeremy Hurst, Peter Sotir Hussey, and Melissa Jee-Hughes. 2000. Health spending and outcomes: Trends in OECD countries, 1960–1998. *Health Affairs* 19(3): 150–57.

Angarola, Robert T., and F. Gail Bormel. 1996. Proposed legislative changes and access to pain medications. *American Pain Society Bulletin* (March/April): 1–5.

Antonovsky, Aaron. 1996. The salutogenic model as a theory to guide health promotion. *Health Promotion International* 11(1): 11–18.

Armstrong, Bruce K. 1985. Epidemiology of cancer in Australia. *Medical Journal of Australia* 142 (January): 124–30.

Armstrong, Karen. 2005. *A short history of myth.* Edinburgh: Canongate.

Ashburn, Michael A. 2001. APS must advocate for policy improvements. *American Pain Society Bulletin* 11(2): 1–3.

Ashby, Michael, Mary Brooksbank, Paul Dunne, and Rod MacLeod. 1996. *Australasian undergraduate medical palliative care curriculum.* Clayton, Victoria: Monash Medical Centre.

Association of Anaesthetists of Great Britain and Ireland and Pain Society. 1997. *Provision of pain services.* [Booklet]. London: Author.

Austoker, Joan. 1988. *A history of the Imperial Cancer Research Fund 1902–1986.* New York: Oxford University Press.

Australasian Medical Gazette. 1906. New South Wales Home for Incurables. 25 (June): 291.

———. 1912. Home for Incurables, Adelaide. 31 (March): 347.

———. 1913. The treatment of cancer. 33 (February): 149–50.

———. 1914. Cancer research scholarship. 35 (June): 518.

Australian and New Zealand College of Anaesthetists (ANZCA). 2003. History of FPM. Retrieved February 15, 2006, from http://www.anzca.edu.au/about/fpmhistory/

Australian and New Zealand Society of Palliative Medicine Newsletter. 1998. President's report 1997. (December): 2.

———. 2000a. New Zealand members. (March/April): 1.

———. 2000b. President's soapbox. (July/August): 1.

———. 2000–2001. President's soapbox. (December/January): 2.

———. 2001a. New Zealand branch report. (October): 3.

———. 2001b. President's soapbox. (May/June): 1.

Australian Cancer Society and Elizabeth Hall. 1995. *Cancer control in Australia: A review of current activities and future directions.* Canberra: Australian Government Publishing Service.

Australian Medical Journal. 1885. Austin hospital. (New series) 7 (March): 139.

Australian Nursing Journal. 1997. Oncology and palliative care: Bridging the gap. 5(4): 26.

Back, Anthony L., and Robert A. Pearlman. 2001. Desire for physician-assisted suicide: Request for a better death? *Lancet* 358(9279): 344–45.

Baker, Robert. 1993. The history of medical ethics. In *Companion encyclopedia of the history of medicine,* vol. 2, ed. W. F. Bynum and Roy Porter, 852–87. New York: Routledge.

Barnett, Pauline, and Kay Smith. 1992. *The organisation and funding of hospice care: An international and New Zealand view.* Wellington, New Zealand: Health Research Services and Personal and Public Health Policy, Department of Health.

Bashford, Alison. 1998. *Purity and pollution: Gender, embodiment, and Victorian medicine.* New York: St. Martin's Press.

Basten, Antony. 1999. The Centenary Institute of Cancer Medicine and Cell Biology. *Medical Journal of Australia* 171 (December): 634–37.

Baszanger, Isabelle. 1998. *Inventing pain medicine: From the laboratory to the clinic.* New Brunswick, NJ: Rutgers University Press.

Bates, Barbara. 1992. *Bargaining for life: A social history of tuberculosis, 1876–1938.* Philadelphia: University of Pennsylvania Press.

Battin, Margaret Pabst. 1995. Suicide. In *Encyclopedia of bioethics,* vol. 5, ed. W. T. Reich, 2444–49. New York: Macmillan Library Reference.

Bauman, Zygmunt. 1992. *Mortality, immortality, and other life strategies.* Stanford, CA: Stanford University Press.

Beckett, T. G. 1902. Treatment of cancer by Roentgen rays. *Australasian Medical Gazette* 21 (September): 450–57.

Beinart, Jennifer. 1987. *A history of the Nuffield Department of Anaesthetics, Oxford, 1937–1987.* New York: Oxford University Press.

———. 1988. The snowball effect: The growth of the treatment of intractable pain in postwar Britain. In *The history of the management of pain: From early principles to present practice,* ed. Ronald D. Mann, 179–200. Park Ridge, NJ: Parthenon Publishing Group.

Bell, Daniel. 1977. Sociology. In *The Fontana dictionary of modern thought,* ed. Allan Bullock and Oliver Stallybrass, 587–89. London: Fontana Books.

Benedek, Thomas G., and Kenneth F. Kiple. 1993. Concepts of cancer. In *The Cambridge world history of human disease,* ed. Kenneth F. Kiple, 102–10. New York: Cambridge University Press.

Bennett, F. O. 1962. *Hospital on the Avon: The history of the Christchurch Hospital 1982–1962.* Christchurch, New Zealand: North Canterbury Hospital Board.

Beresford, Larry, and Stephen R. Connor. 1999. History of the national hospice organization. *Hospice Journal* 14(3/4): 15–31.

Berridge, Virginia. 1996. *AIDS in the UK: The making of policy, 1981–1994.* New York: Oxford University Press.

———. 1999. *Opium and the people: Opiate use and drug control policy in nineteenth- and early twentieth-century England.* New York: Free Association Books.

Berry, R. J., and H. Baillie Johnson. 1979. A place for oncology in medical undergraduate teaching. *Medical Education* 13: 398–400.

Bierstadt, Robert. 1978. Sociological thought in the eighteenth century. In *A history of sociological analysis,* ed. T. Bottomore and R. Nisbet, 3–38. New York : Basic Books.

Billings, J. Andrew. 1998. What is palliative care? *Journal of Palliative Medicine* 1(1): 73–81.

———. 2002. Definitions and models of palliative care. In *Principles and practice of palliative care and supportive oncology,* 2nd ed., ed. A. M. Berger, R. K. Portenoy, and D. E. Weissman, 635–45. Philadelphia: Lippincott, Williams, and Wilkins.

———, and Susan Block. 1997. Palliative care in undergraduate medical education: Status report and future directions. *Journal of the American Medical Association* 278(9): 733–38.

Bird, Beverley, Susan Humphries, and Ann Howe. 1990. *Hospice care in Victoria: A profile of programs and patients in 1988–1989: Report to the Health Department of Victoria.* Bundoora, Victoria, Australia: Aged Care Research Group, La Trobe University.

Blum, Diane. 1999. Overcoming the barriers to cancer pain management: The cancer care pain support and education initiative. *American Pain Society Bulletin* 9(6): 1–5.

Bonica, John J. 1981. Cancer pain. In *Medical complications in cancer patients,* ed. J. Klastershey and M. J. Staquet, 87–115. New York: Raven Press.

———. 1988. Evolution of multidisciplinary/interdisciplinary pain programs. In *Pain centers: A revolution in health care,* ed. Gerald M. Aronoff, 9–32. New York: Raven Press.

Bostrom, Nick. 2003. In defense of posthuman dignity. Retrieved February 15, 2006, from http://www.nickbostrom.com/ethics/dignity.html

Bowden, Keith Macrae. 1974. *Doctors and diggers on the Mount Alexander goldfields.* Maryborough, Victoria, Australia: Hedges and Bell.

Bracken, Patrick J. 2001. Post-modernity and post-traumatic stress disorder. *Social Science and Medicine* 53: 733–43.

Brandt, Allan M., and Martha Gardner. 2000. The golden age of medicine? In *Medicine in the twentieth century,* ed. Roger Cooter and John Pickstone, 21–37. Amsterdam: Harwood Academic Publishers.

Breitbart, William. 1997. Pain in AIDS. In *Proceedings of the 8th World Congress on Pain,* ed. T. S. Jensen, A. Turner, and Z. Wiesenfeld-Hallin. Seattle: International Association for the Study of Pain Press.

———, Barry D. Rosenfeld, Steven D. Pasick, Margaret V. McDonald, Howard Thaler, and Russel K. Portenoy. 1996. The undertreatment of pain in ambulatory AIDS patients. *Pain* 65: 243–49.

Breward, Ian. 1993. *A history of the Australian churches.* Saint Leonards, NSW: Allen and Unwin.

British Medical Association.1988. *Euthanasia: Report of the working party to review the British Medical Association's guidance on euthanasia.* [Report]. London: Author.

Browder, J. Pat, and Richard Vance. 1995. Healing. In *Encyclopedia of bioethics,* vol. 2, ed. W. T. Reich, 1032–38. New York: Macmillan Library Reference.

Brown, David L., and B. Raymond Fink. 1998. The history of neural blockade and pain management. In *Neural blockade in clinical anesthesia and management of pain,* ed. M. J. Cousins and P. O. Bridenbaugh, 3–27. Philadelphia: Lippincott-Raven.

Brownstein, Michael J. 1993. A brief history of opiates, opioid peptides, and opioid reception. *Proceedings of the National Academy of Sciences of the United States of America* 90(12): 5391–93.

Bruera, Eduardo. 1998. Palliative care in Canada. *European Journal of Palliative Care* 5(4): 134–35.

Bryder, Linda. 1988. *Below the magic mountain: A social history of tuberculosis in twentieth-century Britain.* New York: Oxford University Press.

———. 1991. Tuberculosis in New Zealand. In *History of tuberculosis in Australia, New Zealand, and Papua New Guinea,* ed. A. J. Proust, 78–89. Canberra: Brolga Press.

Buckley, Peter. 1998. *Casey House Hospice 1988–1998: A decade of caring.* Toronto: Casey House.

Burge, Frederick, Beverley Lawson, and Grace Johnston. 2003. Trends in the place of death of cancer patients, 1992–1997. *Canadian Medical Association Journal* 168(3): 265–70.

Burleigh, Michael. 1991. Surveys of developments in the social history of medicine III. "Euthanasia" in the Third Reich: Some recent literature. *Social History of Medicine* 4(2): 317–28.

Burns, Rosina. 1968. *Those that sowed: The first religious sisters in Australia.* Sydney: E. J. Dwyer.

Burton, Robert C., and Bruce K. Armstrong. 1997. Daffodils and cancer. *Medical Journal of Australia* 167 (August): 180–81.

Callahan, Daniel. 1990. *What kind of life: The limits of medical progress.* Washington, DC: Georgetown University Press.

———. 1995. *Setting limits: Medical goals in an aging society.* Washington, DC: Georgetown University Press.

———. 1998. *False hopes: Why America's quest for perfect health is a recipe for failure.* New York: Simon and Schuster.

———. 2000. Death and the research imperative. *New England Journal of Medicine* 342(9): 654–56.

———. 2001. Our need for caring. In *The lost art of caring: A challenge to health professionals, families, communities, and society,* ed. L. E. Clifford and R. H. Binstock, 11–24. Baltimore: Johns Hopkins University Press.

Canada NewsWire. 2004. Canadian Pain Coalition launches first annual National Awareness Week to shine spotlight on "epidemic" of pain. Retrieved February 15, 2006, from http://www.newswire.ca/en/releases/archive/October2004/28/c5331.html

Canadian Hospice Palliative Care Association. 2001. Unpublished report, submmitted to the Commission on the Future of Health Care in Canada.

———. 2004. A history. Retrieved February 15, 2006, from http://www.chpca.net/about_us/history.htm

Canadian Strategy for Cancer Control: Palliative Care Working Group. 2002. [Final report]. Retrieved March 14, 2006, from http://209.217.127.72/cscc/pdf/finalpalliativecare Jan2002.PDF

Cancer pain: Report of advisory committee on the management of severe chronic pain in cancer patients. 1984. Ottawa: Minister of Supply and Services of Canada.

Cannadine, David. 1981. War and death, grief and mourning in modern Britain. In *Mirrors of* mortality: Studies in the social history of death,* ed. Joachim Whaley, 187–224. London: Europa Publications.

Cannon, Michael. 1998. *The roaring days.* Mornington, Victoria, Australia: Today's Australia Publishing.

Cantor, David. 1993. Cancer. In *Companion encyclopedia of the history of medicine,* vol. 1, ed. W. F. Bynum and Roy Porter, 537–61. New York: Routledge.

Care of the terminally ill: Report of the working group of the Wellington Health Services Advisory Committee. 1981. Wellington, New Zealand: Wellington Health Services Advisory Committee.

Care of the terminally ill: Report of the working party established by Cancer Foundation of WA, Silver Chain Nursing Association, and Health Department of Western Australia (WA). 1986. Perth: Cancer Foundation of WA, Silver Chain Nursing Association, and Heath Department of WA.

Carlin, Martha. 1989. Medieval English hospitals. In *The hospital in history,* ed. Lindsay Granshaw and Roy Porter, 21–39. New York: Routledge.

Carroll, John. 1986. Where ignorant armies clash by night: On the return of faith and its consequences. In *Conversazione: Seminar on the Sociology of Culture,* 1–13, Bundoora, Victoria, Australia: La Trobe University.

———. 2001. *The western dreaming: The Western world is dying for want of a story.* Sydney: HarperCollins.

———. 2004. *The wreck of Western culture: Humanism revisited.* Melbourne: Scribe Publications.

Cassell, Eric J. 1982. The nature of suffering and the goals of medicine. *New England Journal of Medicine* 806(11): 639–45.

———. 1995. Pain and suffering. In *Encyclopedia of bioethics,* vol. 4, ed. W. T. Reich, 1897–1905. New York: Macmillan Library Reference.

Caton, Donald. 1999. Sacred and secular reactions to pain. In *Pain and suffering in history: Narratives of science, medicine and culture,* 8–11. Los Angeles: History of Pain Symposium, University of California.

Cavenagh, J. D., and F. W. Gunz. 1988. Palliative hospice care in Australia. *Palliative Medicine* 2: 51–57.

Chang, Hui-Ming. 2002. Educating medical students in pain medicine and palliative care. *Pain Medicine* 3(3): 194–96.

Chapman, C. Richard. 2000. Shaping a new century: Our evolving role. *American Pain Society Bulletin* 10(1): 1–4.

Chapman, H. G. 1934. The present position of research about cancer. *Transactions of Australasian Medical Congress* (fourth session): 18–20.

Cherry, Thomas. 1933. Cancer and tuberculosis: A survey of recent work on the causation of cancer. *Medical Journal of Australia* 2 (August): 197–217.

Cica, Natasha. 1997a. Euthanasia: The Australian law in an international context. Part 1: Passive voluntary euthanasia. In *Health Issues Papers,* 59–110. Canberra: Australian Government Publishing Service, Department of the Parliamentary Library.

———. 1997b. Euthanasia: The Australian law in an international context. Part 2: Active voluntary euthanasia. In *Health Issues Papers,* 111–201. Canberra: Australian Government Publishing Service, Department of the Parliamentary Library.

Cimino, James E. n.d. Calvary Hospital Palliative Care Institute. [Information sheet]. Bronx, New York.

City Set on a Hill: Our Lady's Hospice Dublin, 1845–1945. 1945. Dublin: Sisters of Charity.

Clark, David. 1999a. Cradled to the grave? Terminal care in the United Kingdom, 1948–1967. *Mortality* 4(3): 225–47.

————. 1999b. Total pain: Disciplinary power and the body in the work of Cicely Saunders, 1958–1967. *Social Sciences and Medicine* 49: 727–36.

————. 2000a. Palliative care history: A ritual process? *European Journal of Palliative Care* 7(2): 50–55.

————. 2000b. Total pain: The work of Cicely Saunders and the hospice movement. *American Pain Society Bulletin* 10(4): 1–4.

————. 2001. A special relationship: Cicely Saunders, the United States, and the early foundation of the modern hospice movement. *Illness, Crisis, and Loss* 9(1): 15–30.

————. 2002. Between hope and acceptance: The medicalisation of dying. *British Medical Journal* 324 (April): 905–7.

————. 2003. The rise and demise of the Brompton cocktail. In *Opioids and pain relief: A historical perspective,* ed. Marcia L. Meldrum, 85–98. Seattle: International Association for the Study of Pain Press.

————, Helen Malson, Neil Small, Karen Mallett, Bren Neale, and Pauline Heather. 1997. Half full or half empty? The impact of health reform on palliative care services in the UK. In *New themes in palliative care,* ed. David Clark, Jo Hockley, and Sam Ahmedzai, 60–74. Philadelphia: Open University Press.

Clark, David, and Jane Seymour. 1999. *Reflections on palliative care.* Philadelphia: Open University Press.

Clark, John. 1998. President's report. *Newsletter of the Canadian Pain Society* (December): 1–2.

Clarke, Brian. 1996. English-speaking Canada from 1854. In *A concise history of Christianity in Canada,* ed. Terrence Murphy and Roberto Perin, 261–359. New York: Oxford University Press.

Cleary, James, and Misha-Miroslav Backonja. 1996. "Translating" opioid tolerance research. *American Pain Society Bulletin* 6(2): 1–9.

Clendinnen, L. J. 1934. The present status of radium in the treatment of cancer. *Transactions of Australasian Medical Congress* (fourth session): 28–32.

Clow, B. 2001. *Negotiating disease: Power and cancer cure, 1900–1950.* Montreal: McGill-Queen's University Press.

Coates, Alan S. 1998. Cancer control in Australia. *Medical Journal of Australia* 169 (July): 8–9.

Coates, Gordon T. 1982. Palliative care: The modern concept. *Medical Journal of Australia* 2 (November): 503–4.

————. 1985. Treatment for cancer pain. *Medical Journal of Australia* 145 (July): 59–60.

Cohen, Douglas. 1984. The right to live and the right to die. *Medical Journal of Australia* 140 (January): 59–61.

Cole, Roger M. 1991. Medical aspects of care for the person with advanced acquired immunodeficiency syndrome (AIDS): A palliative care perspective. *Palliative Medicine* 5: 96–111.

Cole, Russell. 1965. The problem of pain in persistent cancer. *Medical Journal of Australia* 1 (May): 682–86.

Cole, Thomas R. 1992. *The journey of life: A cultural history of aging in America.* New York: Cambridge University Press.

Colebatch, John H. 1978. Developing role of anticancer drugs in cancer treatment. *Medical Journal of Australia* 1 (March): 265–70.

Comeau, Pauline. 2004. Cancer strategy needed but political will lacking. *Canadian Medical Association Journal* 170(13): 1904.

Connor, J. T. H. 2000. *Doing good: The life of Toronto's General Hospital.* Toronto: University of Toronto Press.

Cooper, David, and John B. Hickie. 2000. HIV medicine. In *The thinkers: A history of the physicians and the development of scientific medicine at St. Vincent's Hospital, Sydney, 1857–1997,* ed. John B. Hickie, 377–387. Caringbah, NSW: Playright Publishing.

Copenhaver, Brian. 1995. Death: Art of dying 1 Ars moriendi. In *Encyclopedia of bioethics,* vol. 1, ed. W. T. Reich, 549–51. New York: Macmillan Library Reference.

Corr, Charles A. 1999. Death in modern society. In *Oxford textbook of palliative medicine,* 2d ed., ed. Derek Doyle, Geoffrey W. C. Hanks, and Neil MacDonald, 31–40. New York: Oxford University Press.

Creed, John Mildred. 1890. *Cremation: A lecture.* Sydney: F. Cunninghame.

———. 1916. *My recollections of Australia and elsewhere, 1842–1914.* London: Herbert Jenkins.

Cremation Society of Victoria Report. 1892. Melbourne: Cremation Society of Victoria.

Cumpston, J. H. L. 1936. The trend of cancer mortality in Australia. *Journal of Hygiene* 36: 95–107.

———. 1989. *Health and disease in Australia: A history,* ed. M. J. Lewis. Canberra: AGPS Press.

Dahl, June L. 1996. State cancer pain initiatives update. *American Pain Society Bulletin* (November/December): 1–3.

———. 2003. The state cancer pain initiative movement in the United States: Successes and challenges. In *Opioids and pain relief: A historical perspective,* ed. Marcia L. Meldrum, 163–73. Seattle: International Association for the Study of Pain Press.

Dalley, David, and John B. Hickie. 2000. Medical oncology and palliative care. In *The thinkers: A history of the physicians and the development of scientific medicine at St. Vincent's Hospital, Sydney 1857–1997,* ed. John B. Hickie, 436–44. Caringbah, NSW: Playright Publishing.

Davies, Betty. 1999. Development in Canada. In *Oxford textbook of palliative medicine,* 2nd ed. Derek Doyle, Geoffrey W. C. Hanks, and Neil MacDonald, 1100–2. Oxford: Oxford University Press.

Davison, Graeme. 1995. Our youth is spent and our backs are bent: The origins of Australian ageism. In *Ageing,* ed. David Walker and Stephen Garton, 40–62. Geelong, Victoria, Australia: Faculty of Arts, Deakin University.

Del Vecchio Good, Mary-Jo. 1991. The practice of biomedicine and the discourse on hope: A preliminary investigation into the culture of American oncology. *Anthropologies of Medicine* 7(91): 121–35.

Department of Health. 2001. *The NHS cancer plan: Making progress.* [Progress report]. London: Author.

Dibley, Florence M. 1991. Home of Peace for the dying 1940–1941. In *The vision unfolding: Deaconess institution 1891–1991,* 16–17. Newtown, NSW: Deaconess Press.

Dominica, Frances. 1999. Development in the United Kingdom. In *Oxford textbook of palliative medicine,* 2nd ed. Derek Doyle, Geoffrey W. C. Hanks, and Neil MacDonald, 1098–1100. New York: Oxford University Press.

Donovan, Merilee Ivers. 1989. A historical view of pain management. *Cancer Nursing.* 12(4): 257–61.

Douglas, Charles D., Ian H. Kerridge, Katherine J. Rainbird, John R. McPhee, Lynne Hancock, and Alan D. Spigelman. 2001. The intention to hasten death: A survey of attitudes and practices of surgeons in Australia. *Medical Journal of Australia* 175: 511–15.

Dow, Derek A. 1991. Springs of charity? The development of the New Zealand hospital system, 1870–1910. In *A healthy country: Essays on the social history of medicine in New Zealand,* ed. Linda Bryder, 44–64. Wellington, New Zealand: Bridget Williams Books.

Dowbiggen, Ian. 2003. *A merciful end: The euthanasia movement in modern America.* New York: Oxford University Press.

Doyle, Derek. 1997. Dilemmas and directions: The future of specialist palliative care. Occasional paper 11. London: National Council for Hospice and Specialist Palliative Care Services.

Drews, Robert S. 1939. History of the care of the sick poor of the city of Detroit (1703–1855). *Bulletin of the History of Medicine* 7: 759–82.

Duffy, John. 1976. *The healers: The rise of the medical establishment.* New York: McGraw-Hill.

———. 1984. American perceptions of the medical, legal, and theological professions. *Bulletin of the History of Medicine* 58(1): 1–15.

Dwyer, Brian. 1998. Not in my wildest imaginings: Changes in practice. Address to the annual general meeting of the Australian and New Zealand College of Anaesthetists, Newcastle, May 6.

Easterbrook, Philippa, and Jeanette Meadway. 2001. The changing epidemiology of HIV infection: New challenges for HIV palliative care. *Journal of the Royal Society of Medicine* 94(9): 442–48.

Edwards, F. G. B., and L. Johnson. 1991. Tuberculosis control in Western Australia. In *History of tuberculosis in Australia, New Zealand, and Papua New Guinea,* ed. A. J. Proust, 51–53. Canberra: Brolga Press.

Elwood, Mark, Brian McAvoy, and John Gavin. 2003. Opportunities to improve cancer care in Australia and New Zealand. *New Zealand Medical Journal* 116 (April): 1–3.

Emanuel, Ezekiel J. 1994. The history of euthanasia debates in the United States and Britain. *Annals of Internal Medicine* 121(10): 793–802.

———. 1999. What is the great benefit of legalizing euthanasia or physician-assisted suicide? *Ethics* 109: 629–39.

Engelhardt, H. Tristram. 1986. From philosophy and medicine to philosophy of medicine. *Journal of Medicine and Philosophy* 11: 3–8.

———. 1990. The birth of the medical humanities and the rebirth of the philosophy of medicine: The vision of Edmund D. Pellegrino. *Journal of Medicine and Philosophy* 15: 237–41.

Ewing, D. P., B. W. McEwen, and L. Atkinson. 1965. Combined chemotherapy and radiotherapy in carcinoma of the lung. *Medical Journal of Australia* 2 (September): 397–400.

Expert Advisory Group on Cancer. 1995. A policy framework for commissioning cancer services: A report by the expert advisory group on cancer to the Chief Medical Officers of England and Wales. Retrieved March 14, 2006, from http://www.dh.gov.uk/assetRoot/04/01/43/66/04014366.pdf

Fainsinger, Robin L. 2000. A century of progress in palliative care. *Lancet* 356 (December): S24.

Farrell, James J. 1982. The dying of death: Historical perspectives. *Death Education* 6: 105–23.

Faulkner, Kathleen W. 1999. Development in the United States. In *Oxford textbook of palliative medicine,* 2nd ed. Derek Doyle, Geoffrey W. C. Hanks, and Neil MacDonald, 1105–6. New York: Oxford University Press.

Feldberg, Georgina D. 1995. *Disease and class: Tuberculosis and the shaping of modern North American society.* New Brunswick, NJ: Rutgers University Press.

Field, David. 1994. Palliative medicine and the medicalization of death. *European Journal of Cancer* 3: 58–62.

Field, M. J., and C. K. Cassell. 1997. *Approaching death: Improving care at the end of life.* Washington, DC: National Academy Press.

Finch, Lynette. 1999. Soothing syrups and teething powders: Regulating proprietary drugs in Australia, 1860–1910. *Medical History* 43(1): 74–94.

Finlay, Ilora. 2001. UK strategies for palliative care. *Journal of the Royal Society of Medicine* 94(9): 437–41.

Foley, Kathleen M. 2003. Advancing palliative care in the United States. *Palliative Medicine* 17: 89–91.

Foster, Zelda, and Inge B. Corless. 1999. Origins: An American perspective. *Hospice Journal* 14(3/4): 9–13.

Frizelle, Frank. 2003. Time for the New Zealand cancer control strategy. *New Zealand Medical Journal* 116 (December): 1–2.

Froggatt, Katherine A. 2001. Palliative care and nursing homes: Where next? *Palliative Medicine* 15: 42–48.

Fye, W. Bruce. 1978. Active euthanasia: A historical survey of its conceptual origins and introduction to medical thought. *Bulletin of the History of Medicine* 52(4): 492–502.

Gallagher, Rollin M. 2002. Pain education and training: Progress or paralysis? *Pain Medicine* 3(3): 196–97.

Gare, Deborah. 2001. *Lady Onslow's legacy: A history of the Home of Peace and the Brightwater Care Group.* Osborne Park, Western Australia: Brightwater Care Group.

Gaudette, Leslie A., Tammy Lipskie, Pierre Allard, and Robin L. Fainsinger. 2002. Developing palliative care surveillance in Canada: Results of a pilot study. *Journal of Palliative Care* 18(4): 262–69.

Gault, E. W., and Alan Lucas. 1982. *A century of compassion: A history of the Austin Hospital.* South Melbourne: Macmillan.

Gelfand, Toby. 1993. The history of the medical profession. In *Companion encyclopedia of the history of medicine,* vol. 2, ed. W. F. Bynum and Roy Porter, 1119–50. New York: Routledge.

George, Rob, and Jo Sykes. 1997. Beyond cancer? In *New themes in palliative care,* ed. David Clark, Jo Hockley, and Sam Ahmedzai, 239–54. Philadelphia: Open University Press.

Gerber, Paul. 1984. Brain death, murder, and the law. *Medical Journal of Australia* 140 (April): 536–37.

Giddens, Anthony. 1994. Living in a post-traditional society. In *Reflexive modernizations: Elites, traditions, and aesthetics in the modern social order,* ed. Ulrich Beck, Anthony Giddens, and Scott Lash, 56–109. Cambridge: Polity Press.

Gilbert, John H.V. 1997. Address to the 8th World Congress on Pain. In *Proceedings of the 8th World Congress on Pain,* ed. T. S. Jensen, J. A. Turner, and Z. Wiesenfeld-Hellin, 17–18. Seattle: International Association for the Study of Pain Press.

Gilligan, J. E., and J. Linn. 1980. Natural death legislation. *Medical Journal of Australia* 2 (November): 473.

Gitlin, Melvin C. 2003. Pain medicine: A contemporary perspective on environmental analysis and strategic planning. *Pain Medicine* 4(3): 213–14.

Glajchen, Myra, and Kimberley Calder. 1998. APS and patient advocacy groups: A partnership whose time has come. *American Pain Society Bulletin* 8(3): 1–2.

Glare, Paul A. 2001. Pain in patients with HIV infection: Issues for the new millennium. *European Journal of Pain* 5(Suppl. A): 43–48.

———, and Stephen Clarke. 2002. The interface of oncology and palliative care in tertiary hospitals: A concept in evolution. *Cancer Forum* 26(1): 6–8.

Glare, Paul A,. and Neil J. Cooney. 1997. HIV and palliative care. In *Managing HIV,* ed. G. Stewart, 119–22. North Sydney: Australian Medical Publishing.

Glare, Paul A., and J. Norelle Lickiss. 2000. Palliative medicine: The way ahead. *Medical Journal of Australia* 173 (November): 452–53.

Glicksman, Myer. 1996. *Palliative care in the hospital setting.* London: National Council for Hospice and Specialist Palliative Care Services.

Glyn Hughes, H. L. 1960. *Peace at the last: A survey of terminal care in the United Kingdom.* [Report]. London: United Kingdom and British Commonwealth Branch of the Calouste Gulbenkian Foundation.

Godden, Judith, and Carol Helmstadter. 2004. Women's mission and professional knowledge: Nightingale nursing in colonial Australia and Canada. *Social History of Medicine* 17(2): 157–74.

Godman, Patrick William. 1995. Attitudes to death in Australia 1788–1994. Ph.D. diss., University of Queensland.

Goldin, Grace. 1981. A protohospice of the turn of the century: St. Luke's House, London, from 1893 to 1921. *Journal of the History of Medicine and Allied Sciences* 36 (October): 383–415.

Goodwin, James S. 1999. Geriatrics and the limits of modern medicine. *New England Journal of Medicine* 340(16): 1283–85.

Goody, Jack. 1975. Death and the interpretation of culture. In *Death in America,* ed. David E. Stannard, 1–8. Philadelphia: University of Pennsylvania Press.

Gourevitch, Danielle. 1969. Suicide among the sick in classical antiquity. *Bulletin of the History of Medicine* 43(6): 501–18.

Granshaw, Lindsay. 1992. The rise of the modern hospital in Britain. In *Medicine in society: Historical essays,* ed. Andrew Wear, 197–218. New York: Cambridge University Press.

Grierson, Janet. 1981. *The deaconess.* London: CIO Publishing.

Griffin, Miriam. 1994. Roman suicide. In *Medicine and moral reasoning,* ed. K. W. M. Fulford, G. R. Gillett, and J. M. Soskice, 106–30. New York: Cambridge University Press.

Griffith, Gareth, and Marie Swain. 1995. *Euthanasia.* Sydney: NSW Parliamentary Library Research Service.

Griffiths, Guy. 1934. Euthanasia. In *Transactions of the Australasian Medical Congress* (fourth session), 161–62. Australia: The Congress.

Grmek, M. D. 1958. *On ageing and old age: Basic problems and historic aspects of gerontology and geriatrics.* The Hague: Uitgeverij Dr. W. Junk.

Gruman, Gerald J. 1966. A history of ideas about the prolongation of life: The evolution of prolongevity hypotheses to 1800. *Transactions of the American Philosophical Society* (New series) 56(9): 5–98.

Gunz, F. W. 1982. Hospices in Australia. *Medical Journal of Australia* 2 (November): 501.

Guthrie, B., M. Nelson, and B. Gazzard. 1996. Are people with HIV in London able to die where they plan? *AIDS Care* 8(6): 709–13.

Hall, J. Storrs. 2005. *Nanofuture: What's next for nanotechnology?* Amherst, NY: Prometheus Books.

Hamersley, H. 1988. Cancer, physics, and society: Interactions between the wars. In *Australian science in the making,* ed. R. W. Home, 197–219. New York: Cambridge University Press.

Harris, Marguerite. 1995. *Hearts to love and hands to save: The story of Calvary Hospital, Hobart.* Lenah Valley, Tasmania: Little Company of Mary, Calvary Hospital.

Harris, Ross D., and Lyn M. Finlay-Jones. 1987. Terminal care in Australia. *Hospice Journal* 3(1): 77–90.

Hart, Harold W. 1980. Some notes on the sponsoring of patients for hospital treatment under the voluntary system. *Medical History* 24 (October): 447–60.

Hastie, Barbara A., Victor L. Kovner, and Betty R. Ferrell. 1998. The California pain summit: Focus on regulatory barriers and medical education. *American Pain Society Bulletin* (8)5: 1–5.

Hayter, Charles R. R. 1998a. The clinic as laboratory: The case of radiation therapy, 1896–1920. *Bulletin of the History of Medicine* 72(4): 663–88.

———. 1998b. Historical origins of current problems in cancer control. *Canadian Medical Association Journal* 158(13): 1735–40.

Henley, Wilton, and Patrick Henley. 1977. The first Auckland hospital. In *The story of Auck-*

land Hospital 1847–1977, ed. David Scott, 7–15. Auckland: Medical History Committee of the Royal Australasian College of Physicians in New Zealand.

Henteleff, Paul D. 1986. Palliative care: A personal review of a decade with death and dying. *Manitoba Medicine* 56: 81–84.

Heyland, Daren K., James K. Lavery, Joan E. Tranmer, S. E. D. Shortt, and Sandra J. Taylor. 2000. Dying in Canada: Is it an institutionalized, technologically supported experience? *Journal of Palliative Care* 16 (October): S10–18.

Hickie, John B. 2000a. The foundation of the division of medicine 1923–1957. In *The thinkers: A history of the physicians and the development of scientific medicine at St. Vincent's Hospital, Sydney, 1857–1997,* ed. John B. Hickie, 128–39. Caringbah, NSW: Playright Publishing.

———. 2000b. St. Vincent's: A teaching hospital. In *The thinkers: A history of the physicians and the development of scientific medicine at St. Vincent's Hospital, Sydney, 1857–1997,* ed. John B. Hickie, 91–114. Caringbah, NSW: Playright Publishing.

Higginson, Irene J., and A. M. McGregor. 1999. The impact of palliative medicine? *Palliative Medicine* 13: 273–74.

Hilden, Joanne M., Bruce P. Himelstein, David R. Freyer, Sarah Friebert, and Javier R. Kane. 2001. End-of-life care: Special issues in pediatric oncology. In *Improving palliative care for cancer,* ed. K. M. Foley and H. Gelband, 161–98. Washington, DC: National Academy Press.

Hodgkinson, Ruth G. 1967. *The origins of the National Health Service: The medical services of the New Poor Law, 1834–1871.* London: Wellcome Historical Medical Library.

Hoffman, Philip C., Ann M. Mauer, and Everet E. Vokes. 2000. Lung cancer. *Lancet* 355 (February): 479–85.

Holmes, M. J. 1925. *Cancer mortality in Australia: A statistical study.* Melbourne: HJ Green Government Printer.

Holmes, Martha Stoddard. 2003. The grandest badge of his art: Three Victorian doctors, pain relief, and the art of medicine. In *Opioids and pain relief: A historical perspective,* ed. Marcia L. Meldrum, 21–34. Seattle: International Association for the Study of Pain Press.

Houlbrooke, Ralph. 1989. Death, church, and family in England between the late fifteenth and early eighteenth centuries. In *Death, ritual, and bereavement,* ed. Ralph Houlbrooke, 25–42. New York: Routledge in association with the Social History Society of the United Kingdom.

Humphreys, C. J. 1999. Undying spirits: Religion, medicine, and institutional care of the dying, 1878–1938. Ph.D. diss., University of Sheffield, South Yorkshire, UK.

Humphry, Derek, and Ann Wickett. 1990. *The right to die: Understanding euthanasia.* Eugene, OR: Hemlock Society.

Ilbery, Peter. 1978. The comprehensive cancer centre. *Medical Journal of Australia* 1 (May): 573–76.

Improving symptom control and end-of-life care for cancer patients requires stronger federal leadership. 2001. Retrieved June 6, 2006, from http://www.soros.org/initiatives/pdia/news/leadership_20010619

Inglis, K. S. 1958. *Hospital and community: A history of the Royal Melbourne Hospital.* Carlton, Victoria, Australia: Melbourne University Press.

Jackson, Avril, and Ann Eve. 1997. In *Hospice care on the international scene,* ed. Cicely Saunders and Robert Kastenbaum, 143–50. New York: Springer.

Jalland, Pat. 1996. *Death in the Victorian family.* New York: Oxford University Press.

———. 2002. *Australian ways of death: A social and cultural history, 1840–1918.* New York: Oxford University Press.

James, C. D. T. 1976. Pain clinics. *Nursing Mirror* 143(24): 56–57.

Jona, J. Leon. 1928. The treatment of inoperable cancer by the injection of a colloidal prepa-ration of various metals—bismuth, lead, copper. *Medical Journal of Australia* 2 (Novem-ber): 587—89.

———. 1929. Corpuscular medication. A new method of administering heavy metals and other elements. The method applied in the treatment of inoperable cancer by the ad-ministration of lead, copper, and bismuth: A progress report. *Transactions of Australasian Medical Congress* (third session): 456–59.

Jones, K. S. 1962. Death and doctors. *Medical Journal of Australia* 2 (September): 329–34.

Jones, Rhys, Adrian Trenholme, Margaret Horsburgh, and Aimee Riding. 2002. The need for paediatric palliative care in New Zealand. *New Zealand Medical Journal* 115(1163) (October): 1–6.

Joranson, David E. 1996. State pain commissions: New vehicles for progress? *American Pain Society Bulletin* (January/February): 1–2.

Joseph, M., Sr. 2001. The Dominican Sisters of Hawthorne: Our history. http://www.hawthorne-dominicans.org/dsh/history. July 27.

Kasap and Associates. 1996. *Report to the palliative care program review.* Canberra: Australian Government Publishing Service.

Kellehear, Allan. 2000. Spirituality and palliative care: A model of needs. *Palliative Medicine* 14: 149–55.

Kelly, Janet J., Susan Y. Chu, James W. Buehler, and the AIDS Mortality Project Group. 1993. AIDS deaths shift from hospital to home. *American Journal of Public Health* 83(10): 1433–37.

Kemp, N. D. A. 2002. *Merciful release: The history of the British euthanasia movement.* New York: Manchester University Press.

Kerr, Colin. 1979. *The Home for Incurables: The first 100 years.* Adelaide, Australia: Lutheran Publishing House.

Kerr, Derek. 1992. Alfred Worcester: A pioneer in palliative care. *American Journal of Hospice and Palliative Care* 9(3): 13–14, 36–38.

———. 1993. Mother Mary Aikenhead, the Irish Sisters of Charity, and Our Lady's Hos-pice for the Dying. *American Journal of Hospice and Palliative Care* 10(3): 13–20.

Kirby, M. D. 1980. The rights of the living and the rights of the dying. *Medical Journal of Aus-tralia* 1 (March): 252–55.

Kliever, Lonnie D. 1995. Death: Western religious thought. In *Encyclopedia of bioethics*, vol. 1, ed. W. T. Reich, 505–12. New York: McMillan Library Reference.

Koh, Eugen. 1988. Voluntary euthanasia. *Medical Journal of Australia* 49 (September): 276.

Kuhse, Helga. 1985a. Euthanasia—again: "Letting die" is not in the patient's best interests: A case for active euthanasia. *Medical Journal of Australia* 143 (May): 610–13.

———. 1985b. To kill or let die? *Medical Journal of Australia* 143 (August): 170–71.

———. 1988. Voluntary euthanasia in the Netherlands. *Medical Journal of Australia* 148 (February): 159.

———, and Peter Singer. 1988. Doctors' practices and attitudes regarding voluntary eu-thanasia. *Medical Journal of Australia* 148 (June): 623–27.

Kunitz, Stephen J. 1991. The personal physician and the decline of mortality. In *The decline of mortality in Europe,* ed. Roger Schofield, David Reher, and Alain Bideau, 248–62. New York: Oxford University Press.

Kurzweil, Ray, and Terry Grossman. 2004. *Fantastic voyage: Live long enough to live forever.* Emmaus, PA: Rodale.

Lamerton, R. 1980. *Care of the dying.* New York: Penguin.

Lancaster, H. O. 1950. Cancer mortality in Australia. *Medical Journal of Australia* 2 (Septem-ber): 501–6.

———. 1958. *Cancer statistics in Australia.* Part 1. *Medical Journal of Australia* 2 (September): 350–56.

Lancet, The. 1994. Their lordships on euthanasia. 343(8895) (February 19): 430–31.

Lander, Harry. 1984. Some medical aspects of euthanasia. *Medical Journal of Australia* 141 (August): 174–77.

Lane, Alan. 1986. Treatment for cancer pain. *Medical Journal of Australia* 144 (March): 334.

Lavery, James V., Joseph Boyle, Bernard M. Dickens, Heather Maclean, and Peter A. Singer. 2001. Origins of the desire for euthanasia and assisted suicide in people with HIV-1 or AIDS: A qualitative study. *Lancet* 358(9279): 362–67.

Lawrence, Christopher. 1985. Incommunicable knowledge: Science, technology, and the clinical art in Britain 1850–1914. *Journal of Contemporary History* 20(4): 503–20.

———. 1998. Still incommunicable: Clinical holists and medical knowledge in interwar Britain. In *Greater than the parts: Holism in biomedicine, 1920–1950,* ed. Christopher Lawrence and George Weisz, 94–111. New York: Oxford University Press.

———, and George Weisz. 1998. Medical holism: The context. In *Greater than the parts: Holism in biomedicine, 1920–1950,* ed. Christopher Lawrence and George Weisz, 1–22. New York: Oxford University Press.

Layland, R., and A. J. Proust. 1991. The Goddard papers. In *History of tuberculosis in Australia, New Zealand, and Papua New Guinea,* ed. A. J. Proust, 27–32. Canberra: Brolga Press.

Leaney, Jennifer. 1989. Ashes to ashes: Cremation and the celebration of death in nineteenth-century Britain. In *Death, ritual, and bereavement,* ed. Ralph Houlbrooke, 118–35. New York: Routledge in association with the Social History Society of the United Kingdom.

Lees, Alan W. 1974. Cancer treatment in the 1970s: The development of oncology centres. *Queen's Nursing Journal* 17 (April): 7–9.

Leet, Martin. 2005. Politics and religion in Australia. *Brisbane Line* (Brisbane Institute) (August 25): 1–3.

Lerner, B. H. 1998. *Contagion and confinement: Controlling tuberculosis along the Skid Road.* Baltimore: Johns Hopkins University Press.

Letter from the president. 2003. *Newsletter of the Canadian Pain Society* (February): 1–3.

Lewis, D. Sclater. 1969. *Royal Victoria Hospital 1887–1947.* Montreal: McGill University Press.

Lewis, Milton. 2003a. *The people's health: Public health in Australia, 1788–1950.* Westport, CT: Praeger Press.

———. 2003b. *The people's health: Public health in Australia, 1950 to the present.* Westport, CT: Praeger Press.

Lickiss, Norelle. 1989. Postgraduate education for palliative care. *Cancer Forum* 13(1): 28–31.

———. 1993. Australia: Status of cancer pain and palliative care. *Journal of Pain and Symptom Management* 8(6): 388–94.

———. 1999. Australia and New Zealand. In *Oxford textbook of palliative medicine,* 2nd ed. Derek Doyle, Geoffrey W. C. Hanks, and Neil MacDonald, 1191–92. New York: Oxford University Press.

———. 2001. Approaching cancer pain relief. *European Journal of Pain* 5(Suppl. A): 5–14.

———. 2005. Draft chapter on history of palliative care in Australia.

Liebeskind, John C., and Marcia L. Meldrum. 1997. John Bonica, world champion of pain. In *Proceedings of the 8th World Congress on Pain,* ed. T. S. Jensen, J. A. Turner, and Z. Wiesenfeld-Hallin, 19–32. Seattle: International Association for the Study of Pain Press.

Lindblom, Ulf. 2001. Patrick D. Wall, 1925–2001. *European Journal of Pain* 5: 343–45.

Lippe, Philipp M. 2000. The decade of pain control and research. *Pain Medicine* 1(4): 286.

Lipton, Sampson. 1990a. Introduction. In *The pain clinic,* ed. Sampson Lipton, Eldon Tunks, and Massimo Zoppi, xxvii–xxxiii. New York: Raven Press.

———. 1990b. Pain: An update. In *The pain clinic,* ed. Sampson Lipton, Eldon Tunks, and Massimo Zoppi, 1–9. New York: Raven Press.

Little, Miles. 1998. Cartesian thinking in health and medicine. In *The tasks of medicine: An ideology of care,* ed. Peter Baume, 75–84. Sydney: MacLennan and Petty.

———. 1999. Assisted suicide and the meaning of life. *Theoretical Medicine and Bioethics* 20: 287–98.

———. 2002. Humanistic medicine or values-based medicine: What's in a name? *Medical Journal of Australia* 177(6): 319–21.

———. 2003. Better than numbers: A gentle critique of evidence-based medicine. *Australian and New Zealand Journal of Surgery* 73: 177–82.

Liu, Maywin. 1998. Anaesthesia and palliative care. *ASA Newsletter* 62(5): 1–3.

Lock, Margaret. 1995. The return of the patient as person: Contemporary attitudes toward the alleviation of suffering in North America. In *History of the doctor-patient relationship,* ed. Y. Kawakata, S. Sokai, and Y. Otsuka, 99–130. Tokyo: Ishyaku Euro-America.

Loeser, John D. 2003. Opiophobia and opiophilia. In *Opioids and pain relief: A historical perspective,* ed. Marcia L. Meldrum, 1–4. Seattle: International Association for the Study of Pain Press.

Loudon, Irvine, and Mark Drury. 1998. Some aspects of clinical care in general practice. In *General practice under the National Health Service, 1948–1997,* ed. Irvine Loudon, John Horder, and Charles Webster, 92–127. London: Clarendon Press.

Lowenthal, Raymond M., and Kerry W. Jestrimski. 1986. Corticosteroid drugs: Their role in oncological practice. *Medical Journal of Australia* 144 (January): 81–84.

Löwy, Ilana. 1995. Nothing more to be done: Palliative care versus experimental therapy in advanced cancer. *Science in Context* 8(1): 209–29.

———. 1996. *Between bench and bedside: Science, healing, and interleukin-2 in a cancer ward.* Cambridge, MA: Harvard University Press.

Ludmerer, Kenneth M. 1999. *Time to heal: American medical education from the turn of the century to the era of managed care.* New York: Oxford University Press.

MacDonald, Neil. 1999. Canada. In *Oxford textbook of palliative medicine,* 2nd ed. Derek Doyle, Geoffrey W. C. Hanks, and Neil MacDonald, 1194–95. New York: Oxford University Press.

———. 1998a. A march of folly. *Canadian Medical Association Journal* 158(13): 1699–1701.

———. 1998b. Palliative care: An essential component of cancer control. *Canadian Medical Association Journal* 158(13): 1709–16.

———, Helen P. Findlay, Eduardo Bruera, Deborah Dudgeon, and Janice Kramer. 1997. A Canadian survey of issues in cancer pain management. *Journal of Pain and Symptom Management* 14(6): 332–42.

MacKay, C.V. 1949. A cancer institute in Victoria. *Medical Journal of Australia* 2 (November): 729.

MacLeod, Rod. 2001. A national strategy for palliative care in New Zealand. *Journal of Palliative Medicine* 4: 70–74.

———. 2002. Caring for children who are dying. *New Zealand Medical Journal* 115(1163): 1–3.

———. 2003. From New Zealand. *Palliative Medicine* 17: 146–47.

MacMahon, E. G. 1973. The pioneers of Lewisham Hospital. *Journal of the Australian Catholic Historical Society* 4: 1–22.

Maddocks, Ian. 1994. A new society of palliative medicine. *Medical Journal of Australia* 160 (June): 670.

————. 1999. Medicine and palliative care. *Medical Journal of Australia* 171 (July): 63–64.

————, and Janet Donnell. 1992. A master's degree and graduate diploma in palliative care. *Palliative Medicine* 6: 317–20.

Magnusson, Roger S. 2002. *Angels of death: Exploring the euthanasia underground.* Melbourne: Melbourne University Press.

Manderson, Desmond. 1993. *From Mr. Sin to Mr. Big: A history of Australian drug law.* New York: Oxford University Press.

Marcus, Kelly Stein, Robert D. Kerns, Barry Rosenfeld, and William Breitbart. 2000. HIV/AIDS-related pain as a chronic pain condition: Implications of a biopsychosocial mode for comprehensive assessment and effective management. *Pain Medicine* 1(3): 260–81.

Martin, Shelley. 2002. The never-ending war against cancer. *Canadian Medical Association Journal* 166(12): 1582.

Mathew, Alison, Sarah Cowley, Julia Bliss, and Gillian Thistlewood. 2003. The development of palliative care in national government policy in England, 1986–2000. *Palliative Medicine* 17: 270–82.

McCauley, Bernadette. 1997. Sublime anomalies: Women religious and Roman Catholic hospitals in New York City, 1850–1920. *Journal of the History of Medicine and Allied Sciences* 52 (July): 289–309.

McCowage, Geoffrey B., Marcus R. Vowels, Rhonda Brown, D'Arcy O'Gorman-Hughes, Leslie White, and Glenn Marshall. 1993. The experience of a single Australian paediatric oncology unit. *Medical Journal of Australia* 159 (October): 453–56.

McCuaig, Katherine. 1982. Tuberculosis: The changing concepts of the disease in Canada 1900–1950. In *Health, disease, and medicine: Essays in Canadian history,* ed. C. G. Roland, 296–307. Toronto: Hannah Institute for the History of Medicine.

McEwen, Brian W., and Frans W. deWilde. 1965. The pain clinic: A clinic for the management of intractable pain. *Medical Journal of Australia* 1 (May): 676–82.

McKenzie, Michael R. 1998. Oncology and palliative care: Bringing together the two solitudes. *Canadian Medical Association Journal* 158: 1702–4.

McManners, John. 1985. *Death and the Enlightenment: Changing attitudes to death among Christians and unbelievers in eighteenth-century France.* New York: Oxford University Press.

Media Release. 1998. The Hon. Dr. Michael Wooldridge, Minister for Health and Family Services, National strategy to improve palliative care. Retrieved March 14, 2006, from http://www.health.gov.au/internet/wcms/publishing.nsf/Content/health-archive-mediarel-1998-mw14898.htm

Medical Journal of Australia. 1914. Cancer in Victoria. 2 (July): 47.

————. 1922. Diathermy and radiotherapy. 2 (September): 342–43.

————. 1931a. Canberra cancer conference. 1 (April): 515–16.

————. 1931b. The Canberra cancer conference. 1 (May): 607–8.

————. 1931c. Cancer organization in Australia. 2 (July): 87–88.

————. 1932. Canberra cancer conference. 1 (May): 697–709.

————. 1933. Canberra cancer conference. 2 (July): 78–92.

————. 1934a. An Australian organization against cancer. 2 (September): 302.

————. 1934b. The Selenide treatment of cancer. 2 (October): 519–20.

————. 1934c. Heroin. 2 (October): 487–88.

————. 1936a. A neuro-hormonal treatment of cancer. 2 (August): 191–93.

————. 1936b. Seventh Australian cancer conference. 2 (August): 236–48.

————. 1937. Australian cancer conference. 2 (August): 234–38.

————. 1944. The future of cancer treatment in Australia. 1 (January): 31–32.

————. 1948. Cancer detection clinic. 2 (August): 192.

————. 1955a. Radiotherapy in the treatment of cancer. 2 (October): 527.

————. 1955b. The treatment of cancer in New South Wales. 2 (November): 913–14.

————. 1956. A special unit for cancer research in New South Wales. 1 (June): 1049–50.

————. 1957a. Consumption of pethidine and morphine. 1 (January): 120–21.

————. 1957b. A special unit for cancer research in New South Wales. 1 (March): 44.

————. 1962. Some clinical observations on breast cancer seen in a radiotherapy department. 2 (August): 204.

————. 1964. The New South Wales State Cancer Council: Research grants. 2 (August): 202.

————. 1966. Surgery and chemotherapy in cancer. 1 (June): 1127–28.

————. 1969. Euthanasia legislation. 1 (May): 987–88.

————. 1972a. The team approach in cancer treatment. 1 (March): 557–58.

————. 1972b. The team approach in cancer treatment. 1 (April): 828.

————. 1974. Cancer centres. 2 (October): 513–14.

————. 1975a. Death in today's society. 2 (July/December): 897.

————. 1975b. New hope in breast cancer treatment. 2 (August): 282.

————. 1976. The problems of legalizing euthanasia—and the alternative. 2 (December): 963–68.

Meldrum, Marcia L. 1999. The founding of the American Pain Society. In *Pain and suffering in history: Papers presented March 13–14 at History of Pain Symposium, University of California, Los Angeles,* 94–97. Los Angeles: University of California.

————. 2003. A capsule history of pain management. *Journal of the American Medical Association* 290(18): 2470–75.

Melzack, R., B. M. Ofiesh, and B. M. Mount. 1979. The Brompton mixture versus morphine solution given orally: Effects on pain. *Canadian Medical Association Journal* 120(4): 435–38.

Melzack, R., J. E. Ofiesh, and B. M. Mount. 1976. The Brompton mixture: Effects on pain in cancer patients. *Canadian Medical Association Journal* 115(2): 125–29.

Memorial Sloan-Kettering Cancer Center. 1998. Dr. Richard Payne named chief of pain and palliative service. Retrieved November 21, 2003, from http://www.mskcc.org/mskcc/html/1246.cfn

Mendelson, George. 1990. Pain 1990: Sixth World Congress on Pain. *Medical Journal of Australia* 153 (October): 406–9.

Metcalf, Donald. 1976. Cancer research for small countries: Why and how? *Medical Journal of Australia* 1 (January): 45–47.

Milton, G. W. 1972. The care of the dying. *Medical Journal of Australia* 2 (July): 177–82.

Mitchell, Ann M. 1977. *The hospital south of the Yarra: A history of Alfred Hospital, Melbourne, from foundation to the nineteen-forties.* Melbourne: Alfred Hospital.

Momeyer, Richard W. 1995. Western philosophical thought. In *Encyclopedia of bioethics,* vol. 1, ed. W. T. Reich, 498–504. New York: Macmillan Library Reference.

Montigny, E. A. 1997. *Foisted upon the government? State responsibilities, family obligations, and the care of the dependent aged in late nineteenth-century Ontario.* Montreal: McGill-Queen's University Press.

Moran, Herbert M. 1946. *In my fashion: An autobiography of the last ten years.* London: Peter Davies.

Morgan, Graeme W. 1996. Development of radiation oncology services in Australia. *International Journal of Radiation Oncology, Biology, and Physics* 36(1): 219–32.

Morris, David B. 1991. *The culture of pain.* Berkeley: University of California Press.

————. 1999. A invisible history of pain: Early nineteenth-century Britain and America. In

Pain and suffering in history: Narratives of science, medicine, and culture, 1–7. Los Angeles: History of Pain Symposium, University of California.

Mount, Balfour M. 1997. The Royal Victoria Hospital palliative care service: A Canadian experience. In *Hospice care on the international scene,* ed. Cicely Saunders and Robert Kastenbaum, 73–85. New York: Springer.

———, J. Ajemian, and J. F. Scott. 1976. Use of the Brompton mixture in treating the chronic pain of malignant disease. *Canadian Medical Association Journal* 115(2): 122–24.

Mullins, George Lane. 1896. Cancer in New South Wales. *Australasian Medical Gazette* 15 (January): 1–8.

Munk, William. 1887. *Euthanasia; or, medical treatment in aid of an easy death.* New York: Longmans, Green.

Murphy, Caroline C. S. 1989. From Friedenheim to hospice: A century of cancer hospitals. In *The hospital in history,* ed. Lindsay Granshaw and Roy Porter, 221–41. New York: Routledge.

Murphy, Terrence. 1996. The English-speaking colonies to 1854. In *A concise history of Christianity in Canada,* ed. Terrence Murphy and Roberto Perin, 105–88. New York: Oxford University Press.

National Action Planning Workshop on End-of-Life Care. March 2–4, 2002. [Report]. Retrieved April 21, 2004, from http://www.hc-sc.gc.ca/english/care/palliative_work shop.html/

National Health and Medical Research Council. 1989. *Management of severe pain: Report of the working party on management of severe pain.* Canberra: Australian Government Publishing Service.

Nelson, Sioban. 2001. *Say little, do much: Nurses, nuns, and hospitals in the nineteenth century.* Philadelphia: University of Pennsylvania Press.

New Zealand Cancer Control Strategy. 2003. Retrieved February 15, 2006, from http://www.moh.govt.nz/moh.nsf/0/3d7504ad140c7ef0cc256d88000e5a16?OpenDocument

New Zealand Ministry of Health. 2002. *Toward a cancer control strategy for New Zealand, Marihi Tauporo.* [Discussion document]. Wellington: Author.

New Zealand Pain Society. 2003. Retrieved November 27, 2003, from http://www.library.ucla.edu.libraries/biomed/iasp/newzealand/

New Zealand Palliative Care Strategy, The. 2001. Wellington, New Zealand: Ministry of Health. Retrieved March 4, 2006, from http://www.moh.govt.nz/moh.nsf/0/65c53a08e9801444cc256e62000aad80?OpenDocument

Newell, Christopher. 1996. Critical reflections on euthanasia and people with disability. *Australian Quarterly* 68(3): 48–58.

Newsletter of the Canadian Pain Society. 2000. Report of editor of journal (January): 3–4.

———. 2003a. Canadian pain coalition. (September): 3–4.

———. 2003b. Letter from the president. (February): 1.

Nicol, Robert. 1994. *At the end of the road: Government, society, and the disposal of human remains in the nineteenth and twentieth centuries.* Saint Leonards, NSW: Allen and Unwin.

North Carolina Pain Initiative. 2001. A statement on the value of opioids for treating people with severe pain. Retrieved November 27, 2003, from http://www.aacpi.wisc.edu/regulatory/nepi.html

Nutton, Vivian. 1992. Healers in the medical marketplace: Toward a social history of Graeco-Roman medicine. In *Medicine in society: Historical essays,* ed. Andrew Wear, 15–58. New York: Cambridge University Press.

O'Callaghan, James P. 2001. Evolution of a rational use of opioids in chronic pain. *European Journal of Pain* 5 (Suppl. A): 21–26.

O'Carrigan, Catherine. 1986. St. Vincent's Hospital, Sydney: Pioneer in nineteenth-century health care. Master's thesis, University of Sydney.

Of life and death: Report of the special Senate committee on euthanasia and assisted suicide. 1995. Ottawa: Senate of Canada.

Oliver, Bobbie. 1992. *Toward a living place: Hospice and palliative care in Western Australia 1977 to 1991.* West Perth: Cancer Foundation of Western Australia.

Otago unveils innovative campaign to advance as a world-class university. 2002. Retrieved March 3, 2006, from http://www.otago.ac.nz/news/news/2002/12e-11-02_press_release.html

Our Lady's Hospice, Harold's Cross. n.d. Dublin: Sisters of Charity.

Pain Society. 1997. *Desirable criteria for pain management programmes.* [Booklet]. London: Author.

———. 2003. What is the Pain Society? Retrieved February 15, 2006, from http://www.painsociety.org/pain_what_is.html

Palliative care week. May 16, 2003. *Kelowna Daily Courier,* Kelowna, British Columbia. Retrieved February 15, 2006, from http://www.sen.parl.gc.ca/scarstairs/PalliativeCare/Fitzpatrick_e.asp

Papper, Emanuel M. 1990. Pain, suffering, and anesthesia in the Romantic period. Ph.D. diss., University of Miami.

Parsinnen, T. M. 1983. *Secret passions, secret remedies: Narcotic drugs in British society, 1820–1930.* Philadelphia: Institute for the Study of Human Issues.

Patterson, James T. 1987. *The dread disease: Cancer and modern American culture.* Cambridge, MA: Harvard University Press.

Perin, Roberto. 1996. French-speaking Canada from 1800. In *A concise history of Christianity in Canada,* ed. Terrence Murphy and Roberto Perin, 199–259. New York: Oxford University Press.

Perron, Marshall. 1996. The rights of the Terminally Ill Act: Conception and birth. Voluntary Euthanasia Society of Victoria, Inc. Retrieved October 1996 from http://home.vicnet.net.au/nvesv/marshall/

Pinell, Patrice. 2000. Cancer. In *Medicine in the twentieth century,* ed. Roger Cooter and John Pickstone, 671–86. Amsterdam: Harwood Academic Publishers.

Pinker, Susan. 2001. New manifesto a "bill of rights" for patients in pain. *Canadian Medical Association Journal* 165(2): 1–2.

Pollard, Brian. 1985. To kill or let die? *Medical Journal of Australia* 143 (July): 48.

———. 1988. Dying: Rights and responsibilities. *Medical Journal of Australia* 149 (August): 147–49.

———. 1998. Interview by Milton Lewis. September 17, Sydney.

———. 2001. Can euthanasia be safely legalized? *Palliative Medicine* 15: 61–65.

———. n.d. PC history in NSW. [Typescript in possession of Milton Lewis, Sydney].

Portenoy, Russell K. 1999. Palliative care: An opportunity for pain specialists. *American Pain Society Bulletin* 9(3): 1–5.

———. 2003. Interview. Developing an integrated department of pain medicine and palliative care. Retrieved March 6, 2006, from http://www2.edc.org/lastacts/archives/archivesJuly01/portfeatureinn.asp

Porter, Roy. 1989a. Death and the doctors in Georgian England. In *Death, ritual, and bereavement,* ed. Ralph Houlbrooke, 77–94. New York: Routledge in association with the Social History Society of the United Kingdom.

———. 1989b. The gift relation: Philanthropy and provincial hospitals in eighteenth-century England. In *The hospital in history,* ed. Lindsay Granshaw and Roy Porter, 149–78. New York: Routledge.

————. 1993. Pain and suffering. In *Companion encyclopedia of the history of medicine,* vol. 2, ed. W. F. Bynum and Roy Porter, 1574–91. New York: Routledge.

————. 1995. *London: A social history.* Cambridge, MA: Harvard University Press.

————. 1996a. Hospitals and surgery. In *The Cambridge illustrated history of medicine,* ed. Roy Porter, 202–45. New York: Cambridge University Press.

————. 1996b. Medical science. In *The Cambridge illustrated history of medicine,* ed. Roy Porter, 154–201. New York: Cambridge University Press.

————. 1996c. What is disease? In *The Cambridge illustrated history of medicine,* ed. Roy Porter, 82–117. New York: Cambridge University Press.

————. 1997. *The greatest benefit to mankind: A medical history of humanity from antiquity to the present.* London: HarperCollins.

————. 1999. Western medicine and pain: Historical perspectives. In *Religion, health, and suffering,* ed. John R. Hinnells and Roy Porter, 364–80. New York: Kegan Paul International.

————, and Dorothy Porter. 1989. *In sickness and in health: The British experience 1650–1850.* London: Fourth Estate.

Poynter, John. 1974. *Alfred Felton.* Great Australians Series. [Booklet]. Melbourne: Oxford University Press.

Principles and provisions of palliative care. 1992. [Joint report of the Standing Medical Advisory Committee and Standing Nursing and Midwifery Advocacy Committee]. London: Her Majesty's Stationery Office.

Procacci, Paolo, and Marco Maresca. 1984. Pain concept in Western civilization: A historical review. In *Recent advances in the management of pain,* ed. Constantino Benedetti, C. Richard Chapman, and Guido Moricca, 1–11. New York: Raven Press.

————. 1998. Historical development of the concept of pain. *Pain Clinic* 10(4): 211–28.

Proctor, Robert N. 1995. *Cancer wars: How politics shapes what we know and don't know about cancer.* New York: Basic Books.

Proust, A. J. 1991. Evolution of treatment. In *History of tuberculosis in Australia, New Zealand, and Papua New Guinea,* ed. A. J. Proust, 147–54. Canberra: Brolga Press.

Providence Health Care. 2003. Holy Family Hospital and the Sisters of Providence. Retrieved February 28, 2006, from http://www.providencehealthcare.org/about_history_holyfamily1.html

Quality End-of-Life Care Coalition. 2003. Ottawa: Canadian Hospice Palliative Care Association.

Quiggan, Pat. 1988. *No rising generation: Women and fertility in late nineteenth-century Australia.* Canberra: Department of Demography, Research School of Social Sciences, Australian National University.

Rawstron, R. E. 2002. *Anaesthesia: Notes on anaesthetics in New Zealand.* Palmerston North, New Zealand: Author.

Reed, Diane. 1987. Community health nursing: A century of progress. In *Proceedings of the first New Zealand conference on the history of medicine in New Zealand and Australian medicine,* ed. R. E. Wright-St. Clair, 123–29. Hamilton, New Zealand: Waikato Postgraduate Medical Society, Waikato Hospital.

Reich, Warren Thomas. 1989. Speaking of suffering: A moral account of compassion. *Soundings* 72(1): 83–108.

————. 1995a. Care: History of the notion of care. In *Encyclopedia of bioethics,* vol. 1, ed. W. T. Reich, 319–31. New York: Macmillan Library Reference.

————. 1995b. Eleven historical dimensions of an ethic of care in health care. In *Encyclopedia of bioethics,* vol. 1, ed. W. T. Reich, 331–36. New York: Macmillan Library Reference.

Reiser, Stanley Joel. 1975. The dilemma of euthanasia in modern medical history: The English and American experience. In *The dilemmas of euthanasia,* ed. John A. Behnke and Sissela Bok, 27–49. New York: Anchor Press/Doubleday.

———. 1978. *Medicine and the reign of technology.* New York: Cambridge University Press.

Report of the inquiry by the Select Committee on Euthanasia, vol. 1. 1995. Darwin, Australia: Legislative Assembly of the Northern Territory.

Rheinberger, Hans-Jorg. 2000. Beyond nature and culture: Modes of reasoning in the age of molecular biology and medicine. In *Living and working with the new medical technologies: Intersections of inquiry,* ed. M. Lock, A. Young, and A. Cambrioso, 19–30. New York: Cambridge University Press.

Richards, Mike. 2000. NHS cancer plan. *Cancer Action* 3 (December): 1–8.

Riley, J. C. 1987. Ill health during the English mortality decline: The friendly societies' experience. *Bulletin of the History of Medicine* 61(4): 563–88.

———. 2001. *Rising life expectancy: A global history.* New York: Cambridge University Press.

Risse, Guenter B. 1999. *Mending bodies, saving souls: A history of hospitals.* New York: Oxford University Press.

Robinson, E. 1994. Undergraduate cancer education around the world. In *Cancer education for undergraduate medical students,* ed. E. Robinson, C. D. Sherman, and R. R. Love, 1–12. Geneva: International Union against Cancer.

Rogers Hollingsworth, J. 1981. Inequality in levels of health in England and Wales, 1891–1971. *Journal of Health and Social Behavior* 22 (September): 268–83.

Roland, Charles G. 1981. The early years of antiseptic surgery in Canada. In *Medicine in Canadian society: Historical perspectives,* ed. S. E. D. Shortt, 237–53. Montreal: McGill-Queen's University Press.

Rosenberg, Charles E. 1987. *The care of strangers: The rise of America's hospital system.* New York: Basic Books.

Royal Cancer Hospital. 1951. *Royal Cancer Hospital, Fulham Road, London, 1851–1951: A short history of the Royal Cancer Hospital prepared for the centenary 1951, The.* London: J. B. Shears and Sons.

Royal Rehabilitation Centre. 1995. *Royal Rehabilitation Centre, Sydney: A condensed history, 1899–1935.* Sydney: Author.

Rumbold, Bruce. 2002. From religion to spirituality. In *Spirituality and palliative care: Social and pastoral perspectives,* ed. Bruce Rumbold, 5–21. New York: Oxford University Press.

Rusden, H. K. 1890. *Cremation: Sanitary necessity.* Melbourne: J. Wing.

Russell, K. F. 1977. *The Melbourne medical school 1862–1962.* Carlton, Victoria, Australia: Melbourne University Press.

Ryan, James, Keith Sutton, and Malcolm Baigent. 1996. *Australasian radiology: A history.* New York: McGraw-Hill.

Sanson-Fisher, R., E. Campbell, P. Ireland, and R. Lovell. 1999. The challenge of setting national cancer control priorities. *Cancer Forum* 23(1): 7–9.

Saunders, Dame Cicely. 1988. The evolution of the hospices. In *The history of the management of pain from early principles to present practice,* ed. R. D. Mann, 167–78. Carnforth, Lancashire: Parthenon Publishing Group.

Schlink, H. H., Clement L. Chapman, and Frederick N. Chenhall. 1947. Cancer statistics from the Royal Prince Alfred Hospital, Sydney. *Medical Journal of Australia* 1 (March): 397–99.

Schmek, Harold M. 1985. Cancer-killing substance moves toward human tests. *Medical Journal of Australia* 143 (November): 150–51.

Schofield, Roger, and David Reher. 1991. The decline of mortality in Europe. In *The decline of mortality in Europe,* ed. Roger Schofield, David Reher, and Alain Bideau, 1–17. New York: Oxford University Press.

Schweder, Richard A., Nancy C. Much, Manomohan Mohapatra, and Lawrence Park. 1997. The "big three" of morality (autonomy, community, divinity) and the "big three" explanations of suffering. In *Morality and health,* ed. A. M. Brandt and P. Rozin, 119–69. New York: Routledge.

Scott, John F. 1981. Canada: Hospice care in Canada. In *Hospice: The living idea,* ed. Cicely Saunders, D. H. Summers, and N. Teller, 176–80. London: Edward Arnold.

———, Neil MacDonald, and Balfour M. Mount. 1999. Palliative medicine education. In *Oxford textbook of palliative medicine,* 2nd ed. Derek Doyle, Geoffrey W. C. Hanks, and Neil MacDonald, 1169–88. New York: Oxford University Press.

Second Annual Report of Austin Hospital. 1883–1884. Melbourne: J. J. Miller.

Seely, John F., and Balfour M. Mount. 1999. Palliative medicine and modern technology. *Canadian Medical Association Journal* 161(9): 1120–21.

Sellers, A. Hardisty. 1940. The contribution of the Ontario cancer clinics to the control of cancer. *Canadian Public Health Journal* 31(2): 72–76.

Sendzuik, Paul. 2003. *Learning to trust: Australian responses to AIDS.* Sydney: University of NSW Press.

Shephard, David A. E. 1993. *Watching closely those who sleep: A history of the Canadian Anaesthetists' Society.* Lewiston, NY: Canadian Anaesthetists' Society.

Shorter, Edward. 1996. Primary care. In *The Cambridge illustrated history of medicine,* ed. Roy Porter, 118–53. New York: Cambridge University Press.

Shortt, S. E. D. 1983–1984. The Canadian hospital in the nineteenth century: An historiographic lament. *Journal of Canadian Studies* 18(4): 3–14.

Siderov, Jim, and John R. Zalcberg. 1994. Prescribing opioids: A painful experience. *Medical Journal of Australia* 161 (November): 515–16.

Siebold, Cathy. 1992. *The hospice movement: Easing death's pains.* New York: Twayne.

Sismondo, Sergio. 2000. Bacon, Francis, 1561–1626. In *Reader's guide to the history of science,* ed. A. Hessenbruch, 65–66. London: Fitzroy Dearborn.

Slack, Paul. 1997. Hospitals, workhouses, and the relief of the poor in early modern London. In *Health care and poor relief in Protestant Europe 1500–1700,* ed. Olle Peter Grell and Andrew Cunningham, 234–51. New York: Routledge.

Small, Neil. 1998. Spirituality and hospice care. In *The spiritual challenge of health care,* ed. M. Cobb and V. Robshaw, 167–82. Edinburgh: Churchill Livingstone.

Smith, Anthony M. 1999. United Kingdom. In *Oxford textbook of palliative medicine,* 2nd ed. Derek Doyle, Geoffrey W. C. Hanks, and Neil MacDonald, 1188–89. New York: Oxford University Press.

Smith, F. B. 1988. *The retreat of tuberculosis 1850–1950.* London: Croom Helm.

Smith, Peter. 1986. Anglo-American religion and hegemonic change in the world system, ca. 1870–1980. *British Journal of Sociology* 37(1): 88–105.

Smith, Peter J. 2000. Should we treat leuchaemia in children? *Medical Journal of Australia* 173 (December): 568–69.

Smith, Wesley J. 1995. Unnecessary tragedy: Assisted suicide comes to Oregon. *Human Life Review* 21(2): 25–40.

Snow, Herbert. 1896. Opium and cocaine in the treatment of cancerous disease. *British Medical Journal* 2 (September): 718–19.

Social Development Committee. 1987. *Report upon the inquiry into options for dying with dignity.* Melbourne: Parliament of Victoria.

Somerville, Margaret A. 1996. Are we just "gene machines" or also "secular sacred"? From new science to a new societal paradigm. *Policy Options* (March): 3–6.

Stannard, David E. 1977. *The Puritan way of death: A study in religion, culture, and social change.* New York: Oxford University Press.

Starr, Kenneth W. 1968. Human cancer prospects, 1967. *Medical Journal of Australia* 1 (April): 733–37.

Stevens, Michael M., and Brian Pollard. 1999. Development in Australia. In *Oxford textbook of palliative medicine,* 2nd ed. Derek Doyle, Geoffrey W. C. Hanks, and Neil MacDonald, 1103–5. New York: Oxford University Press.

Stingl, Michael. 1998. Euthanasia and health reform in Canada. *Cambridge Quarterly of Healthcare Ethics* 7: 348–70.

Stjernsward, Jan, and Noreen Teoh. 1990. The scope of the cancer pain problem. In *Proceedings of the Second International Congress on Cancer Pain: Advances in pain research and therapy,* ed. K. M. Foley, J. J. Bonica, and V. Ventafridda, 7–12. New York: Raven Press.

Stoll, Basil A. 1956. Advanced cancer treated with nitromin. *Medical Journal of Australia* 2 (December): 882–87.

———. 1959. Recent advances in the chemotherapy of cancer. *Medical Journal of Australia* 2 (August): 240–42.

Strassels, Scott. 1998. Summary of recent changes in Massachusetts law. *American Pain Society Bulletin* 8(6): 1–4.

Sullivan, Mark. 1986. In what sense is contemporary medicine dualistic? *Culture, Medicine, and Psychiatry* 10: 331–50.

Supporting Self-Care. The contribution of nurses and physicians. 1997. Retrieved March 7, 2006, from http://www.hc-sc.gc.ca/hcs-sss/pubs/care-soins/1997-self-auto-contribut/index_e.html

Swerdlow, M. 1992. The early development of pain relief clinics in the UK. *Anaesthesia* 47(11): 977–80.

———. 2003. The World Health Organization cancer pain relief program. In *Progress in pain research and management,* ed. Marcia L. Meldrum, 157–61. Seattle: International Association for the Study of Pain Press.

Sydney Morning Herald. 1901. Hospice for the dying. October 25.

Syme, Rodney R. A. 1988. Voluntary euthanasia. *Medical Journal of Australia* 149 (September): 280.

Tattersall, Martin H. N. 1981a. Cancer management in the 1980s. *Medical Journal of Australia* 2 (July): 10–13, 15, 41.

———. 1981b. Pain: Heroin versus morphine. *Medical Journal of Australia* 1 (May): 492.

———, Melina Gattellari, Katie Voigt, and Phyllis N. Butow. 2001. When the treatment goal is not cure: Are patients informed adequately? *Journal of Supportive Care in Cancer* 10: 314–21.

———, and Allen O. Langlands. 1993. Oncology curricula in Australia. *Medical Journal of Australia* 158 (February): 224–25.

Taylor, Richard, Milton Lewis, and John Powles. 1998. The Australian mortality decline: Cause-specific mortality 1907–1990. *Australian and New Zealand Journal of Public Health* 22(1): 37–44.

Taylor-Thompson, Derek. 1992. *Mildmay: The birth and rebirth of a unique hospital.* London: Mildmay Mission Hospital.

Terris, Milton. 1999. National health insurance in the United States: A drama in many acts. *Journal of Public Health Policy* 20(1): 13–26.

Thame, Claudia. 1974. Health and the state: The development of collective responsibility for health care in Australia in the first half of the twentieth century. Ph.D. diss., Australian National University, Canberra, Australia.

Thane, Pat. 2000. *Old age in English history: Past experiences, present issues.* New York: Oxford University Press.

Thompson, Kenneth. 1990. Secularization and sacralization. In *Rethinking progress: Movements, forces, and ideas at the end of the 20th century,* ed. Jeffrey C. Alexander and Piotr Sztompka, 161–81. Boston: Unwin Hyman.

Thomson, David. 1991. The welfare of the elderly in the past: A family or community responsibility? In *Life, death, and the elderly: Historical perspectives,* ed. Margaret Pelling and R. W. Smith, 194–221. New York: Routledge.

Tracy, Sarah W. 1998. An evolving science of man: The transformation and demise of American constitutional medicine, 1920–1950. In *Greater than the parts: Holism in biomedicine, 1920–1950,* ed. Christopher Lawrence and George Weisz, 161–88. New York: Oxford University Press.

Tress, Nora. 1993. *Caught for life: A story of the Anglican Deaconess Order in Australia.* Araluen, NSW: Author and Mission Publications of Australia.

Valent, Paul. 1978. Issues with dying patients. *Medical Journal of Australia* 1 (April): 433–37.

Van der Sluis, I. 1979. The movement for euthanasia 1875–1975. *Janus* 66: 131–72.

van Hooft, Stan. 2002. Toward a philosophy of caring and spirituality for a secular age. In *Spirituality and palliative care: Social and pastoral perspectives,* ed. Bruce Rumbold, 38–50. New York: Oxford University Press.

van Reyk, Paul. 1997. HIV and choosing to die. In *Managing HIV,* ed. G. Stewart, 161. North Sydney: Australasian Medical Publishing.

Vanderpool, Harold Y. 1995. Death and dying: Euthanasia and sustaining life. 1: Historical aspects. In *Encyclopedia of bioethics,* vol. 1, ed. W. T. Reich, 554–63. New York: Macmillan Library Reference.

Virik, Kiran, and Paul Glare. 2000. Pain management in palliative care. *Australian Family Physician* 29(12): 1167–71.

Wald, Florence S. 1997. Hospice's path to the future. In *Death and the quest for meaning: Essays in honor of Herman Feifel,* ed. Stephen Strack, 57–77. Northvale, NJ: Jason Aronson.

Walker, Christine. 1998. Funding Melbourne's hospitals: Some historical moments. *Australian Health Review* 21(1): 29–36.

———. n.d. *Class and the rise of the medical profession in Melbourne's hospitals: 1846–1927.* Melbourne: Chronic Illness Alliance.

Walter, Tony. 2003. Historical and cultural variants on the good death. *British Medical Journal* 327(7408): 218–20.

Ward, Jeanette, and Elaine Henry. 1993. The national cancer prevention policy: Will it sell itself? *Medical Journal of Australia* 159 (October): 502.

Warner, John Harley. 1992. The fall and rise of professional mystery. In *The laboratory revolution in medicine,* ed. A. Cunningham and P. Williams, 110–41. New York: Cambridge University Press.

Watson, J. Frederick. 1911. *The history of the Sydney Hospital from 1811 to 1911.* Sydney: W. A. Gullick, Government Printer.

Wear, Andrew. 1985. Puritan perceptions of illness in seventeenth-century England. In *Patients and practitioners: Lay perceptions of medicine in pre-industrial society,* ed. Roy Porter, 95–99. New York: Cambridge University Press.

———. 1992. Making sense of health and the environment in early modern England. In *Medicine in society: Historical essays,* ed. Andrew Wear, 119–47. New York: Cambridge University Press.

Webling, D. D'Arcy. 1993. "O strong and long-lived death, how cam'st thou in?" Views of euthanasia from the 17th century. *Medical Journal of Australia* 159 (December): 795–96.

Webster, Charles. 2000. Medicine and the welfare state 1930–1970. In *Medicine in the twentieth century,* ed. Roger Cooter and John Pickstone, 125–40. Amsterdam: Harwood Academic Publishers.

Wells, Robert V. 2000. *Facing the "king of terrors": Death and society in an American community, 1750–1910.* New York: Cambridge University Press.

Wigle, Donald T. 1978. Cancer patterns in Canada. *Canadian Journal of Public Health* 69 (March/April): 113–20.

Wildes, Kevin W. 1996. Death: A persistent controversial state. *Kennedy Institute of Ethics Journal* 6(4): 378–81.

———. 2001. The crisis of medicine: Philosophy and the social construction of medicine. *Kennedy Institute of Ethics Journal* 11(1): 71–86.

Wilkinson, Alan. 1997. Changing English attitudes to death in the two world wars. In *The changing face of death: Historical accounts of death and disposal,* ed. Peter C. Jupp and Glennys Howarth, 149–63. New York: St. Martin's Press.

Williams, Simon J., and Michael Calnan. 1996. The "limits" of medicalization? Modern medicine and the lay populace in "late" modernity. *Social Science and Medicine* 42(12): 1609–20.

Wilson, Dottie C., Ina Ajemian, and Balfour Mount. 1978. Montreal (1975): The Royal Victoria Hospital Palliative Care Service. *Death Education* 2 (Spring/Summer): 3–19.

Woodman, Sue. 1998. *Last rights: The struggle over the right to die.* New York: Plenum Trade.

Woodruff, Roger. 1984. Euthanasia for cancer patients: A non-debate. *Medical Journal of Australia* 141 (October): 548–49.

———. 1988. Euthanasia again: Going Dutch. *Medical Journal of Australia* 148 (May): 540.

———. 1996. *Palliative medicine: Symptomatic and supportive care for patients with advanced cancer and AIDS.* Melbourne: Asperula.

Worcester, Alfred. 1977. *The care of the aged, the dying, and the dead.* New York: Arno Press.

Wordley, Dick. 1976. *No one dies alone.* Kogarah, NSW: Australian Creative Workshop for the Little Company of Mary.

World Health Organization. 1995. *National cancer control programs: Policies and managerial guidelines.* Geneva: Author.

———. 1998. *Cancer pain relief and palliative care in children.* [Monograph]. Geneva: Author.

Wright, L. A., and M. Tattersall. 1994. Australian cancer society: Statement on undergraduate cancer education. In *Cancer education for undergraduate medical students,* ed. E. Robinson, C. D. Sherman, and R. R. Love, 103–17. Geneva: International Union against Cancer.

Wylde, R. T. 1890. *A lecture on cremation.* Adelaide, Australia: W. K. Thomas.

Young, John Atherton, Ann Jarvie Sefton, and Nina Webb. 1984. *Centenary book of the University of Sydney Faculty of Medicine.* Sydney: Sydney University Press.

Young, Robert. 1985. Voluntary euthanasia. *Medical Journal of Australia* 142 (January): 166.

Zhukovsky, Donna S., and Myra Glajchen. 2001. Palliative care: Does APS membership need it? *American Pain Society Bulletin* 11(6): 1–4.

INDEX